Targeting
of Drugs

NATO ADVANCED STUDY INSTITUTES SERIES

A series of edited volumes comprising multifaceted studies of contemporary scientific issues by some of the best scientific minds in the world, assembled in cooperation with NATO Scientific Affairs Division.

Series A: Life Sciences

Recent Volumes in this Series

Volume 43 – Advanced Topics on Radiosensitizers of Hypoxic Cells
edited by A. Breccia, C. Rimondi, and G. E. Adams

Volume 44 – Cell Regulation by Intracellular Signals
edited by Stéphane Swillens and Jacques E. Dumont

Volume 45 – Structural Molecular Biology: Methods and Applications
edited by David B. Davies, Wolfram Saenger, and Steven S. Danyluk

Volume 46 – Post-Harvest Physiology and Crop Preservation
edited by Morris Lieberman

Volume 47 – Targeting of Drugs
edited by Gregory Gregoriadis, Judith Senior, and André Trouet

Volume 48 – Neurotransmitter Interaction and Compartmentation
edited by H. F. Bradford

Volume 49 – Biological Effects and Dosimetry of Nonionizing Radiation
edited by Martino Grandolfo, Sol M. Michaelson, and Alessandro Rindi

Volume 50 – Somatic Cell Genetics
edited by C. Thomas Caskey and D. Christopher Robbins

Volume 51 – Factors in Formation and Regression of the Atherosclerotic Plaque
edited by Gustav R. V. Born, Alberico L. Catapano, and
Rodolfo Paoletti

Volume 52 – Chemical Carcinogenesis
edited by Claudio Nicolini

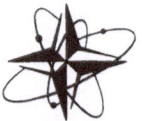

This series is published by an international board of publishers in conjunction with NATO Scientific Affairs Division

A Life Sciences	Plenum Publishing Corporation
B Physics	London and New York
C Mathematical and	D. Reidel Publishing Company
Physical Sciences	Dordrecht, The Netherlands
	and Hingham, Massachusetts, USA
D Behavioral and	Martinus Nijhoff Publishers
Social Sciences	The Hague, The Netherlands
E Applied Sciences	

Targeting of Drugs

Edited by
Gregory Gregoriadis
Judith Senior

Clinical Research Centre
Harrow, United Kingdom

and

André Trouet

International Institute of Cellular and Molecular Pathology
Brussels, Belgium

PLENUM PRESS • NEW YORK AND LONDON
Published in cooperation with NATO Scientific Affairs Division

Library of Congress Cataloging in Publication Data

NATO Advanced Study Institute of Targeting of Drugs (1981: Cape Sounion, Greece)
 Targeting of drugs.

 (NATO advanced study institutes series. Series A, Life sciences; v. 47)
 "Published in cooperation with NATO Scientific Affairs Division."
 Includes bibliographical references and index.
 1. Drugs — Effectiveness — Congresses. 2. Drugs — Vehicles — Congresses. I. Gregoriadis,
Gregory. II. Senior, Judith. III. Trouet, André. IV. Title. V. North Atlantic Treaty
Organization. Division of Scientific Affairs. [DNLM: 1. Drugs — Administration and
dosage — Congresses. 2. Macromolecular systems — Administration and dosage — Con-
gresses. 3. Liposomes — Administration and dosage — Congresses. 4. Vehicles — Adminis-
tration and dosage — Congresses. QV 38 N279t 1981]
RM301.N38 1981   615′.7   82-3822
ISBN-13: 978-1-4684-4243-4   e-ISBN-13: 978-1-4684-4241-0
DOI: 10.1007/978-1-4684-4241-0

Proceedings of a NATO Advanced Study Institute on Targeting of
Drugs, held June 24–July 5, 1981, in Cape Sounion, Greece

© 1982 Plenum Press, New York
Softcover reprint of the hardcover 1st edition 1982
A Division of Plenum Publishing Corporation
233 Spring Street, New York, N.Y. 10013

PREFACE

Successful drug use in biology and medicine is often prejudiced by the failure of drugs that are otherwise active in vitro to act as efficiently in vivo. This is because in the living animal drugs must, as a rule, bypass or traverse organs, membranes, cells and molecules that stand between the site of administration and the site of action. In practice, however, drugs can be toxic to normal tissues, have limited or no access to the target and be prematurely excreted or inactivated. There is now growing optimism that such problems may be resolved by the use of carrier systems that will not only protect the non-target environment from the drugs they carry but also deliver them to where they are needed or facilitate their release there. Carrier systems presently under investigation include antibodies, glycoproteins, cells, reconstituted viruses and liposomes. Recent advances in the chemistry of cell receptor and receptor-recognising molecules, immunology, and natural and artificial membranes have revealed a multitude of ways in which such carrier systems can be modified or improved upon.

This book contains the proceedings of a NATO Advanced Studies Institute on "Targeting of Drugs" held in Sounion, Greece during 24 June - 5 July 1981 and reflects current trends in the use of drug carriers in cancer chemotherapy, anti-microbial and anti-viral therapy, vaccines, genetic engineering, etc. It will be noticed that despite the enthusiasm, vast amount of information amassed and success in experimental animals as experienced by leading investigators in the field, the impact of drug targeting in the clinic has yet to be felt. However, in view of the goal, its complexity and above all the rewards of it being achieved, this must not disappoint the reader (or indeed, delight pessimists!). As formal co-ordinated research programs in targeting are now replacing the pioneer efforts of small, scattered groups, there is considerable hope that targeting will make the use of existing drugs more effective and, ultimately, revolutionize therapy.

We wish to express our appreciation to Drs. Ruth Arnon, A. Evangelopoulos, G.M. Ihler, D. Papahadjopoulos, T. Pataryas and C. Vakirtzi-Lemonias who as members of the international and local committees provided valuable advice and help throughout the planning stages of the Institute, and Mrs. Maria Economou-Karadonti for her continuous interest and moral support. We also thank Mrs. Maureen Moriarty for expert secretarial assistance with the organization of the Institute and Mrs. Pauline Creed for her patience and superb skill in arranging and retyping the manuscripts. The Institute was held under the sponsorship of NATO with partial support from the Hellenic Organization of Tourism, Greece; National Institutes of Health, USA; Novo Industri, Denmark; Olympic Airways, Greece; Rhone Poulenc Belgique SA, Belgium; Sanofi Research, France; and Smith Kline and French Laboratories, USA.

November 1981

                                            Gregory Gregoriadis
                                            Judith Senior
                                            André Trouet

CONTENTS

MACROMOLECULAR CARRIERS

HEPATOCYTE TARGETING OF ANTIVIRAL DRUGS COUPLED TO
GALACTOSYL-TERMINATING GLYCOPROTEINS 1

L. Fiume, C. Busi, A. Mattioli, P.G. Balboni, G. Barbanti-
Brodano and Th. Wieland

TARGETING OF ANTITUMOUR AND ANTIPROTOZOAL DRUGS BY COVALENT
LINKAGE TO PROTEIN CARRIERS 19

A. Trouet, R. Baurain, D. Deprez-De Campeneere, M. Masquelier
and P. Pirson

ANTIBODIES AND DEXTRAN AS ANTI-TUMOUR DRUG CARRIERS 31

R. Arnon

TARGETING OF RADIONUCLIDES AND DRUGS FOR THE DIAGNOSIS AND
TREATMENT OF CANCER 55

T. Ghose, H. Blair, P. Kulkarni, K. Vaughan, S. Norvell and
P. Belitsky

ANTIBODY-TOXIN CONJUGATES AS POTENTIAL THERAPEUTIC AGENTS 83

D. Caird Edwards, P.E. Thorpe and A.J.S. Davies

SELECTIVITY IN CANCER CHEMOTHERAPY 97

T.A. Connors

PARTICULATE AND CELLULAR CARRIERS

DRUG CONJUGATES OF POLYMERIC MICROSPHERES AS TOOLS IN CELL
BIOLOGY 109

I. Pecht, N. Mazurek, A. Petrank and S. Margel

RECONSTITUTED SENDAI VIRUS ENVELOPES AS A VEHICLE FOR THE
INTRODUCTION OF SOLUBLE MACROMOLECULES AND MEMBRANE COMPONENTS
INTO ANIMAL CELLS 125

M. Beigel, G. Eytan and A. Loyter

ERTHROCYTES AS CARRIERS FOR RECOMBINANT CLONED DNA 145

G.M. Ihler

LIPOSOMAL CARRIERS

TARGETING OF LIPOSOMES: STUDY OF INFLUENCING FACTORS 155

G. Gregoriadis, C. Kirby, P. Large, A. Meehan and J. Senior

ANTIBODY-MEDIATED TARGETING OF LIPOSOMES 185

J.N. Weinstein, L.D. Leserman, P.A. Henkart and R. Blumenthal

DELIVERY OF DRUGS IN TEMPERATURE-SENSITIVE LIPOSOMES 203

R.L. Magin and J.N. Weinstein

HYPERTHERMIA-MEDIATED TARGETING OF LIPOSOMES-ASSOCIATED ANTI-
NEOPLASTIC DRUGS 223

M.B. Yatvin, T.C. Cree and J.J. Gipp

LIPOSOMES: FURTHER CONSIDERATIONS OF THEIR POSSIBLE ROLE AS
CARRIERS OF THERAPEUTIC AGENTS 235

B.E. Ryman and G.M. Barratt

CONTENTS

THERAPEUTIC EFFICACY OF CYTOSINE ARABINOSIDE TRAPPED IN
LIPOSOMES 249

E. Mayhew, Y.M. Rustum and F. Szoka

STIMULATION OF HOST RESPONSE AGAINST METASTATIC TUMOURS BY
LIPOSOME-ENCAPSULATED IMMUNOMODULATORS 261

G. Poste, C. Bucana and I.J. Fidler

LIPOSOMES AND THE RETICULOENDOTHELIAL SYSTEM: INTERACTIONS
OF LIPOSOMES WITH MACROPHAGES AND BEHAVIOUR OF LIPOSOMES
IN VIVO 285

R.L. Juliano

IMMUNOADJUVANT PROPERTIES OF LIPOSOMES 301

N. van Rooijen and R. van Nieuwmegen.

ADJUVANT EFFECT OF LIPOSOME PRESENTATION OF SOLUBLE TUMOUR-
ASSOCIATED ANTIGEN 327

D. Gerlier and J.F. Doré

THERAPEUTIC POTENTIAL OF LIPOSOMES AS CARRIERS IN LEISHMAN-
IASIS, MALARIA AND VACCINES 337

C.R. Alving

INTERACTION OF LIPOSOMES WITH CELLS: MODEL STUDIES 355

C. Vakirtzi-Lemonias and K. Sekeris-Pataryas

DEVELOPMENT OF LIPOSOMES AS AN EFFICIENT CARRIER SYSTEM: NEW
METHODOLOGY FOR CELL TARGETING AND INTRACELLULAR DELIVERY OF
DRUGS AND DNA 375

D. Papahadjopoulos, T. Heath, F. Martin, R. Fraley and
R. Straubinger

LIPOSOME-MEDIATED DNA TRANSFER IN EUKARYOTIC CELLS: GENE UPTAKE
AND EXPRESSING IN THE HOST CELL 393

C. Nicolau and C. Sené

CONTRIBUTORS 413

INDEX 419

HEPATOCYTE TARGETING OF ANTIVIRAL DRUGS COUPLED

TO GALACTOSYL-TERMINATING GLYCOPROTEINS

L. Fiume[+], C. Busi[+], A. Mattioli[+], P.G. Balboni[*],
G. Barbanti-Brodano[*] and Th. Wieland[**]

[+]Istituto di Patologia generale, Via San Giacomo
14, I-40126 Bologna, Italy
[*]Istituto di Microbiologia, Via L. Borsari 46
I-44100 Ferrara, Italy
[**]Max-Planck-Institut für Medizinische Forschung
Jahnstrasse 29, D-69 Heidelberg, FRG

INTRODUCTION

This chapter deals with the possibility of specifically introducing inhibitors of DNA synthesis into hepatocytes by conjugation
to galactosyl-terminating glycoproteins which are selectively taken
up by parenchymal liver cells (Morell et al., 1968; Ashwell and
Morell, 1974; Gregoriadis, 1975). This line of research, which was
developed as an approach to the treatment of chronic hepatitis B,
started from the finding (Derenzini et al., 1973) that β-amanitin
after coupling to albumin changed its original target and selectively penetrated into cells of the macrophage system which are very
active in internalising albumin.

AMANITIN-ALBUMIN CONJUGATE

The cyclopeptide amanitins are the main toxins of the toadstool
Amanita phalloides (Wieland, 1968; Wieland and Faulstich, 1978).
They are inhibitors of nuclear RNA-polymerase B (Stirpe and Fiume,
1967; Kedinger et al., 1970; Lindell et al., 1970). The first ultrastructural changes they produce are observed in the nuclei, which
show fragmentation of nucleoli and condensation of chromatin (Fiume
and Laschi, 1965; Marinozzi and Fiume, 1971). In order to obtain an
antiserum against these toxins, β-amanitin was conjugated with rabbit
serum albumin by carbodiimide coupling (Cessi and Fiume, 1969). The
resulting conjugate was highly hepatotoxic. It caused hepatic necrosis by a different mechanism from that of free amanitin

1

(Derenzini et al., 1973). In liver, free amanitin damages only
hepatocytes, while sinusoidal cells are unaffected even after the
administration of high doses of toxin. On the contrary the amanitin-
albumin conjugate produced the typical ultrastructural lesions of
amanitin in sinusoidal cells (endothelial cells and Küpffer cells).
No similar lesions were observed in hepatocytes, at least up to the
dose of 2 LD_{50} of the conjugate.

An aggregated or heavily modified albumin injected into animals
is rapidly endocytosed by cells of the macrophage system, the largest
amount being taken up by liver sinusoidal cells (Kruse and McMaster,
1949; Benacerraf et al., 1957; Haurowitz, 1968; Di Luzio and Morrow,
1971; Buys et al., 1973). It is likely that liver sinusoidal cells
are the target of the amanitin-albumin conjugate because this conjugate, the albumin molecules of which are aggregated and severely
changed (Derenzini et al., 1973), is selectively taken up by these
cells. This conclusion was supported by in vitro experiments which
demonstrated that macrophages are much more sensitive to the conjugate than other cells (Barbanti-Brodano and Fiume, 1973; Fiume and
Barbanti-Brodano, 1974). Moreover with three different cell lines,
a correlation was found between sensitivity to the amanitin-albumin
conjugate and ability to take up $125I$ labelled albumin (Hencin and
Preston, 1979). The conjugate may exert its toxic activity either
directly or by releasing amanitin after penetration into the cells,
thus behaving as a lysosomotropic agent (Trouet et al., 1972; De
Duve et al., 1974). The first possibility cannot be discarded since
the conjugate still inhibits RNA-polymerase B in a cell-free system
although the inhibitory effect of amanitin is decreased after coupling (Fiume et al., 1971; Derenzini et al., 1973; Faulstich and
Trischmann, 1973; Hencin and Preston, 1979). The second mechanism
appears more likely because albumin after penetration into cells is
digested by lysosomal enzymes (Unanue, 1972). It is thus probable
that carrier albumin is similarly digested within lysosomes and that
amanitin, released in a free form, inhibits RNA-polymerase B after
crossing the lysosomal membrane (Derenzini et al., 1973).

INHIBITORS OF DNA SYNTHESIS COUPLED TO ALBUMIN

The finding that the amanitin-albumin conjugate is selectively
toxic for macrophages, prompted us to conjugate inhibitors of DNA
synthesis with albumin as an approach to the treatment of infections
caused by DNA viruses growing in macrophages (Balboni et al., 1976)
and of neoplastic proliferations of these cells (Fiume and Barbanti-
Brodano, 1974). It is indeed possible that other drugs, covalently
linked to albumin, are released in an active form after penetration
of the conjugates into the cells. If these drugs are selective inhibitors of DNA synthesis, the conjugates should hinder the replication of DNA viruses in macrophages without damaging these cells,
which do not divide (Von Furth et al., 1972), and without affecting
normal proliferating cells (bone marrow, gut) which do not take up

albumin. In the same way the conjugates should selectively kill neoplastic proliferating macrophages which display a high albumin uptake
(Gall and Mallory, 1942; Akazaki, 1953; Dunn, 1954).

Two inhibitors of DNA synthesis, 5-fluorodeoxyuridine (FUDR)
and cytosine arabinoside (ara-C), conjugated to rabbit serum albumin
(RSA) by carbodiimide coupling, were found to be released in active
form after penetration of the conjugates in cells cultured in vitro
(Barbanti-Brodano and Fiume, 1974; Balboni et al., 1976). Mice infected with Ectromelia virus, the agent of mousepox, were chosen as
a model to study the antiviral activity of these conjugates in vivo.
Ectromelia virus, when injected intravenously into mice, is ingested
mainly by the Küpffer cells where it starts replication. Then it
infects neighbouring hepatic cells which in turn infect more hepatic
cells after each cycle of growth. The resulting liver necrosis causes
the death of mice (Mims, 1959 a; Mims, 1959 b; Roberts, 1963). FUDR-
RSA and ara-C-RSA, injected in mice during the phase of virus growth
in macrophages, significantly reduced the virus yield in liver whereas free FUDR and ara-C were completely ineffective. Moreover ara-C-
RSA increased the mean survival time of infected mice and the number
of survivors. The conjugates were inactive or only slightly active
if administered 12 or 24 h after infection when the virus replicates
in hepatocytes (Mims, 1959 b; Roberts, 1963). These results indicate
that the conjugates interfere mainly with the phase of virus infection which takes place in liver macrophages*.

INHIBITORS OF DNA SYNTHESIS COUPLED TO GALACTOSYL-
TERMINATING GLYCOPROTEINS

During virus infections in man the growth of DNA viruses in
macrophages occurs only in a pre-symptomatic stage (Fenner and White,
1976), when therapy cannot be started. However the results obtained
with albumin conjugates of ara-C and FUDR suggested a similar approach
for the treatment of human chronic hepatitis B in which the virus
replicates in hepatocytes. Inhibitors of DNA synthesis can be coupled
to glycoproteins which after removal of sialic acid and consequent
exposure of galactosyl residues are selectively taken up by hepatocytes where they are digested in lysosomes (Ashwell and Morell,
1974; Gregoriadis, 1975). If such conjugates behave in parenchymal
liver cells as do albumin conjugates in macrophages, the inhibitors
of DNA synthesis should be selectively concentrated in hepatocytes
and consequently their toxicity for tissues containing dividing cells
should be avoided or reduced.

Trifluorothymidine (F3T), an inhibitor of DNA synthesis, active

_____
*For a review on the biological action of albumin conjugates of
fungal toxins and of inhibitors of DNA synthesis see Fiume et al.,
(1979 a).

in very low doses, was conjugated (Fiume et al., 1979 b) to desialylated fetiun, a carrier which has been previously used to introduce
proteins (Rogers and Kornfeld, 1971) and liposomes (Gregoriadis and
Neerunjun, 1975) into parenchymal liver cells. F_3T was first converted into its glutarate derivative which was subsequently coupled
via its hydroxysuccinimide ester to ϵ-NH$_2$ groups of lysine residues
of asialofetuin (AF). The molar ratio of F_3T to AF in the conjugate
was 8 (50 μg F_3T in 1 mg F_3T-AF). Coupling with F_3T did not change
the ability of AF to interact with specific receptors on the surface
of hepatocytes. Indeed, the clearance of ^{14}C- labelled AF from the
blood of mice was competitively inhibited to the same extent by
F_3T-AF or by an equal amount of non-conjugated AF (Fig. 1). F_3T
and F_3T-AF were injected in mice 44 h after Ectromelia virus infection and their effect on deoxy (5-^{3}H)-cytidine incorporation into DNA
in liver and in bone marrow was determined. Forty-four hours after
infection the largest amount of deoxycytidine incorporation in liver
is probably due to virus DNA synthesis most of which occurs in
hepatocytes (Fiume et al., 1979 b; Fiume et al., 1981). As shown
in Fig. 2, F_3T coupled to AF caused, at the three lower doses, an
inhibition of DNA synthesis in liver more than 3 times higher than
that produced by free drug. On the contrary, the percentage of
inhibition in bone marrow was similar when F_3T was administered
either coupled to AF or as a free drug. These results indicate that,
after injection of the conjugate, F_3T was concentrated in active
form into hepatocytes.

Three possibilities can be considered to explain the inhibition
of DNA synthesis caused by the conjugate in bone marrow.
(1)   Bone marrow cells took up the conjugate. This possibility is
unlikely because the experiments of competition (Fig. 1) indicate
that conjugated AF behaved like native AF which is taken up almost
exclusively (90%) by the liver (Regoeckzi et al., 1978; Regoeckzi
et al., 1980).
(2)   The bond linking F_3T to glutarate in the conjugate was split in
the blood.
(3)   Part of F_3T released from the conjugate in hepatocytes escaped
from these cells into the blood and reached bone marrow cells as a
free drug. To clarify this point the effect of the conjugate on DNA
synthesis in bone marrow was studied in mice with hepatic necrosis
caused by Ectromelia virus or by α-amanitin (Fiume et al., 1979 b).
In these animals the uptake (Fiume et al., 1979 b) and probably the
catabolism of AF by the liver is hindered. Table I shows that DNA
synthesis in bone marrow was not inhibited by F_3T-AF in mice with
hepatic necrosis, whereas free F_3T produced a 50% inhibition as compared with normal controls. These results rule out the first two
possibilities and consequently make it very likely that the inhibition of DNA synthesis in bone marrow of normal and infected mice
was due to F_3T which escaped from hepatocytes after these cells had
taken up the conjugate. This conclusion indicates that, after a
single injection of a conjugate, the drug transported by the carrier

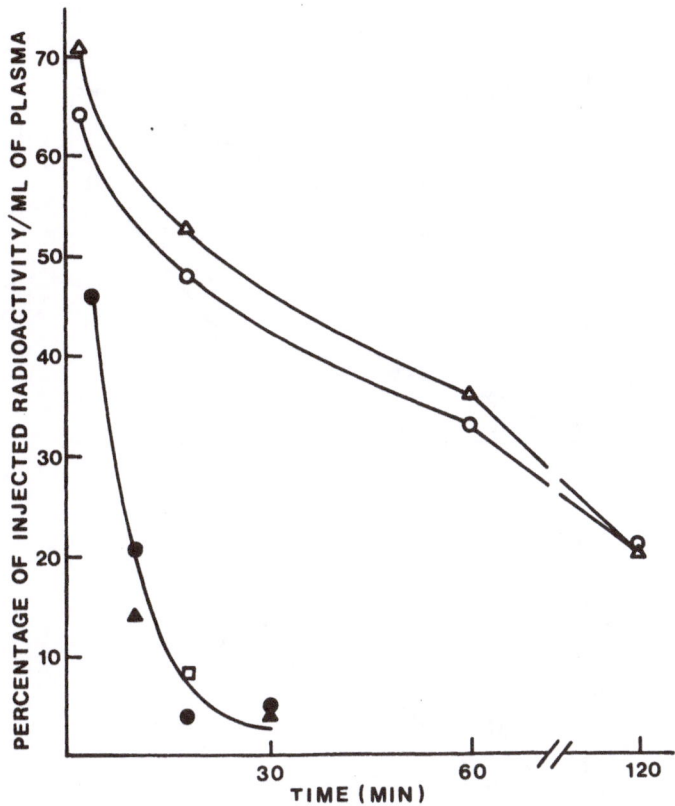

Fig. 1. Blood clearance of ^{14}C - AF (2 μg/g body wt) alone (●)
or in the presence of cold, non-conjugated AF (O),
F$_3$T-AF (△), non-desialylated fetuin (▲) and heat-denatured
rabbit serum albumin (□) (60 μg/g body wt). Each point
represents the mean value of results from 2 animals.
(Reproduced from FEBS Letters (Fiume et al., 1979 b)).

can remain concentrated in target cells only if it is unable to pass
across the external cell membrane as a free molecule. To obtain a
long-lasting targeting of a drug able to cross the cell membrane,
the corresponding conjugate should be administered by continuous
infusion. In this way, the prolonged supply of the conjugate will
maintain a higher drug concentration in target cells than in other
cells.

F3T is not used as a systemic drug in man because of its high
toxicity. In subsequent experiments adenine-9-β-D-arabinofuranoside
(ara-A), which is employed in the treatment of chronic hepatitis B
(Pollard et al., 1978; Chadwick et al., 1978), was coupled to AF
(Fiume et al., 1980). Two different procedures of conjugation were

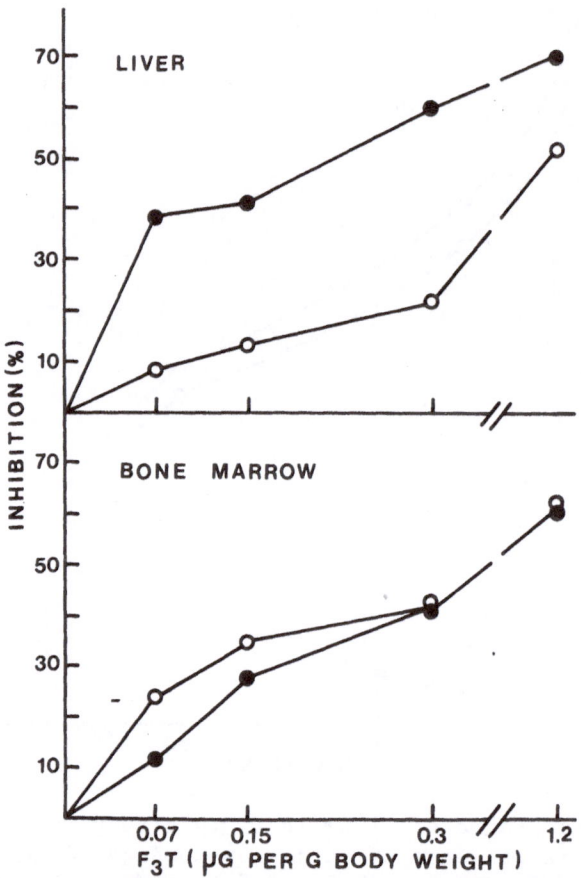

Fig. 2. Inhibition of DNA synthesis by free F_3T (O) or F_3T coupled
to AF (●) in liver and bone marrow of <u>Ectromelia</u> virus infected mice. For each dose of free and conjugated F_3T 2 or
3 experiments were performed. Results (dpm/mg DNA) were
statistically evaluated by means of Student's <u>t</u> test. The
difference between deoxy-(5-^{3}H)-cytidine incorporation into
liver DNA in mice treated with free F_3T or with F3T-AF was
statistically significant for F_3T doses of 0.07, 0.15 and
0.3 μg/g body wt (P<0.001, 0.05 and 0.001 for the 3 doses
respectively). The difference was not statistically significant (P>0.05) for the F_3T dose of 1.2 μg/g body wt.
The difference was not statistically significant for all
the F_3T doses in bone marrow. (Reproduced from FEBS Letters
(Fiume <u>et al</u>., 1979 b)).

TABLE 1

Effect of F_3T-AF and F_3T on deoxy-(5-^{3}H)-cytidine incorporation in bone marrow of normal mice and of mice with liver necrosis

Expt		Compounds	dpm/mg DNA		
1	Normal mice (5)[a]	–	261436 ± 76182		
	Normal mice (5)	F_3T-AF	153228 ± 18056 (41)[b]	P<0.02	
2	Normal mice (5)	–	369721 ± 56586		
	Normal mice (5)	F_3T-AF	203175 ± 39134 (45)	P<0.001	
3	Normal mice (8)	–	290387 ± 56530		
	Mice with hepatic necrosis by Ectromelia virus (7)	F_3T-AF	301983 ± 62928		
4	Normal mice (5)	–	201680 ± 31242		
	Mice with hepatic necrosis by α-amanitin (7)	F_3T-AF	203700 ± 66110		
5	Normal Mice (5)	–	264623 ± 57830		
	Mice with hepatic necrosis by α-amanitin (5)	F_3T-AF	246412 ± 72616 (7)		
6	Normal mice (5)	–	263849 ± 28816		
	Mice with hepatic necrosis by α-amanitin (5)	F_3T	127846 ± 33734 (51)	P<0.001	

[a]Number of mice
[b]Percentage of inhibition

In expt 1-5, F_3T-AF was injected i.v. at 6 g/g body wt corresponding to 0.3 g F_3T. In expt 6 free F_3T was injected i.v. at the dose of 0.3 g/g body wt. In expt 3, F_3T-AF was administered to mice which 80 h earlier had received an i.v. injection of Ectromelia virus (4.0×10^5 p.f.u./g body wt corresponding to 600-times the LD_{50}). In expt 4-6, F_3T-AF or F_3T were injected into mice which 40 h earlier had been injected i.p. with α-amanitin (1.5 g/g body wt). In theIn the groups of Ectromelia viris or α-amanitin treated animals, bone marrow was removed only from those mice showing a macroscopic liver necrosis which was subsequently confirmed by histologic examination. (Reproduced from FEBS Letters (Fiume et al., 1979 b)).

followed. In the first, ara-A glutarate was linked to AF via its
hydroxysuccinimide ester. The conjugated material (ara-A-glut-AF)
emerged from a Sephadex G-75 column in two peaks (A and B). Sodium
dodecyl sulphate-polyacrylamide gel electrophoresis showed that
peak A contained polymers of AF whereas peak B contained the mono-
meric form of AF. The molar ratio of ara-A to AF in both conjugates
(A and B) was 8. In the second procedure ara-A monophosphate (ara-
AMP) was coupled to AF by the use of 1-ethyl-3-(dimethyl-aminopropyl)
carbodiimide. Ara-AMP displays the same antiviral activity as ara-
A (Sidwell et al., 1973); both drugs must be converted to ara-A
triphosphate in order to inhibit DNA synthesis (York and Le Page,
1966; Furth and Cohen, 1967). By carbodiimide coupling ara-AMP is
linked to AF probably by formation of an amide bond between the
ϵ-NH$_2$ group of lysine in AF and the phosphate group of ara-AMP, as
in the analogous reaction in which carbodiimides were used to
conjugate thymidilic acid to albumin (Halloran and Parker, 1966).
The molar ratio of ara-AMP to AF in 3 preparations of ara-AMP-AF
conjugates (I, II, III) ranged from 3.5 to 4. As in the case of
F$_3$T, conjugation with ara-A or ara-AMP did not change the capacity
of AF to interact with the specific receptors on the surface of
hepatocytes. afa-A-glut-AF, ara-AMP-AF, free ara-A and free ara-AMP
were administered to Ectromelia virus-infected mice during the phase
of virus replication in hepatocytes and their effect on (methyl-^{3}H)-
thymidine incorporation into DNA in liver and intestine was determined*. Table 2 shows that free ara-A and ara-AMP produced a
greater inhibition of DNA synthesis in intestine than in liver. On
the contrary ara-A-glut-AF and ara-AMP-AF inhibited DNA synthesis
in liver without producing any significant inhibition in the intestine. A comparable inhibition of DNA synthesis in liver was produced
by conjugated ara-A and ara-AMP at doses 2-4 times lower than those
of the free drugs. These results indicate that, after injection of
the conjugates, ara-A and ara-AMP were concentrated in an active
form in hepatocytes. In the case of ara-AMP-AF the ester bond
linking phosphate to ara-A may be broken down in hepatocyte lysosomes
so that it cannot be excluded that the drug released from the conjugate was ara-A and not ara-AMP. A drawback for a clinical use of
conjugates prepared with AF is the scarcity of fetuin which is

---

*Before the administration of free or conjugated ara-A and
ara-AMP, mice were injected with 2'-deoxycoformycin (dCF) which is
an inhibitor of ara-A deaminiation (Borondy et al., 1977; Plunkett
et al., 1979). Administration of dCF was necessary because ara-A is
more than 100 times less active in rodents than in primates due to
its more rapid metabolism in the former species (Whitley et al.,
1975). In fact doses of ara-A and ara-AMP up to 5 μg (19 nmol) and
10 μg (29 nmol)/g body wt, respectively, did not produce any significant inhibition of DNA synthesis in liver and intestine of Ectromelia
virus-infected mice. dCF administered alone to Ectromelia virus infected mice was ineffective on DNA synthesis in liver and intestine.

TABLE 2

Inhibition of DNA synthesis in liver and intestine of Ectromelia virus-infected mice after inject-ion of free or conjugated ara-A and ara-AMP.

Exp. no	Compound injected	ara-A administered (nmol/g body wt)	Inhibition of DNA synthesis (%) Liver	Intestine
1	ara-A	13.1	42 P<0.001[b]	60 P<0.001
2	ara-A	18.7	58 P<0.005	68 P<0.001
3	ara-AMP	8.6	57 P<0.005	60 P<0.001
4	ara-AMP	17.2	66 P<0.001	77 P<0.001
5	ara-AMP	34.5	77 P<0.001	89 P<0.001
6	ara-A-glut-AF(A)	5.6(33)[a]	38 P<0.02	15 n.s.
7	ara-A-glut-AF(B)	1.9(11)	26 P<0.05	8 n.s.
8	ara-A-glut-AF(B)	5.6(33)	43 P<0.01	16 n.s.
9	ara-AMP-AF(I)	1.8(22)	38 P<0.005	0
10	ara-AMP-AF(II)	1.1(15)	44 P<0.001	0
11	ara-AMP-AF(II)	2.2(30)	59 P<0.001	19 n.s.
12	ara-AMP-AF(III)	2.8(42)	53 P<0.005	13 n.s.

a   In parentheses the amount of conjugate injected (in μg/g body wt).

b   Results were statistically evaluated by means of Student's t-test. The difference was considered not statistically significant (n.s.) for P>0.05.

(Reproduced from FEBS Letters (Fiume et al., 1980))

isolated from fetal calf serum. Also other naturally occuring glycoproteins, which after desialylation are selectively taken up by hepatocytes, can be obtained only in relatively small amounts. Since
proteins, after coupling to thioglycoside of D-galactose (Krantz et
al., 1976) or to lactose (Wilson, 1978; Hubbard et al., 1979), bind
to the hepatic receptor for asialoglycoproteins and are internalised
in hepatocytes*, experiments were performed (Fiume et al., 1981) to
assess whether lactosaminated serum albumin (L-SA), which can be
easily obtained in large amounts, can substitute for AF as hepato-
tropic drug carrier. Lactosaminated rabbit (L-RSA) and human (L-HSA)
serum albumin were prepared by reductive amination with cyanobor-
hydride (Gray, 1974; Schwartz and Gray, 1977). ara-AMP was conjugated to L-SA by carbodiimide coupling. One L-RSA-ara-AMP and
threeL-HSA-ara-AMP conjugates were prepared. The molar ratios sugar/
albumin and ara-AMP/albumin of the conjugates are reported in Table
3. L-SA-ara-AMP conjugates interacted with the hepatic receptor for
asialoglycoproteins; in fact they competitively inhibited blood
clearance of ^{14}C-AF in mice. Free ara-A and ara-AMP, as well as
coupled ara-AMP, were administered to Ectromelia virus-infected mice
as in previous experiments, and their effect on thymidine incorporation into DNA in liver, intestine and bone marrow was determined**.
As shown in Table 3 free ara-A and ara-AMP inhibited DNA synthesis
to the same extent in liver and intestine; they produced a smaller
inhibition in bone marrow. On the contrary inhibition of DNA
synthesis caused by ara-AMP coupled to L-SA was higher in liver than
in intestine where in some experiments thymidine incorporation was
completely unaffected. Conjugated ara-AMP did not interfere with DNA

---

*Some years ago it was supposed that the amanitin-albumin con-
jugate entered liver parenchymal cells after binding of the amanitin
group to a receptor involved in transporting β-amanitin into the hepatocytes (Fiume, 1969). This led us to consider more generally the
possibility of facilitating the cellular penetration of a large
molecule - e.g., a protein - by conjugating it with a smaller molecule for which a binding site exists on the cell membrane (Fiume,
1969; Fiume et al., 1971). It was later observed that the amanitin-
albumin conjugate enters into sinusoidal liver cells and not into
hepatocytes (Derenzini et al., 1973); however the facilitation hypothesis received experimental support by independent experiments which
showed that proteins, after coupling to small sugar molecules,
penetrates selectively into cells which possess surface receptors
for the coupled carbohydrates (Rogers and Kornfeld, 1971; Wilson,
1978; Wilson et al., 1979; Youle et al., 1979).

**In these experiments, in order to inhibit ara-A deamination
9-erythro-(2-hydroxyl-3 nonyl) adenine (EHNA) (Plunkett et al.,
1979) instead of dCF was used. EHNA, administered alone to Ectromelia virus-infected mice, did not affect thymidine incorporation
in liver, intestine or bone marrow.

Table 3

Inhibition of DNA synthesis in liver, intestine and bone marrow of _Ectromelia_ virus-infected mice after injection of free ara-A, ara-AMP and conjugated ara-AMP.

Compound injected	ara-A (nmol/g body wt)	Inhibition of DNA synthesis (%)		
		Liver	Intestine	Bone marrow
ara-A	9.4	45(S)	44(S)	0
ara-A	13.0	50(S)	55(S)	25(S)
ara-AMP	34.5	50(S)	61(S)	43(S)
$L_{25.5}$-RSA-ara-$AMP_{4.0}$	1.0(20.7)+	30(S)	0	ND**
$L_{25.5}$-RSA-ara-$AMP_{4.0}$	2.0(41.5)	53(S)	23(S)	ND
$L_{21.6}$-HSA-ara-$AMP_{7.5}$	1.6(16.6)	21(NS)*	0	0
$L_{21.6}$-HSA-ara-$AMP_{7.5}$	4.2(43.5)	43(S)	0	0
$L_{21.2}$-HSA-ara-$AMP_{10.9}$	4.9(35)	50(S)	19(NS)	2(NS)
$L_{23.2}$-HSA-ara-$AMP_{11.2}$	4.0(28.2)	48(S)	0	0
$L_{23.2}$-HSA-ara-$AMP_{11.2}$	4.8(35)	58(S)	18(NS)	0

+ In parenthesis the amount of conjugate injected (in μg/g body wt).
* Results were statistically evaluated by means of Student's t test. The difference was considered statistically significant (S) or not significant (ÑS) for P $<$ or $>$ 0.05 respectively.
** ND = Not done.

synthesis in bone marrow. A comparable inhibition of DNA synthesis
in liver was produced by doses of conjugated ara-AMP lower than
those of free drugs. These results indicate that L-SA can work as
carrier for selectively transporting ara-AMP into hepatocytes.

In chronic hepatitis B, ara-A, administered alone or in combination with interferon, inhibits viral replication (Pollard et al.,
1978; Merigan and Robinson, 1978; Chadwick et al., 1978; Bassendine,
1980) and in some patients brings about a disappearance of Dane particles from blood (Pollard et al., 1978; Merigan and Robinson, 1978)
and liver (Merigan and Robinson, 1979). However, ara-A produces
side effects, such as gastro-intestinal and neurological disturbances
which may necessitate discontinuation of therapy (Sacks et al., 1979);
moreover it causes a marked lymphocytopenia (Hafkin et al., 1979)
which may affect the outcome of the treatment since successful anti-
viral therapy appears to require the cooperation of host immune response. Selective concentration of ara-A or ara-AMP into hepatocytes
as achieved by coupling these drugs to L-SA, should reduce the side
effects and improve the efficacy of the treatment. Since ara-A and
ara-AMP pass across the external cell membrane, the conjugates should
be administered by continuous infusion in order to assure a prolonged
hepatocyte targeting of the drugs (see above). This does not represent a disadvantage because also free ara-A is given by continuous
infusion in the treatment of chronic hepatitis B (Pollard et al.,
1979; Chadwick et al., 1978) as well as of infections caused by
other DNA viruses (Whitley et al., 1975). A drawback in the clinical
use of these conjugates could be their immunogenicity. In further
experiments we will study this problem and assess whether laboratory
animals produce antibodies against conjugates prepared with homologous lactosaminated albumin and infused intravenously. The finding
that galactosyl terminal albumins are not bound to macrophages
(Stahl et al., 1978), and the evidence that molecules which are not
taken up by these cells are either poor immunogens or not immunogenic
at all (Benacerraf and Unanue 1979), make it possible that antibodies against these conjugates will not be produced.

ACKNOWLEDGEMENTS

Part of authors' work reported in this chapter was supported by
funds from Consiglio Nazionale delle Ricerche, Progetto Finalizzato
Virus (grants no 77.00244.84 and 78.00339.84) and Progetto Finalizzato Controllo Crescita neoplastica (grants no 79.00626 and
80.01545/96).

REFERENCES

Akazaki, K., 1953, Tumors of the reticulo-endothelial system, Acta
     Path, Jap. 3:24.
Ashwell, G., and Morell, A.G., 1974, The role of surface carbohy-
     drates in the hepatic recognition and transport of circulating

glycoproteins, Adv. Enzymol., 41:99.

Balboni, P.G., Minia, A., Grossi, M.P., Barbanti-Brodano, G., and
    Fiume, L., 1976, Activity of albumin conjugates of 5-fluoro-
    deoxyuridine and cytosine arabinoside on poxviruses as a lyso-
    somotropic approach to antiviral chemotherapy, Nature, 264:181.

Barbanti-Brodano, G., and Fiume, L., 1973, Selective killing of
    macrophages by amanitin-albumin conjugates, Nature New Biology,
    243:281.

Barbanti-Brodano, G., and Fiume, L., 1974, In-vitro effect of a 5-
    fluorodeoxyuridine albumin conjugate on tumour cells and on
    peritoneal macrophages, Experientia, 30:1180.

Bassendine, M.F., 1980, Adenine arabinoside, in:"Virus and the liver",
    Bianchi, L., Sickinger, K., Gerok, W., and Stalder, G.A., eds,
    MTP, Lancaster.

Benacerraf, B., Biozzi, G., Halpern, B.N., Stiffel, C., and Mouton,
    D., 1957, Phagocytosis of heat-denatured human serum albumin
    labelled with ^{131}I and its use as a means of investigating
    liver blood flow, Br. J. Expl. Pathol., 38:35.

Benacerraf, B., and Unanue, E.R., 1979, "Textbook of Immunology"
    Williams and Wilkins, Baltimore, London.

Borondy, P.E., Chang, T., Maschewske, E., and Glazko, A.J., 1977,
    Inhibition of adenosine deaminase by co-vidarabine and its
    effect on the metabolic disposition of adenine arabinoside
    (vidarabine), Ann, NY Acad. Sci. 284:9.

Buys, C.H., Marieke, G.L., Elferink, J.M., Bouma, J.M., Gruber,
    M., and Nieuwenhuis, P., 1973, Proteolysis of formaldehyde-
    treated albumin in Küpffer cells and its inhibition by
    suramin, J. Reticuloend. Soc., 14:209.

Cessi, C., and Fiume, L., 1969, Increased toxicity of β-amanitin
    when bound to a protein, Toxicon, 6:309.

Chadwick, R.G., Bassendine, M.F., Crawford, E.M., Thomas, H.C., and
    Sherlock, S., 1978, HBsAg-positive chronic liver disease:
    inhibition of DNA polymerase activity by vidarabine, Brit.
    Med. J., 2:531.

De Duve, C., De Barsy, Th., Poole, B., Trouet, A., Tulkens, P.,
    and Van Hoof, F., 1974, Lysosomotropic agents, Biochem.
    Pharmacol. 23:2495/

Derenzini, M., Fiume, L., Marinozzi, V., Mattioli, A., Montanaro,
    L., and Sperti, S., 1973, Pathogenesis of liver necrosis
    produced by amanitin-albumin conjugates, Lab. Invest., 29:150.

Di Luzio, N.R., and Morrow, H.S., 1971, Comparative behaviour of
    soluble and particulate antigens and inert colloids in reti-
    culoendothelial-stimulated or depressed mice, J. Reticuloend.
    Soc., 9:273.

Dunn, T.B., 1954, Normal and pathologic anatomy of the reticular
    tissue in laboratory mice, with a classification and discuss-
    ion of neoplasms, J. Natl. Cancer Inst., 14:1281.

Faulstich, H., and Trischmann, H., 1973, Toxicity and inhibition of
    RNA polymerase by α-amanitin bound to macromolecules by an azo
    linkage, Hoppe-Seyler's Z. Physiol. Chem., 354:1395.

Fenner, F., and White, D.O., 1976, "Medical Virology", Academic
    Press, New York, San Francisco, London.
Fiume, L., 1969, Penetration of a β-amanitin-rabbit-albumin conju-
    gate into hepatic parenchymal cells, Lancet, II:853
Fiume, L., and Barbanti-Brodano, G., 1974, Selective toxicity of
    amanitin-albumin conjugates for macrophages, Experientia, 30:76.
Fiume, L., Busi, C., Mattioli, A., Balboni, P.G., and Barbanti-
    Brodano, G., 1981, Hepatocyte targetting of adenine-9-β-D-
    arabinofuranoside 5'-monophosphate(ara-AMP) coupled to lacto-
    saminated albumin, FEBS Lett., in press.
Fiume, L., Campadelli-Fiume, G., and Wieland, Th., 1971, Facilitated
    penetration of amanitin-albumin conjugates into hepatocytes
    after coupling with fluorescein, Nature New Biol., 230:219.
Fiume, L., and Laschi, R., 1965, Lesioni ultrastrutturali prodotte
    nelle cellule parenchimali epatiche dalla falloidina e dalla
    α-amanitina, Sperimentale, 115:288.
Fiume, L., Mattioli, A., Balboni, P.G., and Barbanti-Brodano, G.,
    1979 a, Albumin conjugates of fungal toxins and of inhibitors
    of DNA synthesis, in: "Drug Carriers in Biology and Medicine"
    G. Gregoriadis ed., Academic Press, London, New York, San
    Francisco.
Fiume, L., Mattioli, A., Balboni, P.G., Tognon, M., Barbanti-Brondano
    G., De Vries, J., and Wieland, Th., 1979 b, Enhanced inhibition
    of virus DNA synthesis in hepatocytes by trifluorothymidine
    coupled to asialofetuin, FEBS Lett., 103:47.
Fiume, L., Mattioli, A., Busi, C., Balboni, P.G., Barbanti-Brodano,
    G., De Vries, J., Altmann, R., and Wieland, Th., 1980,
    Selective inhibition of Ectromelia virus DNA synthesis in
    hepatocytes by adenine-9-β-D-arabinofuranoside (ara-A) and
    adenine-9-β-D-arabinofuranoside 5'-monophosphate (ara-AMP)
    coupled to asialofetuin, FEBS Lett., 116:185.
Furth, J.J., and Cohen, S.S., 1967, Inhibition of mammalian DNA
    polymerase by 5'-triphosphate of 9-β-D-arabinofuranosyladenine,
    Cancer Res., 27:1528.
Gall, E.A., Mallory, T.B., 1942, Malignant lymphoma. A clinico-
    pathologic survey of 618 cases, Am. J. Path., 18:381
Gray, G.R., 1974, The direct coupling of oligosaccharides to
    proteins and derivatized gels, Arch. Biochem. Biophys.,
    163:426.
Gregoriadis, G., 1975, Catabolism of glycoproteins in: "Lysosomes
    in Biology and Pathology (4)", J.T. Dingle, and R.T. Dean,
    eds. North Holland Publishing Co., Amsterdam, Oxford and
    American Elsevier Publishing Co., New York.
Gregoriadis, G., and Neerunjun, E.D., 1975, Homing of liposomes
    to target cells, Biochem. Biophys. Res. Commun., 65:537
Hafkin, B., Pollard, R.B., Tiku, M.L., Robinson, W.S., and Merigan,
    T.C., 1979, Effects of interferon and adenine arabinoside
    treatment of hepatitis B virus infection of cellular immune
    responses, Antimicrobial Agents and Chemotherapy, 16:781.
Halloran, M.J., and Parker, C.W., 1966, The preparation of nucleo-

tide protein conjugates: carbodiimides as coupling agents, J. Immunol., 96:373.

Haurowitz, F., 1968,"Immunochemistry and the biosynthesis of anti-bodies,"Interscience, New York.

Hencin, R.S., and Preston, J., 1979, Differential inhibition of cultured cell types by α-amanitin bovine serum albumin conjugates, Mol. Pharmacol., 16:961.

Hubbard, A.L., Wilson, G., Ashwell, G., and Stukenbrok, H., 1979, An electron microscope autoradiographic study of the carbohydrate recognition systems in rat liver. I. Distribution of ^{125}I-ligands among the liver cell types, J. Cell Biol., 83:47.

Kedinger, C., Gniazdowski, M., Mandel, J.L., Gissinger, F., and Chambon, P., 1970, α-Amanitin: a specific inhibitor of one of two DNA-dependent RNA polymerase activities from calf thymus, Biochem. Biophys. Res. Commun., 38;165

Krantz, M.J., Holtzman, N.A., Stowell, C.P., and Lee, Y.C., 1976, Attachment of thioglycosides to proteins: Enhancement of liver membrane binding, Biochemistry, 15:3963.

Kruse, H., and McMaster, P.D., 1949, The distribution and storage of blue antigenic azoproteins in the tissues of mice, J. Exp. Med., 90:425.

Lindell, Th., Weinberg, F., Morris, P.W., Roeder, R.G., and Rutter, W.J., 1970, Specific inhibition of nuclear RNA-polymerase II by α-amanitin, Science, 170:447.

Marinozzi, V., and Fiume, L., 1971, Effects of α-amanitin on mouse and rat liver cell nuclei, Exp. Cell. Res., 67:311.

Merigan, T.C., and Robinson, W.S., 1978, Antiviral therapy in HBV infection, in: "Viral hepatitis" Vias, G.N., Cohen, S.N., Schmid, R., eds., The Franklin Institute Press, Philadelphia.

Mims, C.A., 1959 a, The response of mice to large intravenous injections of Ectromelia virus. I. The fate of injected virus, Br. J. Expl. Pathol., 40:533.

Mims, C.A., 1959 b, The response of mice to large intravenous injection of Ectromelia virus. II. The growth of virus in the liver, Br. J. Expl. Pathol., 40:543.

Morell, A.G., Irvine, R.G., Sternlieb, I., Scheinberg, I.H., and Ashwell, G.A., 1968, Physical and chemical studies on ceruloplasmin, J. Biol. Chem., 243:155.

Plunkett, W., Alexander, L., Cubb, S., and Loo, T.L., 1979, Comparison of the activity of 2'-deoxycoformicin and erythro-9-(2-hydroxy-3-nonyl)adenine in vivo, Biochem. Pharmacol., 28:201.

Pollard, R.B., Smith, J.L., Neal, E.A., Gregory, P.B., Merigan, T.C., and Robinson, W.S., 1978, Effect of vidarabine on chronic hepatitis B virus infection. J. Am. Med. Ass., 239:1648.

Regoeczi, E., Chindemi, P.A., Hatton, M.W.C., and Berry, L.R., 1980, Galactose-specific elimination of human asialotransferrin by the bone marrow in the rabbit, Arch. Biochem. Biophys., 205:76.

Regoeczi, E., Debanne, M.T., Hatton, M.W.C., and Koj, A., 1978, Elimination of asialofetuin and asialorosomucoid by the intact rat. Quantitative aspects of the hepatic clearance mechanism, Biochim. Biophys. Acta, 541:372.

Roberts, J.A., 1963, Histopathogenesis of mousepox: III Ectromelia virulence, Br. J. Expl. Pathol., 44:465.

Rogers, J.C., and Kornfeld, S., 1971, Hepatic uptake of proteins coupled to fetuin glycopeptide, Biochem. Biophys. Res. Commun. 45:622.

Sacks, S.L., Smith, J.L., Pollard, R.B., Sawhney, V., Mahol, A.S., Gregory, P., Merigan, T.C., and Robinson, W.S., 1979, Toxicity of vidarabine, J. Am. Med. Ass. 241:28.

Schwartz, B.A., and Gray, G.R., 1977, Proteins containing reductively aminated disaccharides. Synthesis and chemical characterisation Arch. Biochem. Biophys., 181:542.

Sidwell, R.W., Allen, L.B., Huffman, J.H., Khwaja, T.A., Tolman, R.L., and Robinson, R.K., 1973, Anti DNA virus activity of the 5'-nucleotide and 3', 5'-cyclic nucleotide of 9- -D-arabinofuran-osyladenine, Chemotherapy, 19:325.

Stahl, P.D., Rodman, J.S., Miller, M.J., and Schlesinger, P.H., 1978, Evidence for receptor-mediated binding of glycoproteins, glyco-conjugates, and lysosomal glycosidases by alveolar macrophages, Proc. Natl. Acad. Sci. USA, 75:1399.

Stirpe, F., and Fiume, Lk., 1967, Effect of α-amanitin on ribonuc-leic acid synthesis and on ribonucleic acid polymerase in mouse liver nuclei, Biochem. J., 105:779.

Trouet, A., Deprez-De Campeneere, D., and De Duve, C., 1972, Chemo-therapy through lysosomes with a DNA-daunorubicin complex, Nature New Biology, 239:110.

Unanue, E.R., 1972, The regulatory role of macrophages in antigenic stimulation, Adv. Immunol., 15:95.

Van Furth, R., Cohn, Z.A., Hirsch, J.G., Humphrey, J.H., Spector, W.G., and Langevoort, H.L., 1972, The mononuclear phagocyte system: a new classification of macrophages, monocytes, and their precursor cells, Bull. Wld. Hlth. Org., 46:845.

Whitley, R.J., Ch'ien, L.T., Buchanan, R.A., and Alford, C.A. Jr., 1975, Studies on adenine arabinoside. A model for antiviral chemotherapeutics, Persp. Virol., 9:315.

Wieland, Th., 1968, Poisonous principles of mushrooms of the genus Amanita, Science, 159:946.

Wieland, Th., and Faulstich, H., 1978, Amatoxins, phallotoxins, phallolysin, and antamanide: the biologically active components of poisonous Amanita mushrooms, Crit. Rev. Biochem., 5:185.

Wilson, G., 1978, Effect of reductive lactosamination on the heptic uptake of bovine pancreatic ribonuclease A dimer, J. Biol. Chem., 253:2070.

Wilson, G., Eidelberg, M., and Michalak, V., 1979, Selective hepatic uptake of synthetic glycoproteins, J. Gen. Physiol., 74:495.

York, J.L., and Le Page, G.A., 1966, A proposed mechanism for the action of 9-β-D-arabinofuranosyl-adenine as an inhibitor of the growth of some ascites cells, Can. K. Biochem. Physiol., 44:19.

Youle, R.J., Murray, G.J., and Neville, D.M., 1979, Ricin linked to monophosphopentamannose binds to fibroblast lysosomal hydrolase receptors, resulting in a cell-type-specific toxin, Proc. Natl. Acad. Sci. USA, 76:5559.

TARGETING OF ANTITUMOUR AND ANTIPROTOZOAL DRUGS BY COVALENT LINKAGE TO PROTEIN CARRIERS

André Trouet, Roger Baurain, Danièle Deprez-De Campeneere, Michèle Masquelier & Philippe Pirson

Laboratory of Physiological Chemistry
Université Catholique de Louvain and International Institute of Cellular and Molecular Pathology
Brussels, Belgium

The possibility of directing drugs selectively to their cellular targets was considered for the first time by Paul Ehrlich at the beginning of this century. It is, however, only since about twenty years that developments in biology and medicine have incited an increasing number of laboratories to try to translate this dream into reality. One of the most promising and most explored approaches is the linkage of very active but toxic pharmacological agents to carriers which will transport and target these selectively to sites of action.

Targeting through the use of carriers relies on the assumption that the carrier will recognise selectively the target site and interact with it so as to allow the transported drug to become active. Targeting of a drug requires first of all that the drug should be linked to the carrier in a stable manner, and that as a consequence, the drug should remain associated with the carrier all along its way through the body from the site of administration to the site of interaction with the target. This implies a resistance of the link between the drug and the carrier to the various enzymatic and physicochemical conditions prevailing in the bloodstream and the extracellular fluids. This stability implies also that the drug should remain inactive as long as it is associated with its carrier since otherwise it would be able to exert its action before reaching the target. A corollary of this stability requirement is that there should be a mechanism by which the drug will be activated after reaching its destination. When considering the cell biological aspects of this problem of activation, four possible sites can be distinquished. The first and most

19

promising one is the lysosomal compartment; it concerns carriers which
after having reached the target cell surface, are endocytozed, concentrated inside the lysosomes wherein the drugs could be released.
A second possible site is extracellular, close to the cell surface
and would involve the activation of the drug through the enzymes of
the plasma membrane or the enzymes which are released by the target
cells in the surrounding extracellular space. As a third possibility,
the carrier would be unable to penetrate the cell and promote the
intracytoplasmic penetration of the transported drug by allowing its
transmembrane passage; this would mostly concern liposomes and possibly some toxins. A fourth site of activation would be intracellular
for carriers which can enter cells by permeation across the cell
membrane. In the latter case, it must be realised that the selectivity of the carried drug will not be determined by a selective cell
uptake of the drug carrier which will enter any cell type. Alkylating
agents have, for example, been linked to steroid hormones reacting
with cytoplasmic receptors present in breast and prostatic tumours.[1]
The carried drug, however, remained active and it is at present
difficult to think of an intracellular process which would allow antitumour drugs linked to steroid hormones to become activated upon
reaction of the hormones with their receptor.

The great majority of carriers tested are of macromolecular
nature and are supposed to interact specifically with the cell surface
in order to be endocytozed. In this category one finds DNA, liposomes, red blood cell ghosts, lectins, synthetic polymers, nanocapsules and various proteins, such as glycoproteins, polypeptidic
hormones and antibodies.[2] In the remaining part of this paper, we
will deal only with carriers of macromolecular or corpuscular nature.
These carriers have to fulfill a further set of criteria, such as
appropriate interaction with the target cells, degradability and last
but not least selectivity (Table 1).

Endocytosis and transfer into the lysosomal compartment is the
major and up to now unique practical route by which carriers (lysosomotropic carriers) can deliver their drugs intracellularly. Only
some liposome types have been claimed to deliver their content by
fusion with the cell membrane and direct penetration of their drugs
into the cytoplasm. Although some slight evidence in favour of such
a mechanism could be obtained in in-vitro conditions using cells in
culture, it has not yet been proven to occur even at low frequency
in vivo.[3]

In order to avoid the problem of lysosomal overloading, the
carrier should be degradable and all carrier types fulfil this criteria, except the nanocapsules, the in-vivo degradability of which
still remains questionable.[4] The size of the carrier plays also a
determinant role in the targeting of drugs to tissues or cells separated from the injection site or the bloodstream by anatomical
barriers such as the capillary walls or the blood-brain barrier.

Table 1. Criteria to be fulfilled by a lysosomotropic
          drug–carrier conjugate

The carrier should be:

1. selective for the target cell surface,

2. endocytozed by the target cell and be transferred
   into the lysosomal compartment,

3. degradable,

4. non–immunogenic,

5. permeable to the anatomical barriers separating the
   administration site and the target.

The drug should be resistant to lysosomal enzymes and pH.

The drug–carrier conjugate should be:

1. stable in the bloodstream and extracellular spaces,

2. pharmacologically inactive,

3. sensitive to the lysosomal enzymes or pH such that
   it can be released in an active form,

4. non–immunogenic.

Size will play an important role with regard to the capillary walls
when one considers that the capillary structures of tissues vary
extensively. Capillary walls are very incomplete with discontinuous
basal membrane and endothelial lining in the liver, spleen and bone
marrow. They become increasingly important with a continuous basal
membrane and a complete endothelial lining in various other tissues
culminating in the impermeable blood–brain barrier.

     The carrier–drug conjugate should also be non–immunogenic and
this seems to be one of the major problems of the immunotoxins which
are conjugates of antibodies and toxins of plant or bacterial
origin.[5]

     The intralysosomal activation step adds three supplementary
conditions; the carrier should be endocytozed after reaction with
the cell membrane and reach the lysosomes subsequently, the drug
should be released from the carrier in an active form through the
action of lysosomal enzymes or the acidic pH prevailing in the
lysosomes and the drug itself should be resistant to the action of
the lysosomal enzymes and pH.

     Finally, the most important quality of a carrier is that of
recognising and interacting selectively with a target cell. For

antitumour drugs obvious candidates are antibodies directed against
tumour specific antigens, differentiation and embryonic antigens
found on the surface of tumour cells; one should also consider peptide
hormones reacting with some tumour cell types. An absolute selectivity will perhaps be difficult to achieve for all the cancer cell
types but it should be remembered that important advances in cancer
chemotherapy can be made by endowing toxic agents with a level of
selectivity depending not so much on a specific penetration into the
target cells but more on preventing their penetration in one or
several normal cell types which are very sensitive to the toxic effects
of the drugs. As carriers for antiprotozoal drugs one should consider
glycoproteins which are known to be taken up by macrophages of the
reticuloendothelial system or, as we will see later, by hepatocytes.

Keeping in mind these theoretical considerations we have tried
to develop a method for the covalent linkage of the antitumour drug
daunorubicin (DNR) to protein. DNR was chosen because like its
analogue doxorubicin, it is a very potent antitumour agent and because
we know from our previous work with DNA complexes that DNR and DOX
are resistant to lysosomal hydrolases and acidic pH.[6] Serum albumin
(SA) was chosen as a test protein carrier not for its selectivity
properties but for practical reasons of availability. It was used to
test whether a suitable technique for linking DNR to proteins could
be developed, which would then later be used to link DNR to selective protein carriers such as antibodies, polypeptide hormones and
glycoproteins.

DNR was in a first step linked to succinylated SA by an amide
bond formed between the DNR aminogroup and the carboxylic side chain
group of the protein in presence of water soluble carbodiimide (ECD)
as condensing agent. SA was first extensively succinylated in order
to prevent the formation of SA polymers in the presence of ECD. The
reversibility of this linkage by the action of lysosomal hydrolases
was tested in vitro by incubating the conjugates in the presence of
a purified lysosomal extract. The liberation of intact DNR was then
determined by HPLC and fluorometry.[7] After 10 hours of incubation
(Table 2) only 2% of the protein-linked drug could be detected as a
free and intact DNR. This result was not unexpected since the amide
bond is probably protected from an attack by the hydrolytic enzymes
due to the steric hindrance effect of the carrier protein. Moreover,
this bond is not in an α position with regard to an asymmetric carbon
which makes it a poor substrate for peptidases and proteases. In
order to cicumvent these problems we decided to intercalate amino-
acids between DNR and the protein. Leucine was chosen as the aminoacid adjacent to DNR since preliminary studies had shown that leucyl-
DNR was hydrolysed rapidly into DNR by lysosomal hydrolases.[8] The
spacer arm was increased to form a di, tri or tetrapeptide by altern-
ating leucine and alanine in order to maintain a sufficient water
solubility and a good sensitivity to hydrolytic enzymes. The four
types of SA-DNR conjugates with a spacer arm varying from one amino-

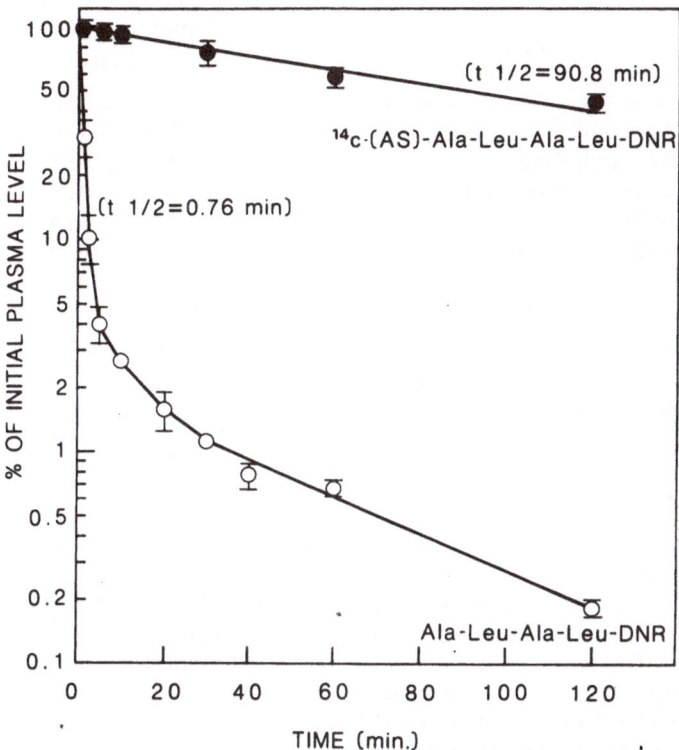

Fig. 1.   Plasma disappearance of tetrapeptide daunorubicin free or
          linked to succinylated serum albumin, after i.v. injection
          into mice.

DBA$_2$ mice received i.v. [14]C-(SA)-Ala-Leu-Ala-Leu-DNR(●)
or Ala-Leu-Ala-Leu-DNR (O) at a dose corresponding to 7 mg
DNR/kg. Succinylated serum albumin was labelled with [14]C
before linking to DNR derivative. TCA-insoluble radioactivity was followed in the plasma and drugs were analysed
by HPLC and fluorometry.
Mean $\pm$ S.D. values of 2 separate assays are given.

TABLE 2

Lysosomal hydrolysis of conjugates of DNR linked
directly or through a peptide spacer arm to
succinylated serum albumin.*

Conjugate	DNR released % ± S.D.
(SA)–DNR	2.6 ± 0.4
(SA)–Leu–DNR	5.0 ± 0.8
(SA)–Ala–Leu–DNR	8.0 ± 0.9
(SA)–Leu–Ala–Leu–DNR	59.5 ± 2.3
(SA)–Ala–Leu–Ala–Leu–DNR	74.1 ± 0.5

DNR linked to succinylated serum albumin (SA) delivered through
a peptide spacer arm was incubated for 10 hours at 38°C, pH 5.5
in the presence of lysosomal enzymes purified from rat liver. The
amount of DNR released was detected by high pressure liquid chromatography and fluorometry and expressed as a percentage of the
total fluorescence.

acid to a tetrapeptide were then incubated with lysosomal hydrolases
and the release of intact DNR determined as described before (Table
2). The amount of active DNR released in vitro from the conjugates
remains very low when one aminoacid or a dipeptide is used as a
spacer arm. The amount of DNR released increases however, very
significantly when a tripeptide or tetrapeptide spacer arm is intercalated between DNR and the protein, 74% of DNR being released in
this latter case after 10 hours.

The stability of the SA–tetrapeptide–DNR conjugate in serum was
checked by incubating for 24 hours at 37° in the presence of 95% calf
serum. Only 3% of the conjugated DNR was released in these experimental conditions. We have also followed the plasma disappearance
in mice of SA–tetrapeptide–DNR after i.v. injection at a DNR dose of
7 mg/kg. SA was labelled with ^{14}C before binding of DNR and the
amount of TCA insoluble radioactivity in the plasma was determined
for up to 2 hours after injection (Fig. 1). The protein carrier has
a half–life of 91 min and since no free drug could be detected in the
samples we can assume that no DNR was released from the conjugate
in vivo. As a control, free DNR–tetrapeptide was injected i.v. and
found to display a biphasic plasma clearance curve with a first phase
half–life of 0.76 min.

We have tested finally the chemotherapeutic activity of the
various SA–DNR conjugates on the L1210 leukemia in mice. In these
experiments, leukemic cells and drugs were given i.p. and the
survival curves of such an experiment are shown in Fig. 2. These

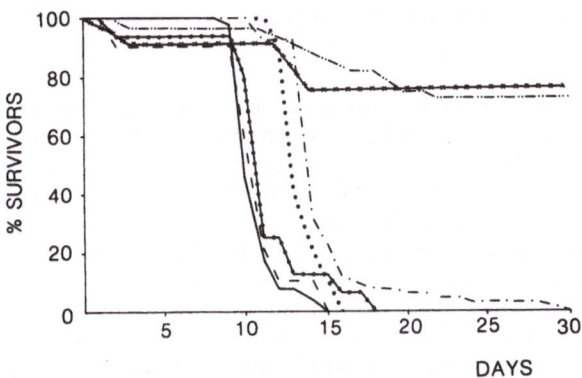

Fig. 2.   Survival of mice bearing i.p. L1210 leukemia after i.p.
treatment with various succinylated serum albumin–DNR
conjugates.

10^4 L1210 cells were inoculated i.p. on day 0 into DBA$_2$
mice. Drugs were administered by the same route on days 1
and 2 at the optimal tolerated dose (2 mg/kg for free DNR;
7.5 mg DNR/kg for the conjugates).

—: control mice; ·–·–·: DNR; •–•–•:SA–DNR; – – – :SA;Leu–DNR;
•••SA-Ala-Leu-DNR; ✗✗✗: SA-Leu-Ala-Leu-DNR; –"– SA-Ala-Leu-
Ala-Leu-DNR. Each curve corresponds to at least 2 pooled
experiments.

in-vivo experiments were performed in order to check whether the in-vitro criteria for the lysosomal reversibility of the SA-DNR bond could be confirmed in an in-vivo assay, and not to test the carrier potentialities of succinylated SA. Free DNR at the maximum tolerated dose of 2 mg/kg is marginally active whereas DNR linked directly to SA or through the intercalation of leucine has no therapeutic effect at 7.5 mg/kg in DNR. The SA-dipeptide-DNR conjugate induces a slight increase in life span similar to that of DNR but without any long-term survivors. In close parallel with the in-vitro data of Table 2, the therapeutic activity increases strikingly when a tri- or tetra-peptide spacer arm is intercalated between SA and DNR. In these conditions, more than 70% of the animals survive 30 days after the inoculation of leukemic cells.

We have thus developed a method for linking anthracyclines such as DNR to proteins. This linkage remains stable in the presence of serum and in plasma but can be hydrolyzed by lysosomal enzymes both in vitro and in vivo allowing the release of DNR. Several methods for conjugating DNR to protein carriers described before make use of gluteraldehyde or ECD as condensing agents[9], of periodate oxidation[10] and of leucyl-arginyl-glucopyranosyl as a spacer arm.[11] However, the conjugates thus obtained were sometimes active on cells in vitro and either inactive or not tested in in-vivo conditions. In the development of effective and selective antitumour drug-carrier conjugates the main effort must now be devoted to finding protein carriers possessing selective affinity for tumour cells and to determine whether by using such selective carriers, chemotherapy will be able to become the real effective answer to the problem of cancer.

We have, however, attempted to explore in vivo the selectivity potentialities of cell specific carriers by linking the antimalarial agent Primaquine (PQ) to a hepatocyte-selective glycoprotein via a tetrapeptide spacer arm and by testing the chemotherapeutic effect of this conjugate on the exoerythrocytic or hepatic stage of the murine Plasmodium berghei infection. In malaria, after inoculation by mosquitoes the infectious sporozoites invade the hepatocytes wherein they multiply and develop into schizonts which then invade the blood and the erythrocytes. The importance of the hepatic stage of the infection is greatest in malaria caused by Plasmodium vivax and Plasmodium ovale, since these protozoa can remain in a dormant state in the hepatocytes as hypnozoites and induce recurrences of the disease in absence of exposure to infected mosquitoes. One of the most active drugs against this liver stage of infection is PQ, the usefulness of which as a causal prophylactic agent is, however, restricted by its toxicity. Since, on the other hand, glycoproteins such as asialoglycoproteins with galactose terminal residues, are selectively recognised and endocytozed by hepatocytes[12], successful targeting of PQ by linking to a hepatocyte-specific carrier should result not only in a reduction of toxicity of PQ as observed when PQ is entrapped in liposomes[13], but also in an increase of its chemotherapeutic activity due to a more selective uptake by the target cells.

Asialofetiun (ASF) with less than 10% of its original content in sialic acid was obtained by treatment of calf fetuin with Clostridium perfringens neuraminidase. The tetrapeptide derivative of PQ (Ala-Leu-Ala-Leu-PQ), obtained as described previously[14] was linked to the amino side chain of ASF with the intercalation of a succinyl group (ASF-tetrapeptide-PQ). A drug/protein molar ratio varying between 5 and 8 was consistently obtained. As a control, the tetrapeptide derivative of PQ was also linked to ASF extensively succinylated (up to 85% of lysines) prior to conjugation. This succ-ASF-tetrapeptide-PQ was characterized by a drug/protein molar ratio varying between 5 and 6.

PQ, ASF-tetrapeptide-PQ and succ-ASF-tetrapeptide-PQ were tested against the experimental murine malaria. Plasmodium berghei sporozoites were injected i.v. in TB$_{ESP}$ mice and the different drugs given i.v. 3 hours after. The therapeutic results are expressed in terms of increase in life span and long term survivors and reported in Table 3. We give as a comparison the chemotherapeutic results obtained with PQ included in small multilamellar vesicles.[13] With free PQ the highest non toxic dose is 25 mg/kg, resulting in an ILS value in excess of 320% and inducing only 50% long term survivors. PQ is thus unable to exert experimentally a causal prophylactic effect after one i.v. injection. As described before[13], PQ entrapped in liposomes is less toxic than PQ but not more active and 100% cure of the animals can be obtained at a dose of 60 mg/kg. The results are quite different with ASF-tetrapeptide-PQ since this conjugated form of PQ is more active than free PQ inducing 100% long term survivors at a dose of 25 mg/kg. In contrast and as expected from the drug-carrier concept, when PQ is linked to a highly modified carrier such as succinylated ASF it becomes less active than even the free drug. This latter result suggests very strongly that when linked to a carrier which has most probably lost its specificity for the hepatocytes, PQ is to a lesser extent taken up by these cells than when given as a free drug. These results provide us the first evidence in favour of the possibility of targeting drugs in in-vivo conditions. The comparison between the results obtained with liposomes and with ASF are particularly interesting since liposomes by conveying PQ to liver and spleen have mainly an effect on the toxicity of PQ by decreasing its uptake by sensitive tissues.[13] The concentration of PQ in hepatocytes themselves seems not to be increased after administration of PQ entrapped into liposomes because they are mostly taken up by the Küpffer cells. Although further experiments are needed to substantiate and to complete the presented data, the higher activity of ASF-tetrapeptide-PQ is most probably due to a high hepatocyte concentration of PQ resulting from the targeting effect of ASF and from its intracellular uptake by endocytosis.

TABLE 3

Antimalarial activity of primeaquine and
asialofetuin-primaquine conjugates [a]

DRUG	Dose [b] (mg/kg)	ILS (%)	LTS/N [c]	CPD$_{50}$ [d]
Controls	-	0	0/223	-
PQ	6.25	46	0/6	22.5
	12.5	58	11/33	
	15.0	166	10/23	
	20.0	110	25/55	
	25.0	>320	50/94	
	30.0 [e]	91	2/9	
ASF-Ala-Leu-Ala-Leu-PQ	6.25	100	1/12	12.8
(MR = 7)	10.0	170	5/12	
	12.5	160	7/16	
	15.0	>400	7/12	
	20	>400	5/6	
	25	>400	12/12	
Succ-ASF-Ala-Leu-Ala-Leu-PQ				
(MR = 5.4-6.0)	6.25	26	0/7	38.5
	12.5	68	0/7	
	25	68	1/7	
	35	>163	4/7	
	50	>163	5/8	
Liposomes-PQ	20	109	4/14	26.7
	25	255	9/18	
	30	273	10/20	
	40	>355	21/24	
	60	>355	8/8	
	70	>355	12/12	

[a]Drugs were given intravenously 3 hours after inoculation of the
P.berghei sporozoites in male TB$_{ESP}$ mice

[b]Doses are expressed as mg PQ diphosphate equivalents/kg body weight

[c]Long term survivors per number of treated mice

[d]Dose curing 50% of treated mice (causal prophylactic dose 50%)

[e]Toxic dose

MR= Drug/protein molar ratio

In conclusion, we think that the stage is set for the final step which could bring the drug carrier concept into clinical application. This final step will be the most difficult one for antitumour drugs since it will require the search for, and the development of, carriers selective for tumour cells. This will be needed for every cell type and problems such as those of immunogenicity and accessibility will have to be carefully analysed and solved before it becomes possible to test the clinical validity of the drug carrier concept. The same ultimate step should be easier for targeting drugs towards cells such as hepatocytes or macrophages which possess receptors for selective glycoproteins. The possible indications for these carriers are anti-infectious drugs directed against malaria protozoa or viruses invading hepatocytes or against bacteria and protozoa which are harboured at some or all stages of their cycle in the cells of the reticuloendothelial system.

ACKNOWLEDGEMENTS

This work was supported by the Caisse Generale d'Epargne et de Retraite, Brussels (Belgium) and by the Rhône-Poulenc, S.A., Paris (France). This investigation also received financial support from the U.M.D.P./WORLD BANK/WHO Special Program for Research and Training in Tropical Diseases.

REFERENCES

1. M.E. Wall, G.S. Abernethy and F.I. Carroll, The effects of some steroidal alkylating agents on experimental animal mammary tumour and leukemia systems, J. Med. Chem. 12: 810 (1969)
2. G. Gregoriadis, Targeting of drugs, Nature, 265:407 (1977)
3. G. Poste, The interaction of lipid vesicles (liposomes) with cultured cells and their use as carrier for drugs and macro-molecules, in: "Liposomes in Biological Systems", G. Gregoriadis and A.C. Allison, eds., John Wiley & Sons, Chichester (1980)
4. J. Kreuter and P. Speiser, In vitro studies of poly(methyl meta-crylate) adjuvants, J. Pharm. Sci. 65: 1624 (1976)
5. F. Moolten, S. Zajdel and S. Cooperband, Immunotherapy of experi-mental animal tumors with antitumor antibodies conjugated to diphteria toxin or ricin, Ann.N.Y. Acad. Sci. 277: 690 (1976)
6. A. Trouet, D. Deprez-De Campeneere and C. de Duve, Chemotherapy through lysosomes with a DNA-daunorubicin complex, Nature, 239: 110 (1972)
7. R. Baurain, D. Deprez-De Campeneere and A. Trouet, Determination of daunorubicin, doxorubicin and their fluorescent metabol-ites by high-pressure liquid chromatography: plasma levels in DBA2 mice, Cancer Chemother.Pharmacol. 2: 11 (1979)
8. M. Masquelier, R. Baurain and A. Trouet, Amino acid and dipeptide derivatives of daunorubicin: I. Synthesis, physico-chemical properties and lysosomal digestion, J. Med. Chem. 23: 1166

(1980)
9. E. Hurwitz, R. Levy, R. Maron, M. Wilchek, R. Arnon and M.
    Sela, The covalent binding of daunomycin and adriamycin to
    antibodies, with retention of both drug and antibody activ-
    ities, Cancer Res. 35: 1175 (1975)
10. E. Hurwitz, R. Maron, R. Arnon, M. Wilchek, and M. Sela,
    Daunomycin-immunoglobulin conjugates, uptake and activity
    in vitro, Eur. J. Cancer, 44: 1213 (1978)
11. M. Monsigny, C. Kieda, A-C. Roche and F. Delmotte, Preparation
    and biological properties of a covalent antitumor drug-arm-
    carrier (DAC conjugate), FEBS Lett. 119:181 (1980)
12. A.G. Morell, G. Gregoriadis, I.H. Scheinberg, J. Hickman and
    G. Ashwell, The role of sialic acid in determining the
    survival of glycoproteins in the circulation, J. Biol.
    Chem., 246: 1461 (1971)
13. P. Pirson, R.F. Steiger and A. Trouet, Liposomes in the chemo-
    therapy of experimental murine malaria, Ann. Trop. Med.
    Parasitol, 74: 383 (1980)
14. A. Trouet, P. Pirson, R.F. Steiger, M. Masquelier, R. Baurain
    and J. Gillet, Development of new derivatives of primaquine
    by association with lysosomotropic carriers, Bull. WHO,
    59: 449 (1981)

ANTIBODIES AND DEXTRAN AS ANTI-TUMOUR DRUG CARRIERS

Ruth Arnon

Department of Chemical Immunology
The Weizmann Institute of Science
Rehovot 76100, Israel

INTRODUCTION

The approach described herewith is an attempt to use antibodies directed towards tumor-associated antigens or other polymers or macromolecules, as carriers for cytotoxic anti-cancer agents in order to improve the effectiveness of cancer chemotherapy.

Among the presently used means for treatment of cancer, chemotherapy, namely treatment with suitable drugs, constitutes a major and indispensable therapeutic approach, used in addition to surgery, radiotherapy and, to a lesser extent, immunotherapy. The advantage of chemotherapy is that it can be used effectively for disseminated, as well as localized, cancer. However, the cytotoxic drugs which are effective in killing neoplastic cells usually have detrimental effects also on normal cells, particularly the rapidly proliferating ones of the gastrointestinal tract and bone marrow, and cancer chemotherapy is ultimately limited by the toxicity of the drugs to these normal tissues, especially when employed in high dosages. One possible approach for increasing the effectiveness of antitumor drugs would be to find methods of altering their distribution in the body so as to increase their local concentration at the tumor sites, while a lower systemic concentration is maintained. In this way the selectivity of their toxicity for the tumor cells might be enhanced.

Paul Ehrlich (1906) was the first to suggest that molecules with an affinity for certain tissues might be able to serve as carriers of cytotoxic agents, concentrating them on the appropriate target cells in vivo. Various macromolecules have been shown to localize in tumor cells in vivo and were tested as possible carriers for cytotoxic drugs (Isliker et al., 1969). With the development of tumor immunology,

31

several investigators have sought to use antibodies to antigenic
determinants expressed preferentially on tumor cells as carriers of
cytotoxic agents. It is still open to question whether genuinely
tumor-specific antigens do exist. However, without going too deeply
into this problem, it is clear that antibodies, either polyclonal or
monoclonal, can be prepared which can distinguish between tumor cells
and normal ones in a selective fashion, and may thus be adequate by
virtue of this selectivity.

Either complexes or covalent conjugates of drugs with immunoglobulins and antibodies have been employed for treatment of tumors.
The resulting conjugates and complexes were shown to have selective
toxicity towards cells recognized by the antibodies, as discussed in
recent reviews (Arnon, 1979; O'Neil, 1979). For example, chlorambucil
has been linked non-covalently to antitumor antibodies and the complex
has been found to kill the target tumor cells more efficiently than
either the free drug or the antibody alone (Ghose et al., 1972;
Szekerke et al., 1972; Flechner, 1973). In two other studies (Davies
and O'Neil, 1973, 1974; Rubens and Dulbecco, 1974) it was shown that
similar effects could be obtained by administering the free drug and
the antibody separately. It is thus possible that when the drug is
administered as a non-covalent complex with antibody it dissociates
in vivo and acts separately and synergistically with the antibody,
as also suggested by Segerling et al. (1974).

The strategy described here is the use of conjugates in which
the drug is bound chemically to the carrier. It has been previously
shown that cytotoxic drugs of low molecular weight may retain their
activity after covalent linkage to macromolecules. Thus, methotrexate
was bound by an azo bond to hamster immunoglobulin (Mathe et al,
1958) as well as to fibrinogen and human serum albumin (HSA)
(Magnenat et al., 1969). The resulting conjugates possessed significant activity, as did conjugates of a methyl hydrazine derivative
with fibrinogen and albumin (Magnenat et al., 1969), or conjugates of
several nitrogen mustards with proteins and synthetic polypeptides
(Szekerke et al., 1967). We have reported previously that daunomycin
bound to antibodies yields a biologically active conjugate (Hurwitz
et al., 1975). Recently, with the development of hybridoma technology
for preparation of monoclonal antibodies (Kohler and Milstein, 1976),
an increasing number of scientists have tried to use them as carriers
for cytotoxic agents, with varying degree of success (Gilliland et
al., 1981; Krolick et al., 1980; Youle and Neville, 1980; Blythman et
al., 1981).

The drugs we have used (Hurwitz et al., 1975; Levy et al., 1975)
are mainly the antitumor antibiotics, daunomycin and adriamycin, two
of the most useful chemotherapeutic cancer agents presently available
(Frei, 1972; O'Bryan et al., 1973). Daunomycin has been complexed
or conjugated to several macromolecular carriers in the last decade,
for the purpose of targeted local delivery. Thus, Trouet et al.

(1972) complexed it with DNA that served as a lysosomotropic agent;
Kitao and Hattori (1977) used Concanavalin A as a carrier for daunomycin, assuming that it will bind specifically to particular carbo-
hydrate-bearing cells; and Varga et al. (1977) have prepared a
Melanotropin-daunomycin conjugate, and demonstrated that it showed
receptor-mediated cytotoxicity towards melanoma cells in tissue
culture.

In our experiments the drugs were bound in a covalent manner to
antibodies, either conventional or monoclonal, specific towards
several experimental murine tumors. A prerequisite for the success
of the whole approach is that both the drug and the antibodies will
retain their activity when the two are linked. Results presented
here will illustrate the retained activity and selective cytotoxicity
of such conjugates both in vitro and in vivo.

THE TUMOR SYSTEMS

Our investigations have been concerned with several tumor
systems:

1) Bone marrow derived lymphatic leukemia - A dimethylbenzan-
thracene-induced leukemia in SJL/J mice (Haran-Ghera and Peled, 1973),
maintained by subcutaneous passage in syngeneic mouse strains. The
cells of this leukemia bear immunoglobulin on their surface and are,
therefore, referred to as B-leukemia cells.

2) Plasmacytoma RPC5 - A mineral oil induced plasmacytoma in
BALB/c mice (Potter and Robertson, 1960), maintained by subcutaneous
passage in BALB/c mice.

3) A Moloney virus induced lymphoma (YAC) - Developed by Klein
and Klein (1964) in A/J mice. It appears usually as a lymphoma in
the ascitis form, and is maintained by passage in A/J mice.

4) Lewis lung carcinoma (3LL) - A spontaneous tumor which grows
in C57BL/6J mice (Seguira and Stock, 1955), with patterns of progression resembling those of human neoplasms. It grows at the site of
transplantation (usually intra-footpad) or subcutaneously as a local
primary tumor (L-3LL), and after 2-3 weeks develops as visible
metastatic foci (M-3LL) in the lungs.

5) A leukemia (38C 13) - Produced in C3H/eB mice (Haran-Ghera
and Peled, 1973) by induction with 7,12-dimethylbenzanthracene.

ANTIBODY PREPARATIONS

The carriers used for attachment of the drugs are antibodies
directed towards the various tumors, raised in either rabbits, goats
or syngeneic mice. In various experiments use was made of either

the immunoglobulin fraction (Ig) of the respective antisera, purified antibodies obtained from them, or monoclonal antibody products of suitable hybridomas:

Anti-YAC was produced in rabbits or in a goat by injection of a soluble papain digest of the YAC cell membrane (Hurwitz et al., 1978b). Xenogeneic antibodies were purified from the sera by absorption and elution from glutaraldehyde-fixed YAC cells. Monoclonal anti-YAC antibodies were also produced, by using spleen cells of syngeneic mice immunized with whole YAC cells for hybridization. The resultant hybridoma (KH3-4) was of the IgM class (Eshhar et al. 1980).

Anti-3LL sera were produced in rabbits and in syngeneic mice by repeated injections of 3LL cells (Hurwitz et al., 1979). The xenogeneic sera were rendered specific by in vivo absorptions in syngeneic mice. Monoclonal antibodies were prepared from immunized rat spleen, hybridized with the mouse myeloma (NSI). The respective hybridoma line (6B) was of the IgG class.

Anti-38C leukemia was produced by injecting a goat with a 38C 13 cell surface IgM (Bergman and Haimovich, 1977). The serum was rendered specific by adsorbing out all the goat anti-mouse antibodies, except those directed to the cell surface IgM.

The Ig fractions were prepared by precipitation with ammonium sulphate, at 33% saturation from goat and rabbit sera, and at 43% saturation from mouse sera.

DRUG-ANTIBODY CONJUGATES

The conjugates used in this study contained four different drugs - daunomycin (Dau), adriamycin (Adr), methoetrexate (MTX), and platinum compounds (Pt), which were covalently linked to the various immunoglobulin or antibody preparations either directly or via a linking polymer. The individual conjugates used in the various experiments are described in the following.

1) Conjugates of daunomycin and adriamycin. Two different binding procedures were used for binding the drugs to the immunoglobulins: (a) The direct binding procedure. Periodate oxidation of the drugs was performed to cleave the bond between C_3 and C_4 of the amino sugar. This produced carbonyl groups capable of reacting with free amino groups on the protein, and the resulting Schiff-base linkages were subsequently reduced with sodium borohydride (Hurwitz et al., 1975). (b) Linking of daunomycin or adriamycin to immunoglobulins via a dextran bridge. Dextran was oxidized by periodate. The polyaldehyde dextran was reacted first with daunomycin for 20 hr at room temperature and then with the antibody for 20 hr at 4°C. The product was then reduced by $NaBH_4$, using 15-30%

of the amount required for total reduction of the aldehyde groups on
the oxidized dextran. These conditions were used since reduction was
necessary for stabilization of the conjugate, but more rigorous reducing conditions caused damage to both the drug and the antibody. The
antibody-dextran-daunomycin was separated from free drug and drug-
dextran conjugates by gel filtration. The binding through dextran
resulted in increased substitution of antibody by drug, from about
4-6 M/M by the direct binding to as much as 50 M/M, without significa-
cant loss of antibody activity. On the other hand, binding of
daunomycin via dextran caused a more drastic reduction in the drug
activity than the direct binding, but this could be compensated for
by increasing the concentration of the drug-conjugate or by prolonging the incubation time with the cells, after which 90%-95% cytotoxicity could eventually be achieved. The antibody and drug activities of the conjugates are summarized in Table 1.

The chemical nature of the bond formed between polyaldehyde-
dextran and daunomycin has not been elucidated. When the drug was
bound by non-hydrolyzable linkages, the resulting conjugates lost
completely the drug activity in vitro (Hurwitz et al., 1980). It is
assumed, therefore, that the dextran aldehyde groups form oxazolidine
derivatives with the drug's sugar amino group and its vicinal hydroxy
group, or that unreduced Schiff bases are formed.

In contrast to the daunomycin, the adriamycin-polyaldehyde
derivatives prepared under similar conditions were either inactive
or of very low activity. A different method of linkage was therefore
introduced in which the NH_2-sugar of the drug was left intact: The
drug was bound to a hydrazine derivative of dextran via its keto
group (carbon 13) (Hurwitz et al., 1980), and the antibodies were
attached to the hydrazone-dextran derivative by 0.1% glutaraldehyde.
The reduction of this bond, by equivalent amounts of $NaCNBH_3$, could
be performed before or after the binding of adriamycin. This
derivative maintained very high drug activity and at least 50% of the
antibody activity (Table 1).

MTX-antibody conjugates. In this case as well, two different
conjugates were prepared: a) In the first one the drug was linked
directly to the antibodies using water soluble carbodiimide. The
degree of substitution in different preparations was 6-8 moles MTX
per mole antibody, and its pharmacological activity in the conjugates
was retained almost to the full extent. The antibody activity in the
MTX-antibody conjugate was about 75% of the original antibody activity as determined for the conjugate MTX-anti-ovalbumin using the
precipitin assay. Higher degree of drug substitution resulted in
more drastic loss of antibody activity. b) In order to obtain a
higher degree of drug substitution without affecting the antibody
activity, the MTX was bound to the antibody via a bridge of copolymer
of glutamic acid and lysine, p(G-L), of M.W. 18,700 (with a ratio of
Glu:Lys 4.7:1, prepared according to Katchalsky and Sela, 1958).

Table 1. Activity of Daunomycin-immunoglobulin Conjugates

Antibody	Drug	Method of Binding	Extent Substitution M/M	Pharmacological Activity[a]	Antibody Activity[b]
Anti-RPC5 (rabbit)	Dau	Direct	5	-	77
Anti-B-leukemia (rabbit)	Dau	Direct	2;6	86	50;30
Anti-YAC, Ig (goat)	Dau	Via dextran	30	53	70
Anti-YAC, Ig	Adr	Via Hydrazine		100	50
Anti-YAC, Ig (goat)	MTX	Via p(G-L)	63	100	50
Anti-YAC, Ig (goat)	Pt	Direct	10	>100	100
Anti-YAC, purified antibody (goat)	Dau	Via dextran	25	48	73
Anti-YAC hybridoma	Dau	Via dextran	500	12	
Anti-YAC hybridoma	MTX	Via p(G-L)	250	83	
Anti-YAC hybridoma	Pt	Direct	10	>100	100
Anti-3LL (rabbit)	Dau	Direct	5	85	N.D.

Antibody	Drug	Method of Binding	Extent Substitution M/M	Pharmacological Activity[a]	Antibody Activity[b]
Anti-3LL (mouse)	Dau	Direct	4	78	N.D.
Anti-3LL hybridoma	Dau	Via dextran		47	
Anti-3LL hybridoma	MTX	Via p(G-L)	44,77	100	80

[a] Drug activity of the conjugate is expressed as % of that of the free drug and was measured by inhibition of ^{3}H-uridine or ^{3}H-thymidine incorporation in the case of daunomycin and adriamycin, or ^{3}H-deoxy-uridine incorporation in the case of methotrexate.
[b] Antibody activity of the conjugate is expressed as % of that of the unmodified antibody or Ig and was measured by complement dependent cytoxicity for anti-RPC-5, anti-B leukemia, and for some of the anti-YAC conjugates. The others were tested by direct or indirect binding assays.

The binding procedure consisted of two steps, each performed with water-soluble carbodiimide. In the first step the drug was bound to the copolymer in a dimethylformamide-water mixture. The yield of bound drug in this step is about 20%. In the second step this MTX-substituted copolymer was linked to the antibody preparations, in most cases monoclonal antibodies. The mixture containing the carbodiimide reagent was allowed to react in PBS for 2 hrs at room temperature and then fractionated on Sephadex to remove unbound drug. The yield of this step with respect to bound MTX was 70% and the degree of substitution in the conjugates varied from 45 to 250 mole/mole in the different preparations. The drug activity of the antibody-bound MTX was well preserved (from 80 to 100%) and the antibody activity in the conjugate was 50-80% of the original activity (Table I).

Platinum-antibody conjugates. Platinum (Pt) was complexed to Ig with the intention of reconstructing a product similar to the anti-cancer drug cis-diamino platinum dihydrochloride-(Cis-DDP), with a built-in specific carrier. These complexes were formed by direct reaction of the antibody with the platinum salt K_2PtCl_4 (Hurwitz et al., 1981). The drug activity in the complexes, both the Pt-goat anti-YAC Ig and Pt-mouse anti-YAC hybridoma, was much higher than that of Cis-DDP which was used for comparison and the antibody activity, as measured by antigen-binding, was also fully maintained (Table 1). The complement fixation capacity in some of the preparations was significantly diminished; it should be noted, however, that the decrease in complement mediated cytotoxicity, which might be due to the blocking of the complement binding site, need not interfere with the capacity of such complexes to serve as drug-carriers.

In-vitro activity determinations. The antibody activity was measured by one or more of the following techniques. (a) complement mediated cytotoxicity. (b) Indirect binding assays using as a second antibody ^{125}I-goat-anti-mouse (Fab')$_2$. (c) Direct binding assays with ^{125}I or ^{35}S labeled antibodies or with radioactively labeled antigens.

The pharmacological activity of the drugs or their antibody conjugates was measured by inhibition of synthesis of DNA-precursors, DNA or RNA (Hurwitz et al., 1975). Thus, the activity of daunomycin and adriamycin was estimated by their inhibition of ^3H-uridine or ^3H-methylthymidine incorporation; platinum salt or its Ig-complexes was evaluated by the inhibition of ^3H-methylthymidine incorporation; the activity of methotrexate (MTX) and its conjugates was determined by the inhibition of ^3H-deoxy-uridine incorporation.

THE SPECIFIC·CYTOTOXIC EFFECTS OF THE CONJUGATES IN VITRO

In preliminary studies with a model antibody system, anti-BSA, it was possible to demonstrate that drugs can be covalently bound to antibodies without losing their toxic effect on cells, and without a drastic curtailment of the antibody activity (Hurwitz et al., 1975). The next step was to determine whether the drugs bound to antibodies against individual tumours show preferential cytotoxicity against their specific target cells. This point was investigated with the daunomycin conjugates of anti-RPC-5 and anti-B-leukemia. To reveal their specificity they were allowed to attach to the target cells during a short incubation in vitro, after which the cells were washed to remove non-specific proteins and their drug conjugates, and then examined for residual drug effect by following the RNA synthesis, as expressed in percent inhibition of incorporation of ^{3}H−uridine. For the purpose of comparing the cytotoxicity effected by the same material on different target cells, experiments were carried out with aa concentration of daunomycin-antibody conjugate which is capable of effecting 60% inhibition of uridine incorporation.

The results depicted in Fig. 1 illustrate the specificity of the cytotoxic effects of the conjugates. Thus, in the RPC-5 system the conjugate in which the daunomycin was linked to anti-RPC-5 exerts 60% cytotoxicity, whereas the conjugate daunomycin-anti-B leukemia causes less than 20% inhibition of uridine incorporation. Opposite results were obtained in the B-leukemia system where the daunomycin-anti-B leukemia conjugate was highly effective in contrast to the conjugate with the anti-RPC-5. The conjugate in which the daunomycin was attached to the irrelevant anti-BSA is non-effective in either system under the experimental conditions. Free daunomycin inhibited uridine incorporation in both systems, although less efficiently than the specific conjugate.

In view of the assumption that xenogeneic antibodies might be used for drug-antibody conjugates if employed for cancer therapy, several advantages could be envisaged for the use of Fab dimers (Nisonoff et al., 1960), rather than intact antibodies (Arnon, 1979). We have therefore investigated whether Fab' dimers, derived by pepsin digestion of the Ig fraction of anti-YAC will also be effective as covalent carriers for daunomycin (Hurwitz et al., 1976).

The specific cytotoxicity of daunomycin-anti-(Fab')$_2$ conjugate was tested as in the previous experiments, by exposing the tumor cells to drug-bound (Fab')$_2$ fractions, or the free drug, for only 5 min. The cells were then washed to remove reactants that were unbound to the cells, and the toxicity of the daunomycin remaining in contact with the cells was assessed by the inhibition of ^{3}H − uridine incorporation. As can be seen from the results (Table 2), daunomycin-anti-YAC was twice as active as either the conjugate with the unrelated (Fab')$_2$ of anti-BSA or the free drug. Thus it is apparent that, according to the criteria used hitherto for the intact immunoglobulins, the Fab' dimer of the immunoglobulin is as efficient as the intact antibody molecule, and the removal of the Fc did not impair the capacity of the antibodies to act as carriers for anti-tumor drugs.

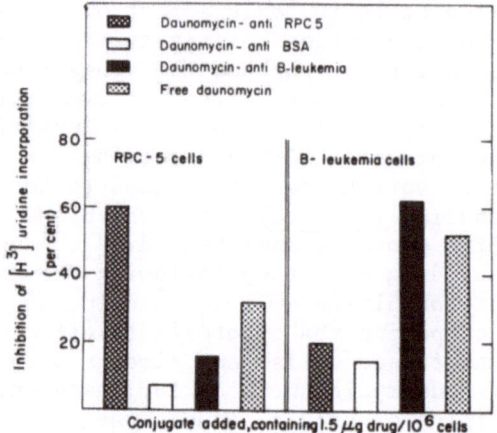

Fig. 1.   The specific cytotoxicity of daunomycin immunoglobulin
          conjugates. The assay was performed by incubating the
          drug-antibody conjugate with the particular cells toward
          which the antibody is directed for a short period (5 min).
          After washings, incubation was continued and inhibition
          of ^{3}H-uridine incorporation of the cell bound conjugates
          was tested.

          As already mentioned. it is advantageous to remove the Fc por-
tion of the immunoglobulins, for several reasons: it should decrease
the immunogenicity of the antibody, which is an important feature
when heterologous antibodies are used; it will shorten the persistence time of any unreacted drug-conjugate in the blood circulation,
and it will decrease the danger of any complement-mediated cytotoxicity affecting normal cells in the host animal. Indeed, we have
observed that the general toxicity of the $(Fab')_2$ is much weaker than
that of intact IgG. Thus, mice in the control groups injected with
a 5 mg dose of the anti-tumor IgG showed high mortality within 24 hr
and the surviving animals appeared rather sick, whereas mice injected
with a similar dose of the Fab' dimer preparation appeared normal and
healthy. This is not surprising, since within the scope of this
work, the function of the carrier antibody is just to guide the drug
to its target cells, and the only activity required of it is the
antigen-binding activity which is supposed to be retained in full in
the $(Fab')_2$.

          A system of particular interest is the Lewis lung carcinoma
(3LL). This tumor has patterns of progression similar to those of
human neoplasma - it grows in C57BL mice at the site of transplantation as a local primary tumor (L-3LL) and after 2 to 3 weeks develops
as visible metastatic foci (M-3LL) in the lungs. Our studies with

TABLE 2

Specific Cytotoxicity of Daunomycin
Linked to Anti-YAC (Fab')$_2$[a]

YAC Cells Incubated With	Extent Substitution M/M	Ab Activity	% Inhibition of ^{3}H−uridine Incorporation
Daunomycin−anti−YAC	16	74	60, 56
Daunomycin−anti−BSA	14	85	36, 34
Free daunomycin			33, 16

[a]YAC cells were exposed to the various daunomycin preparations for
5 min following which the washed cells were assayed for inhibition
of ^{3}H−uridine incorporation. When allowed to react with the
cells for 3 hr, both preparations exhibited the full pharmacological
activity of the drug.

this tumor (Hurwitz et al., 1979) were aimed at establishing the
extent of interaction of cells from the local and the metastatic
tumor with anti-3LL antibodies and their daunomycin conjugates. For
this purpose both rabbit and syngeneic antibodies were investigated.
The immunoglobulin (Ig) isolated from rabbit antiserum against the
L-3LL reacted with the M-3LL to the same extent as with the homologous
L-3LL, and showed almost no activity with normal syngeneic cells.
Antibodies against L-3LL prepared in syngeneic mice also reacted
similarly with L-3LL and M-3LL; they thus seemed suitable as
carriers for drugs.

Experiments with the daunomycin conjugate of this anti-3LL
showed that both L-3LL and M-3LL cells are able to take up the material. Thus, incubation of the cells with either the free drug or the
drug conjugate, at a concentration of 5 μg/ml of daunomycin, caused
90% inhibition of ^{3}H−uridine incorporation. The specificity of
this inhibition is demonstrated in Figure 2. In these experiments
as well, the cells were incubated with daunomycin or its conjugates
for 5 minutes at 4°C, and were then washed to remove any unbound
material before further incubation for 4 hours at 37°C. Under these
conditions free daunomycin inhibited only at high concentration (over
20 μg/ml), whereas the daunomycin−anti−3LL was much more effective,
causing 50% inhibition at 4 μg/ml).

These results seem particularly promising in view of the fact
that specific anti-3LL hybridoma (6B) is capable of localizing preferentially in the lungs of mice bearing 3LL metastases, as compared
to other tissues of the same mice or to lungs of normal mice (Fig.3).
The hybridoma products, labelled with [75]Se (by incorporation of the
label into the 6B cells), showed high specific accumulation in the
lungs, a 31-39 fold increase, as compared to other organs. This did
not occur in lungs of healthy mice. Such local delivery of the drug,
combined with high pharmacological activity of the drug retained in
the conjugate, is encouraging as a basis for a therapeutic approach.

THE MODE OF ACTION OF CONJUGATES IN VITRO

The mode of action of antibody-drug derivatives was studied with
conjugates of daunomycin. The chemotherapeutic activity of daunomycin
attached to antibody or other specific and nonspecific macromolecules
demands the ability of the conjugates either to release the drug upon
contact with the cell, or to penetrate the cell and release the drug
intracellularly, or - alternatively - to penetrate the cell and the
nucleus and possibly perform its activity in the macromolecular form.
We have performed some experiments designed to elucidate the mechanism
of action of the conjugates, namely, measuring the uptake of labeled
materials by the YAC cells (Hurwitz et al., 1978a). The label was
introduced by using [3]H - borohydride during the preparation of the
conjugate, and is, therefore, present exclusively at the macromolecular conjugates and not in the free drug.

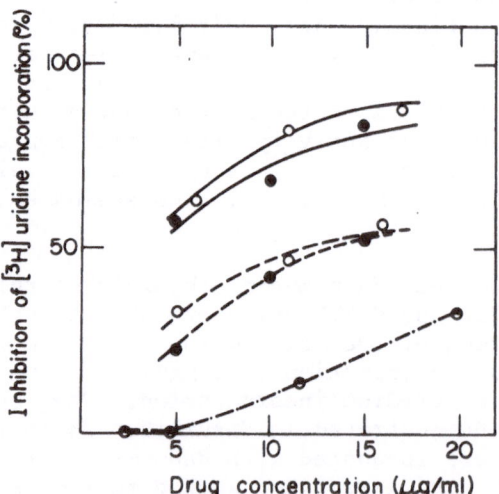

Fig. 2.   The specific cytotoxicity of daunomycin linked to syngeneic
           anti-3LL Ig. Daunomycin-C57BL anti-3LL Ig (————),
           daunomycin-normal Ig (-----) or free daunomycin (-.-.-.-.)
           were added to monolayers of 10^5 cell/well L-3LL (o) or M-3LL(•).

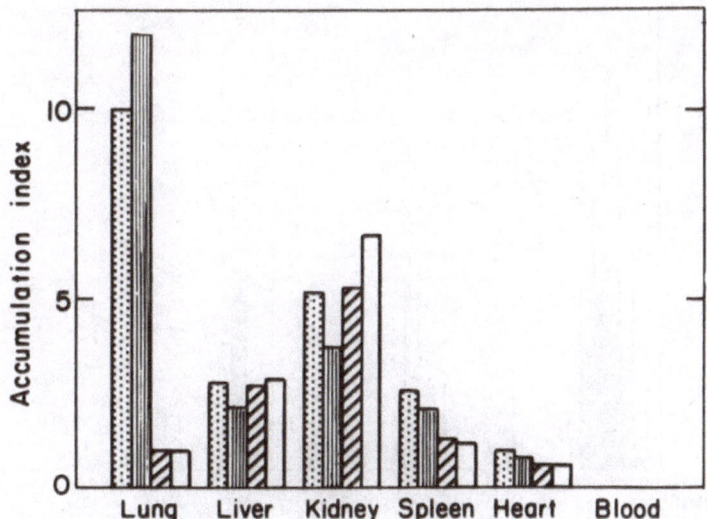

Fig. 3.   The <u>in vivo</u> distribution of ^{75}Se labeled anti-3LL (6B) vs
^{75}Se-anti-DNP (SPE). The labeled hybridomas were injected
into metastasis-bearing mice or their normal controls.
After 20 hr the mice were killed and the radioactive content of various tissues was determined. The results are
presented as the accumulation index, namely the ratio of
the cpm per g tissue to the cpm per ml blood. ▦ 6B in
metastatic mice; ▥ 6B in normal mice; ▨ SPE in
metastatic mice; ▭ SPE in normal mice.

    The uptake of daunomycin and its conjugates by YAC cells or by
normal cells (rat splenocytes) is depicted in Figure 4. It is expressed as percentage of uptake of the total radioactivity added to
a fixed number of cells. The distribution of daunomycin or
daunomycin-conjugates in the membranes or the cytoplasm, and its
possible attachment to the nucleus, were measured as a function of
time of incubation. As can be seen, the free drug penetrated the
cells very rapidly. The accumulation of the drug in or on the
nuclei (shaded areas in the figure) paralleled its uptake by the
intact cells and amounted roughly to two thirds of it.

    Daunomycin-antibody conjugates, whether directly bound or <u>via</u>
a dextran bridge, penetrated into the YAC cells and attached to their
nuclei, although at a much lower rate than that of the free drug.
Daunomycin bound directly to antibodies entered the cells at higher
levels than when bound through dextran or when the drug was bound
to normal Ig. The optimal concentrations were similar to those
obtained for free drug without a noted dependence on the amount of
antibody in the preparation. The accumulation of drug on the nuclei
was parallel at all times tested to the extent of uptake by the whole

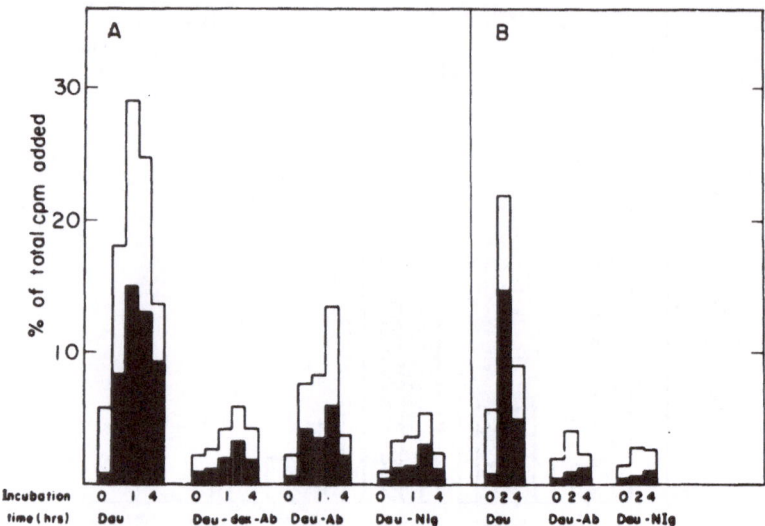

Fig. 4.   The in vitro uptake of daunomycin and its conjugates by
           YAC cells (A) and normal rat lymphocytes (B) measured as
           a function of time. Measurements of uptake were made at
           zero time, after 0.5, 1, 2, 3 and 4 hr following the
           addition of drug. The total drug accumulation in the
           cells is denoted by the open bars, whereas the nuclear
           incorporation by shaded areas.

cells, amounting to half to two thirds of its value. We have not
tested whether the conjugates have penetrated the nucleic or were
just attached to them.

     In normal non-related cells (rat splenocytes) the uptake of free
drug was lower than that by the tumor cells. The daunomycin conjugates with either anti-YAC antibodies or normal Ig (linked directly),
were taken up at low rates and did not differ from each other. This
was expected since these cells do not bind goat anti-YAC.

     Daunomycin linked directly to antibody could enter the nucleus
in the conjugate form, or, alternatively, it might be released from
the carrier by lysosomic enzymes prior to its penetration into the
nucleus. The labeling method used would not have enabled us to
differentiate between these two alternatives. However, when daunomycin is linked to antibody through dextran and labelled at the
reduction step, most of the radioactive label is in the dextran
bridges. The finding of the label in or on the nucleus, even though
there are no dextranases in lysosomes, gives weight to the possibility that a large conjugate is capable of entering the cell and
approaching the nucleus.

The data reported above neither put forward nor prove a particular mechanism for the cytotoxic activity of large molecular weight, covalent complexes of daunomycin. It is possible that the free drug, released from the complexes in situ, is the compound that performs the cytotoxic activity. However, our results demonstrate that such complexes are able to reach the nucleus, provided that they show some affinity to the cell surface. In view of these findings the possibility of using either anti-tumor antibodies or their Fab dimers as a carrier for anti-cancer drugs should have significant potential.

IN-VIVO STUDIES

The next and most important step in the evaluation of the drug conjugates is the test of their ability to prevent in vivo the development of tumors. We have investigated the effect of daunomycin bound to anti-tumor antibodies, mainly with the tumor system of the YAC Moloney virus induced lymphomas (Hurwitz et al., 1978b) and the Lewis lung carcinoma (Hurwitz et al., 1979). The effect was assessed by the suppression of tumor growth, as indicated by prolongation of the life span of the mice, and by the prevalence of long term survivors.

The in vivo studies of efficacy of the conjugates with the 3LL tumor system presented some difficulties since all three anti-cancer drugs used in our investigations, namely, daunomycin, adriamycin and methotrexate, were found ineffective against the 3LL tumor. They did not prevent or delay tumor development when injected shortly after intrafootpad transplantation of the tumor cells, or in conjunction with the amputation of the leg bearing the tumor. Thus, they were ineffective in delaying the median survival of the tumor bearing mice, or in prevention the development of metastates.

Notwithstanding this negative response, we have tested the in vivo activity of the antibody-conjugates, in anticipation that the possible localization of the drug at the tumor site might increase their anti-cancer potential. However, the conjugates tested, using monoclonal antibodies, did not lead to positive therapeutic effects.

Much better results were obtained in studies with the YAC lymphoma. In this system we used conjugates prepared with either the Ig fraction of the antisera, the purified antibodies from it, or monoclonal antibodies. All the conjugates were prepared by linking the drug via a dextran bridge. Thus their content of daunomycin was approximately 25 M/M, allowing the use of relatively high drug doses in the systemic treatment. Groups of 5 to 10 mice were transplanted with 10^5 tumor cells and then treated with the appropriate drug conjugates (Ig fraction of antiserum or purified antibodies), with control groups including free drug, conjugates of drug and normal Ig, mixtures of drug and antibodies, and antibodies alone. The tumor

cells were transplanted i.p., the drug and drug-antibodies were
injected i.v., usually 2 days and in some experiments 5 days following the implantation of tumor cells.

The effect in vivo of dau-dex-anti-YAC, either with the Ig
fraction or with purified antibodies, as compared to daunomycin, was
indicative of an advantage of the conjugate over the free drug at
high doses (p $<$ 0.05) (Hurwitz et al., 1978b). A similar effect, was
sometimes obtained by using the drug conjugated to normal immunoglobulin or just to dextran. However, at the lower drug doses the
results demonstrated an advantage of the conjugate of the specific
antibody over that with normal immunoglobulin. The purified antibodies themselves had a small but reproducible effect in delaying the
onset of the tumor (Table 3).

It would be logical to assume that a conjugate of the drug with
specific monoclonal antibody might be more efficient than a conjugate
with polyclonal antibodies. We, therefore, repeated the experiment
with the specific anti-YAC hybridomas. As mentioned above, our monoclonal anti-YAC antibodies KH$_{3-4}$, which showed specificity to the YAC
cells and did not react with any normal A/J tissue, was of the IgM
class. Hence its daunomycin conjugate, although prepared in an
identical procedure to the other dau-dex-antibody conjugates, contained 500 moles of daunomycin per mole of antibody (Table 1). It
was therefore disappointing to observe that its in vivo effect was
not highly beneficial. As can be seen from the results presented in
Table 3, the conventional goat anti-YAC antibodies are much more
effective as drug carriers than the monoclonal antibodies. Under the
conditions of this particular experiment, in which the transplantation
of the tumor was subcutaneous instead of intraperitoneal, the drug
bound to the goat anti-YAC was more efficient than the free drug
or other conjugates even at a low dose. The conjugate with the monoclonal antibodies on the other hand, was not more effective than a
conjugate with a non-relevant protein.

The reason for the lower efficacy of the conjugate with the
monoclonal anti-YAC antibodies is not yet clear. It is possible that
this particular hybridoma product, although quite specific in its
in vitro binding to the tumor cells and not to normal lymphocytes, is
not an effective drug carrier because of its IgM nature. On the other
hand, it may well be that monoclonal antibodies, by and large, could
not function as carriers, in spite of their improved specificity,
because of their ability to recognize only very few determinants on
the cell surface. Xeno-antibodies, on the other hand, while less
specific, are able to recognize and react with a whole array of surface antigens and could thus be more potent in their binding and
cytotoxic abilities. A mixture of several specific monoclonal antibodies may prove to be the optimal reagent in the future.

TABLE 3

The in vivo[a] effect of daunomycin conjugates to mouse monoclonal anti-YAC in comparison to daunomycin conjugate with goat anti-YAC purified antibodies.

Treatment[b]	Drug mg/kg	Ab mg/kg	% Survival
PBS	–	–	0
Daunomycin	12	–	60
	17	–	60
Dau–dex–KH$_{3-4,10}$[c]	12.5	100	20
	20	200	83
Dau–dex–X63[d]	12.5	75	20
	22	250	80
Dau KH$_{3-4,10}$	12.5	250	0
Dau–dex anti-YAC (Ab)	12.5	50	100
Dau + anti-YAC (Ab)	12.5	100	60
Anti-YAC (Ab)	–	100	20

[a]YAC cells, 10^5 in 0.5 ml PBS were injected subcutaneously into mole A/J mice (10 weeks old).
[b]Treatment was given i.v. on day 3.
[c]KH$_{3-4,10}$, an anti-YAC IgM obtained from a cloned mouse-mouse hybridoma.
[d]X63, the original IgG produced by the NSI myeloma, serves as normal Ig.

DAUNOMYCIN–DEXTRAN CONJUGATE

This conjugate was prepared originally as a control for the previously described daunomycin-dextran-antibody conjugates, using a very similar method of preparation (Bernstein et al., 1978): Periodate-oxidized dextran T-10 (M.W. 10,000) or T-40 (M.W. 40,000) is first prepared using different ratios of NaIO$_4$ to dextran for

different degrees of oxidation (varying from 25% to 75%). After
dialysis and lyophilization, daunomycin is added to the solution of
the oxidized dextran in ratios varying from 1:5 to 1:1, and the
reaction products are reduced with 15-30% of equimolar amounts of
$NaBH_4$ (optimal conditions, since too extensive reduction has a damaging effect on the drug). In spite of the partial reduction the
products are reproducible and are stable over a period of at least
several months.

Unexpectedly, this conjugate showed cytotoxic activity towards
the tumor cells when tested both in vitro and in vivo. The results
of in vitro experiments (performed with 10^6 YAC cells) have shown
that at low drug doses, the activity of the conjugate, as compared
with the free drug, was reduced. However, by increasing the concentration of the conjugate or prolonging the incubation period from 2
to 4 hours, maximal cytotoxic effect (80-90%) can be reached, similar
to that seen with the free drug. It was therefore considered important to evaluate this conjugate for in vivo therapeutic effect, even
though it did not contain specific antibodies. It was previously
shown that high-molecular weight carriers which are not in any way
specific for tumor cells may still serve as carriers for chemotherapeutic drugs. The known high endocytic activity of several neoplasms
is probably responsible for the preferred uptake of the drug in the
macromolecular form (Isliker et al., 1964). Various attempts were
made to employ this approach with covalently linked (Szekerke et al.,
1972) and not covalent combinations of complexes (Trouet et al.,
1972; De Duve et al., 1974; Trouet et al., 1974), as summarized by
Gregoriadis (1977). Dextran itself has been used previously as a
carrier for various hormones and drugs in an attempt to prolong their
action and to stabilize them in vivo (Molteni and Scrollini, 1977).

We have evaluated the effect of daunomycin-dextran conjugates
in vivo in the YAC system according to the suppression of tumor
development, as assessed by the prolongation of survival of mice
after previous transplantation of the tumor cells (Bernstein et al.,
1978). The results presented in Fig. 5 demonstrate the efficacy of
the conjugate. At low drug doses (less than 15 mg/kg) the free drug
was more effective than the conjugate, probably due to the partial
loss of drug activity upon binding. However, at higher doses (20-25
mg/kg), when the free drug is toxic, the conjugate was very effica-
cious, inducing 100% prevention of tumor development, even when
administered five days following the tumor challenge.

In-Vivo Toxicity of Daunomycin-dextran Conjugates

From the data reported above it is apparent that by conjugation
to dextran the toxicity of daunomycin is diminished. In view of the
crucial importance of the issue of toxicity of anti-cancer drugs and
its ramification on their applicability, it was of interest to compare the toxicity of the free and macromolecularized daunomycin in a

Fig. 5.   Therapeutic effect of
daunomycin-dextran
compared with that of
the free drug. Mice
were given transplants
of 10^5 tumor cells i.p.
The treatment (to 10
mice/group) was given
i.v. either 2 days (A)
or 5 days (B) after the
tumor inoculation.
Daunomycin dextran:
150 μg (○), 400 μg (△)
or 500 μg (□).
Daunomycin: 150 μg (○),
300 μg (▲) or 450 μg
(■), PBS (+).

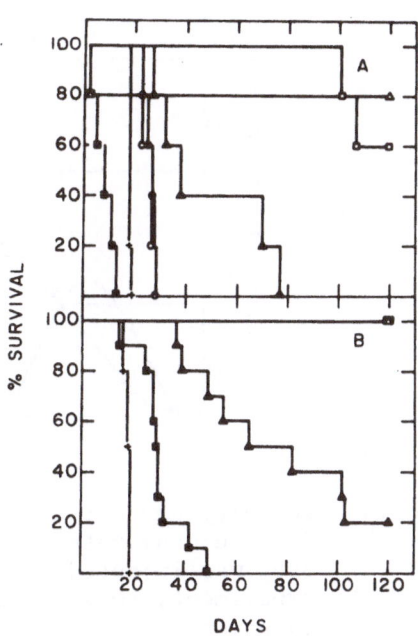

more detailed manner.

Recent studies (Levi-Schaffer et al., 1981) have demonstrated
that both the acute and sub-acute toxicity of daunomycin-dextran
conjugate are much lower than that of the free drug. Thus, as shown
in Fig. 6, its LD_{50} is almost 3 fold higher than that of free
daunomycin and so are the values of the therapeutic indices. Consequently, in the case of daunomycin-dextran conjugate there is a
range of drug concentration (between 22 and 24 mg/kg) in which there
is no mortality of mice either from drug toxicity or from tumor, in
mice inoculated with YAC cells. This could be considered as a
"safe region".

The lower toxicity was manifested also after multiple admini-
strations, of the optimal therapeutic dose. After four injections
we obtained full survival of the mice treated with the daunomycin-
dextran conjugate, as compared with very high mortality (90-100%) of
the mice similarly treated with the free drug.

The most dramatic difference was observed by the histological
examinations, which demonstrated that free daunomycin is extremely
detrimental and causes massive atrophy of spleen, and bone marrow,
with damage to liver and heart tissue as well. In contrast, the
daunomycin-dextran conjugate had hardly any damaging effect, either
immediately after or even two months following 4 injections of the

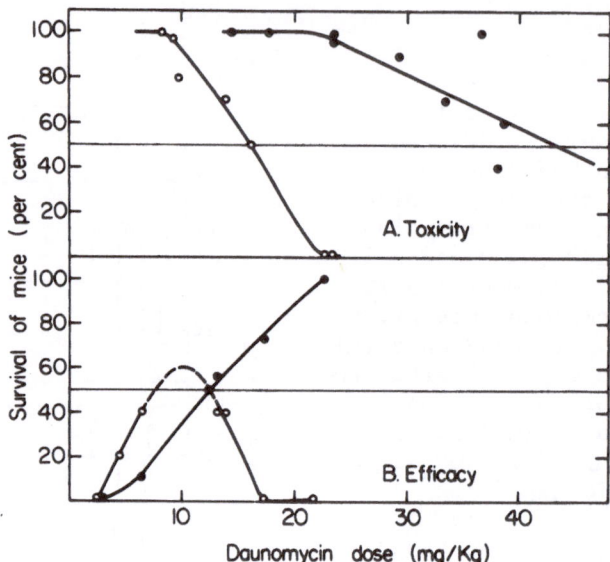

Fig. 6.   Toxicity and efficacy of free daunomycin (o) and its
           dextran conjugate (●). In the toxicity experiments the
           drug was injected into untreated mice, and in the efficacy
           experiment, to mice prechallenged with 10^5 cells of YAC
           lymphoma.

therapeutic dose. It should be emphasized that almost no damage was
observed in the heart muscle tissue, a finding which might be of
importance in view of the known cardiotoxicity of daunomycin that is
manifested as a cumulative effect after repeated doses (Gillagoda et
al., 1976). Dextran has several advantages as a carrier for chemotherapeutic drugs (Bernstein et al., 1978): It is a non-degradable
polymer and can thus prolong the half-life of the drug in vivo. It
is also known as a blood volume expander (Gronwall and Ingelman,
1955), a feature indicating its suitability for human use. The findings that it lowers the toxicity of daunomycin encourages the conti-
nuation of the investigations in this direction.

CONCLUDING REMARKS

     The results reported here indicate that antibodies may serve as
carriers for anti-cancer drugs to the tumor cells. It is still too
early to decide whether this approach will develop into a therapeutic
procedure for treatment of cancer. The main difficulty anticipated
is the preparation of suitable antibodies which will be specific
only for the tumor cells and will not interact at all with normal
tissue. These antibodies should be immunospecifically purified so
as to avoid the presence of high amounts of irrelevant immunoglobulins. With the rapid development of the hybridoma technology it is

hopeful that the preparation of monospecific adequate anti-tumour antibodies might become feasible in the near future, and that in the right combination they might serve as potential carriers for improvement of chemotherapy. Concomitantly, the use of other carriers, such as dextran, might also prove beneficial, and although lacking the feature of specificity, they might still manifest several advantages as drug carriers.

REFERENCES

Arnon, R., 1979, Anti-tumor antibodies as carriers for anti-cancer drugs, in:"Tumor-associated antigens and their specific immune response", F. Spreafico and R. Arnon, eds., Academic Press, New York.

Bergman, Y., and Haimovich, J., 1977, Characterization of a carcinogen-induced murine B lymphocyte cell line of C3H/eB origin, Eur. J. Immunol. 7: 413.

Bernstein, A., Hurwitz, E., Maron, R., Arnon, R., Sela, M., and Wilchek, M., 1978, Higher antitumor efficacy of daunomycin when linked to dextran: in vivo and in vitro studies, J. Natl. Cancer Inst. 60: 379.

Blythman, H.E., Casellas, P., Gros, O., Gros, P., Jansen, F.K., Paolucci, F., Pau, B., and Vidal, H., 1981, Immunotoxins: hybrid molecules of monoclonal antibodies and a toxin subunit specifically kill tumor cells, Nature 290: 145.

Davies, D.A.L., and O'Neil, G.J., 1973, In vivo and in vitro effects of tumor specific antibodies with chlorambucil, Br. J. Cancer 28: Suppl. I, 285.

Davies, D.A.L. and O'Neil, G.J., 1974, Protection of mice against syngeneic lymphomata, II, Collaboration between drugs and antibodies, Br. J. Cancer 30: 305.

De-Duve, C., De Barsy, T., Poole, B., Trouet, A., Tulkens, P., and van Hoof, F., 1974, Lysosomotropic agents, Biochem. Pharmacol. 23: 2495.

Ehrlich, P., 1906, "Collected Studies on Immunity", Vol II, John Wiley, New York.

Eshhar, Z., Hurwitz, E., and Hadas, E., 1980, Production of hybridomas secreting monoclonal antibodies against components of normal and malignant cells, in: "New Developments With Human and Veterinary Vaccines", Alan R. Liss Inc., New York.

Flechner, I., 1973, The cure and concomitant immunization of mice bearing Ehrlich ascites tumors by treatment with an antibody-alkylating agent complex, Eur. J. Cancer 9: 741.

Frei, E., 1972, Prospects for cancer chemotherapy, Cancer 30: 1656.

Ghose, T., Norvell, S.T., Guclu, A., Cameron, D., Bodurtha, A., and MacDonald, A.S., 1972, Immunochemotherapy of cancer with chlorambucyl carrying antibody, Br. Med. J. 3: 495.

Gillagoda, A.C., Mannuel, C., Tan, C.T.C., Wollner, V., Steinberg,

S.S., and Murphy, M.L., The cardiotoxicity of adriamycin and daunomycin in children, Cancer 37: 1070.

Gilliland, D.G., Stepelewski, Z., Collier, R.J., Mitchell, K.F., Chang, T.H., and Koprowski, H., 1981, Antibody-directed cytotoxic agents: use of monoclonal antibody to direct the action of toxin A chains to colorectal carcinoma cells, Proc. Natl. Acad. Sci. U.S.A. 77: 4539.

Gregoriadis, G., 1977, Targeting of drugs, Nature 265: 407.

Gronwall, A., and Ingelman, B., 1944, Untersuchungen uber dextran und sein verhalten bei parenteraler Zufuhr, Acta Physiol. Scand, 7: 97.

Haran-Ghera, N., and Peled, A., 1973, Thymus and bone marrow derived lymphatic leukemia in mice, Nature 241: 396.

Hurwitz, E., Maron, R., Arnon, R., and Sela, M., 1975, The covalent binding of daunomycin and adriamycin to antibodies with retention of both drug and antibody activities, Cancer Res. 35: 1175.

Hurwitz, E., Maron R., Arnon, R., and Sela, M., 1976, Fab dimers of anti-tumor immunoglobulins as covalent carriers of daunomycin, Cancer Biochem. Biophys. 1: 197.

Hurwitz, E., Maron, R., Arnon, R., Wilchek, M., and Sela, M., 1978a, Daunomycin-immunoglobulin conjugates, uptake and activity in vitro, Eur. J. Cancer 14: 1213.

Hurwitz, E., Maron, R., Bernstein, A., Wilchek, M., Sela, M., and Arnon, R., 1978b, The effect in vivo of chemotherapuetic drug antibody conjugates in two murine experimental tumor systems, Int. J. Cancer 21: 747.

Hurwitz, E., Schechter, B., Arnon, R., and Sela, M., 1979, Binding of anti-tumor immunoglobulins and their daunomycin conjugates to the tumor and its metastases, In vitro and in vivo studies with Lewis Lung Carcinoma, Int. J. Cancer 24: 461.

Hurwitz, E., Wilchek, M., and Pita, J., 1980, Soluble molecules as carriers for daunorubicin, J. Applied Biochem. 2: 25.

Hurwitz, E., Kashi, R., and Wilchek, M., 1981, Platinum complexed anti-tumor immunoglobulins specifically inhibit DNA synthesis of tumor cells, submitted.

Isliker, H., Cerottini, J.C., Jaton, J.-C., and Magnenat, G., 1969, Specific and non-specific fixation of plasma proteins in tumors, in: "Chemotherapy of Cancer", Elsevier, Amsterdam.

Katchalski, E., and Sela, M., 1958, Synthesis and chemical properties of poly-α-amino acids, Adv. Prot. Chem. 8: 243.

Kitao, T., and Hattori, K., 1977, Concanavalin A as a carrier of daunomycin, Nature 265: 81.

Klein, E., and Klein, G., 1964, Antigenic properties of lymphoma induced by Moloney agent, J. Natl. Cancer Inst. 32: 547.

Köhler, G., and Milstein, C., 1976, Derivation of specific antibody producing tissue culture and tumor lines by cell fusion, J. Immunol. 6: 511.

Krolick, K.A., Villemez, C., Isakson, P., Uhr, J.W., And Vitetta,E.S., 1980, Selective killing of normal or neoplastic B cells by antibodies coupled to the A chain of ricin, Proc. Natl. Acad. Sci. USA. 77: 5419.

Levi-Schaffer, F., Bernstein, A., Meshorer, A., and Arnon, R., Reduced toxicity of daunomycin by conjugation to dextran, Cancer Treatment Reports, in press.

Levy, R., Hurwitz, R., Maron, R., Arnon, R., and Sela, M., 1975, The specific cytotoxic effects of daunomycin conjugated to antitumor antibodies, Cancer Res. 35: 1182.

Magnenat, R., Schidler, R., and Isliker, H., 1969, Transport d'agents cytostatiques par le proteines plasmatiques. III. Activite antitumorale in vitro de conjugues cytostatique-azoproteines, Eur. J. Cancer 5: 33.

Mathe, G., Tran, B.L., and Bernard, J., 1958, Essai sur la leucemie 1210 de la souris d'une combinaison par diazotazion d'ametho-pterine et de γ-globulines de hamsters porteurs de cette leucemie par hetergreffe, Compt. Rend. 246: 1626.

Molteni, E.L., and Scrollini, F., 1977, Methode pour prolonger l'action des medicaments par la formation de composés macromoleculaires, Eur. J. Med. Chem. 9: 618.

Nisonoff, A., Wissler, F.C., Lippman, L.N., and Woernley, D.L., 1960, Separation of univalent fragments from bivalent rabbit antibody molecule by reduction of disulfide bonds, Arch. Biochem. Biophys. 89: 230.

O'Bryan, R.M., Luce, J.K., Talky, R.W., Gottlieb, J.K., Baker, L.H., and Bonadonna, G., 1973, Phase II evaluation of adriamycin in human neoplasia, Cancer 32: 1.

O'Neill, G.J., 1979, The use of antibodies as drug carriers, in: "Drug Carrier in Biology and Medicine", G. Gregoriadis, ed., Academic Press, London.

Potter, M., and Robertson, C.L., 1960, Development of plasma-cell neoplasms in BALB/c mice after intraperitoneal injection of paraffin-oil adjuvant, heat-killed staphylococcus mixtures, J. Natl. Cancer Inst. 25: 847.

Rubens, R.D., and Dulbecco, R., 1974, Augmentation of cytotoxic drug action by antibodies directed at cell surface, Nature 248: 81.

Segerling, M., Ohanian, S.H., and Borsos, T., 1974, Effect of metabolic inhibitors on killing of tumor cells by antibody and complement, J. Natl. Cancer Inst. 53: 1411.

Sequira, K., and Stock, C.C., 1955, Studies in a tumor spectrum. III. The effects of phosphoramides on the growth of a variety of mouse and rat tumors, Cancer Res. 15: 38.

Szekerke, M., Wade, R., and Whisson, M.E., 1967, Some serum protein nitrogen mustard complexes with high chemotherapeutic selecti-vity, Nature, 215: 1303.

Szekerke, M., Wade, R., and Whisson, M.E., 1972, The use of macro-molecules as carriers of cytotoxic groups. I. Conjugates of nitrogen mustards with proteins, polypeptidyl proteins and polypeptides, Neoplasma 19: 179.

Trouet, A., Deprez-de Campeneere, D., and De Duve, C., 1972, Chemotherapy through lysosomes with a DNA-daunorubicin complex,

    Nature 239: 110.
Trouet, A., Deprez-de Campeneere, D., De Smedt-Molengreaux, M.,
    Attasi, G., 1974, Experimental leukemia chemotherapy with
    a "lysosomotropic" adriamycin-DNA complex, Eur. J. Cancer 10:
    405.
Varga, J.M., Asato, N., Lande, S., and Lerner, A.B., 1977,
    Melanotropin-daunomycin conjugate shows receptor-mediated
    cytotoxicity in cultured murine melanoma cells, Nature 267:
    56.
Youle, R.J., and Neville, Jr., D.M., 1980, Anti-thy-1,2 monoclonal
    antibody linked to ricin is a potent cell type specific toxin,
    Proc. Natl. Acad. Sci. USA 77: 5843.

TARGETING OF RADIONUCLIDES AND DRUGS FOR THE DIAGNOSIS AND TREATMENT OF CANCER

T. Ghose[a], H. Blair[b], P. Kulkarni[a], K. Vaughan[c],
S. Norvell[d], and P. Belitsky[e]

Departments of Pathology[a] and Biochemistry[b]
Dalhousie University; Department of Chemistry
Saint Mary's University, Halifax, N.S., Canada
B3H 3C3;[c] Departments of Surgery[d] and Urology,[e]
Dalhousie University, Halifax, N.S., Canada, B3H 4H7

INTRODUCTION

The application of antibody-linked agents in the diagnosis and treatment of cancer is based on two findings. First, a variety of membrane-bound tumor-associated antigens (TAA) has been serologic- ally defined for both animal and human tumors[1,2]. Antibodies against many of thse antigens selectively localise in the target tumor in vivo[1,3,4,5]. Second, methods are available for linking agents to immunoglubulin molecules with retention of agent and anti- body activities[1,3].

In this chapter we shall deal mainly with our experience in applying antibodies to targeting of chemotherapeutic agents in cancer treatment. We will also discuss the evidence or localisa- tion of antiTAA antibodies in tumors and the use of labelled anti- bodies for the detection and possible therapy of cancer.

TARGETING OF CHEMOTHERAPEUTIC AGENTS BY ANTIBODIES

For rational application in chemotherapy, drug-antibody con- jugates must exhibit a greater chemotherapeutic index than either drug or antibody alone. We were first able to obtain such active conjugates by linking chlorambucil to xenogeneic antitumor anti- bodies against several mouse tumors[6-9]. These conjugates were more effective tumor inhibitors both in vivo and in vitro than the indi- vidual agents used separately, or together but unlinked[8]. The effectiveness of noncovalently linked chlorambucil-antitumor globulin

conjugates is supported by reports of other investigators[10-12].
Since publication of these papers and articles describing the action
of diphtheria toxin linked to antibodies[13], a number of laboratories
have studied other agents and antibodies against different cellular
components.

Table 1 A & B gives selected examples of cytotoxic agents that
have been linked to antibodies and have been shown to be more effective tumor inhibitors than equimolar or equitoxic doses of the agent
and/or antibody. (For a detailed discussion and references before
1978 see reference 1). In brief, the general finding has been that
cytocidal amounts of drug can be delivered to target tumor cells
both _in vitro_ and _in vivo_ using specific antibody molecules or their
fragments as carriers. Moreover, this superior tumor inhibitory
effect has been observed for agents with different modes of anti-
tumor activity (e.g. DNA alkylation or intercalation, enzyme
inhibition, cell surface modification). However, the basis of the
superior tumor inhibition by antibody-linked agents and the applicability and effectiveness of this approach to eradicating human
cancer cells remains to be assessed. Our own experience concerning
the production, assay and testing of several different drug-antibody
conjugates follows.

Chlorambucil

When chlorambucil (CBL) was noncovalently bound to antitumor
globulins, it retained alkylating activity without impairing the
immunological reactivity of the immunoglobulin[33]. Such antitumor
globulin-linked CBL inhibited the mouse Ehrlich ascites carcinoma
and EL4 lymphoma more effectively than did CBL alone, antibody alone,
or comparable amounts of CBL bound to nonspecific immunoglobulins[6,7].
In a preliminary clinical trial, patients with disseminated malignant melanoma survived longer after treatment with antimelanoma
globulin-bound CBL than did a comparison group with dimethyltriazen-
oimidazole carboxamide[34,35]. Initial analysis of data from our ongoing double-blind randomized study supports this conclusion
(unpublished observations). Superior inhibition by CBL-antibody
conjugates both _in vitro_ and _in vivo_ has been attributed to tumor-
specific localisation and endocytosis subsequent to capping[36,37].
Other possible contributing factors include drug-antibody synergism
and a depot effect governed by the rate of release of active drug
from the conjugate. However, it has been demonstrated that these
results, either _in vivo_ or _in vitro_, cannot be explained merely by
synergism between CBL and antitumor globulins[8,12]. More recently,
we used ECDI to link CBL covalently to antitumor IgG with retention
of alkylating and antibody activities. Both covalent and noncovalent
conjugates were more effective in treating tumor-inoculated C57BL/6J
mice than the drug alone, the antitumor IgG alone, or the drug
linked to non-tumor specific IgG[9].

Trenimon (2,3,5-tris (1-aziridinyl)-p-benzoquinone)

We studied the action of the alkylating agent Trenimon on subcutaneous transplants of the H6 hepatoma in A/J mice. Hepatoma-inoculated mice were given various combinations of conjugates, free Trenimon and IgG. Our results demonstrated that linkage of Trenimon to IgG lowered the drug's systemic toxicity with comparative retention of its antitumor activity. This action was potentiated by antihepatoma IgG whether Trenimon was directly linked to IgG or free antihepatoma IgG was administered along with Trenimon conjugated to nonspecific rabbit IgG[18].

Adriamycin

We have used a multivalent intermediary, dextran T-40, to obtain a ternary conjugate of adriamycin:dextran:goat antirenal carcinoma IgG in the molar ratio 47:2:1, which retained both drug and antibody activities. When administered to BALB/c mice bearing intrarenal adenocarcinoma, it prolonged survival more than did adriamycin, free or linked to dextran only[32].

Methotrexate

Methotrexate (MTX) is widely used to treat human cancer[38]. Before preparing conjugates of MTX and antibodies against TAA, we carried out model studies of its binding to rabbit anti-BSA IgG and found that an active ester procedure employing N-hydroxysuccinimide (NHS) was more effective than previous methods[14,15]. This method yielded reasonable amounts of conjugate while retaining adequate antibody activity and DHFR inhibitory capacity. Ten moles of MTX per mole of IgG could be incorporated with retention of 90% of the anti-BSA activity of an equivalent weight of unconjugated IgG and with recovery of 70% of the original protein.

The demonstrated superiority of the active ester method for producing active conjugates led us to use this technique to link MTX to a rabbit IgG antibody against the mouse EL4 lymphoma[15]. Conjugates containing 13 moles of MTX per mole of IgG retained their reactivity with EL4 cells when subjected to membrane immunofluorescence assay. When tumor-inoculated mice (10^4 EL4 cells per animal) were injected with this conjugate, 1, 4 and 7 days after tumor inoculation (MTX dose: 4 mg per kg per injection), they survived significantly longer than mice treated with equivalent amounts of drug alone, antitumor IgG alone, drug followed by antitumor IgG, or drug linked to nontumor specific IgG[15] (Fig. 1). Eight of 11 mice treated with this MTX-antiEL4 IgG conjugate have thus far survived tumor-free for over 100 days (not shown). We are now trying to establish the optimal conjugate dose, therapeutic schedule, and the maximum tumor load that can be eradicated.

Table 1A. Agent-antibody conjugates exhibiting tumor inhibition either in vitro or in vivo that were superior to agent or antibody alone - direct linkage.

Agent	Method of linkage	Test system and Ab	Comments
Methotrexate (MTX)	Carbodiimide or N-hydroxy-succin-imide	BALB/c mice; i.p.EL4 lymphoma; rabbit IgG Ab treat i.p.	Increase in toxicity and chemotherapeutic index.MTX-linked to antiTAA IgG more eff-ective than free agents, their synergistic effect, or MTX-linked to nontumor specific IgG[14,15].
MTX	Mixed anhydride of MTX	C3H mice; i.p. ovarian carcinoma; rabbit Y globulin	Conjugate prolonged survival compared with control agents[16]. In our experience[14,15] and that of Latif et al.[17] exposure of MTX to acetic anhydride under conditions specified produces inactivation of MTX. Conjugates containing active MTX obtained by NHS and ECDI mediated linkage are 100% lethal to mice at these dose levels.
Chlorambucil	Non-covalent	BALB/c mice; Harding Passey melanoma; rabbit IgG Ab	Confirms previous results that chlorambucil-immune IgG complex was more effective tumor inhibitor in vivo than individual free agents or their synergistic effect[12].
Chlorambucil	Carbodiimide	C57BL/6J mice; EL4 lym-phoma; rabbit IgG Ab	Covalent conjugate more effective tumor inhibitor in vivo compared to free agents but less effective than non-covalent conjugate[9].

Agent	Method of linkage	Test system and Ab	Comments
Trenimon (2,3,5-tris (1-aziridinyl) -p-benzoqui- none)	Partial re duction of IgG with dithio- threitol	A/J mice; H6 hepa- toma; rabbit igG Ab	Binding of Trenimon to IgG reduced its toxicity allowing administration of larger doses; this led to increased therapeutic effectiveness. Trenimon linked to antibody IgG was more effect- ive tumor inhibitor than Trenimon-linked to nontumor specific IgG[18].
Neocarzino- statin	Carbodiimide	Human leukemia cell line NALL-i (acute lymphoblastic leukemia); rabbit IgG Ab	Inhibition of NALL-I cells in vitro[19].
Adriamycin/ Daunomycin	Gluteraldehyde (Daunomycin)	Mouse hepatoma cells BW-7756; unspecified antibody to alpha foetoprotein	Inhibition of tumor cells in vitro[20].
Adriamycin/ Daunomycin	Gluteraldehye	Strain 13 of guinea pigs; Methylchol- anthrene induced sarcoma (MC-D); goat IgG antibody against guinea pig fibrin	Conjugate more effective than free drug after intratumoral injection in vivo but not more effective than free drug again- st MC-D cells in vitro[21].
Diptheria toxin (Fragment A)	N-succinimidyl-3- (pyridyldithio) propionate	Human colorectoral cell lines in culture; mouse hybridoma derived IgG Ab	Specific cytotoxicity to appropriate antigen carrying cell lines in vitro[22].

(continued)

Table 1A. (continued)

Agent	Method of linkage	Test system and Ab	Comments
Diphtheria toxin (Fragment A)	Reaction of S-sulfonated fragment A with Fab-SH	Mouse lymphoma (L1210); rabbit IgG Ab	Cytotoxicity toward L1210 cells in vitro[23].
Diphtheria toxin (Fragment A)	Chlorambucil mixed anhydride	Human lymphoblastoid cell lines CLA4 and Daudi; horse anti-human lymphocyte globulins (both intact IgG and its Fab2 fragment)	IgG and Fab2 conjugates equally toxic in vitro to antigen-containing cells but not to antigenically unrelated cells[24,25].
Ricin (Fragment A)	N-Succinimidyl-3-(2-pyridyldithio) propionate[24]	Human colorectal carcinoma cell lines in culture; mouse hybridoma-produced Ab	Toxic to appropriate antigen-bearing cells in culture[23].
Ricin (Fragment A)	N-Succinimidyl-3-(2-pyridyldithio) propionate[24].	Murkne B cells (normal/neoplastic) in culture; affinity purified rabbit IgG Ab or hybridoma produced Ab to: mouse μ chain; other mouse immunoglobulins subclasses; idiotypes of mouse B cell tumor BCL1	Conjugates specifically cytotoxic to appropriate antigen-bearing cells in vitro[26].

Agent	Method of linkage	Test system and Ab	Comments
Ricin (Fragment A)	3-(2-pyridyldithio) propionic acid on conjugation with carbodiimide	Mouse T cell leukemia WEH1-7 (Thy 1,2 antigen); mouse hybridoma produced IgM Ab	Specific cytotoxic effect in vitro, prolongation of survival after treatment of tumor-bearing mice[27].
Ricin (Fragment A)	3-(2-pyridyldithio) propionic acid on conjugation with carbodiimide	TNP coated HeLa cells; rabbit antiDNP IgG	More toxic to TNP coated HeLa cells than unmodified HeLa cells in vitro[28].
Ricin (Fragment A)	m-maleimidobenzoyl-N-hydroxysuccinimide in conjunction with partial disulfide reduction	Mouse EL4 cells; monoclonal rat IgG 2b Ab to Thy 1,2 antigen.	Selective toxicity to Thy 1,2 antigen bearing cells in vitro[29].
Ricin (Fragment A)	5,5'-dithio-bis-(2-nitro-benzoic acid) after reductive cleavage.	Human B cells; Fab fragment specific for human immunoglobulin.	Selective toxicity to Ig positive cells in vitro[30].

Table 1B. Agent-antibody conjugates exhibiting tumor inhibition either *in vitro* or *in vivo* that were superior to agent or antibody alone – linkage via intermediaries

Agent	Intermediary	Method of linkage	Test system and Ab	Comments
PDM	polyglutamate	(i) carbodiimide	See ref. 1	see ref. 1
	dextran	(ii) carbodiimide (i) CN Br (ii) glutaraldehyde	See ref. 1	See ref. 1
Daunomycin	dextran	periodate	Mouse Yac lymphoma *in vivo* (tumor ip/drug i.v.); rabbit IgG Ab	At high doses, daunomycin dextran–antitumor IgG conjugate superior to free drug but not to drug linked to dextran or via dextran to non-specific IgG. At low doses daunomycin dextran–antitumor IgG conjugate is more effective tumor inhibitor than daunomycin dextran–nonspecific IgG conjugate[31].
Daunomycin	dextran	periodate	Human myelo-sarcoma line K562 xeno-grafted in nude mice; goat anti-K56 γ globulins	Linkage to dextran reduced the toxicity of daunomycin. Dauno-mycin dextran–antitumor Ig was less effective than mixture of Ig and daunomycin[17].

Agent	Intermediary	Method of linkage	Test system and Ab	Comments
Daunomycin	dextran	periodate	BALB/c mice; intrarenal syngeneic graft of renal carcinoma treat i.v.; goat IgG Ab	Linkage of adriamycin to dextran or via dextran to immunoglobulins reduced toxicity allowing administration of conjugates containing larger amounts of the drug. At high dose levels adriamycin-dextran-antitumor IgG was more effective tumor inhibitor than equimolar amounts of adriamycin administered as dextran conjugate or as adriamycin-dextran-nonspecific IgG conjugate, or than the LD10 dose of free adriamycin[32].
Chlorambucil	dextran	(i) CN Br (ii) glutaraldehyde	Human myelosarcoma line K562 xenografted in nude mice; goat anti K562 γ-globulins.	Chlorambucil-dextran-antitumor IgG conjugate was the most effective tumor inhibitor _in vivo_. It was marginally superior to the chlorambucil-dextran conjugate and antitumor IgG administered unlinked[17].

Conjugation using the water soluble carbodiimide 1-ethyl-3-(3-dimethylaminopropyl) carbodiimide (ECDI), while more prone to side reactions and losses by protein precipitation, should also produce amide-linked MTX-IgG. It is therefore interesting to compare tumor inhibition by ECDI-and-NHS-produced conjugates at equimolar dose levels. Figure 1 shows additional survival curves for the groups of tumor-inoculated mice treated with a conjugate synthesized following the ECDI procedure. At a dose of 4 mg per kg of MTX in conjugate form administered daily for five days, there was no difference in the survival between groups of tumor-inoculated mice receiving NHS- or ECDI-produced conjugates. These data show that the MTX incorporated by ECDI is equally effective as the MTX incorporated using the NHS-based procedure despite the lower yield of recoverable conjugate and the somewhat lower amount of drug incorporated by ECDI. This result is not unexpected since both procedures should yield amide-linked MTX conjugates.

LINKAGE OF CHEMOTHERAPEUTIC AGENTS FOR ANTIBODY MEDIATED TARGETING

An ideal binding method should retain chemical groupings essential for drug and antibody activities, allow maximal drug incorporation, and make the drug available in active form at the target site. It is important to learn which agents will be active when administered as antibody conjugates and which linkages will provide greatest inhibition. In this way, optimal drug-linkage combinations can be identified and guiding principles developed for this approach to cancer therapy. There are two categories of binding methods; binding drugs directly to antibodies, and binding them through appropriate spacer intermediaries. Direct binding has several advantages compared with binding using intermediaries i.e. less chemical manipulation with reduced risk of side reactions and minimal increase in the size of the molecule. However, the small number of available reactive groups in IgG for linkage limits incorporation if antibody activity is to be retained.

Direct Linkage to Antibodies

Linkage methods frequently employed in this field have been those based on reagents such as water soluble carbodiimides and glutaraldehyde (see Table 1) because of the availability of carboxyl and amino groups in the targeting antibody and frequently also in the cytotoxic agent. Studies that have compared different linkage groups in the same system are rare. One exception is the study of cytotoxicity carried out by Sela's group[39] in which conjugates of daunomycin and IgG to be compared were prepared by three methods producing different kinds of linkages: glutaraldehyde (Michel-type adduct), periodate-borohydride (secondary amine) and a water soluble carbodiimide (amide). Relative cytotoxicity as measured by uptake of labelled uridine decreased in the order given; the amide-linked drug was almost completely inactive[39].

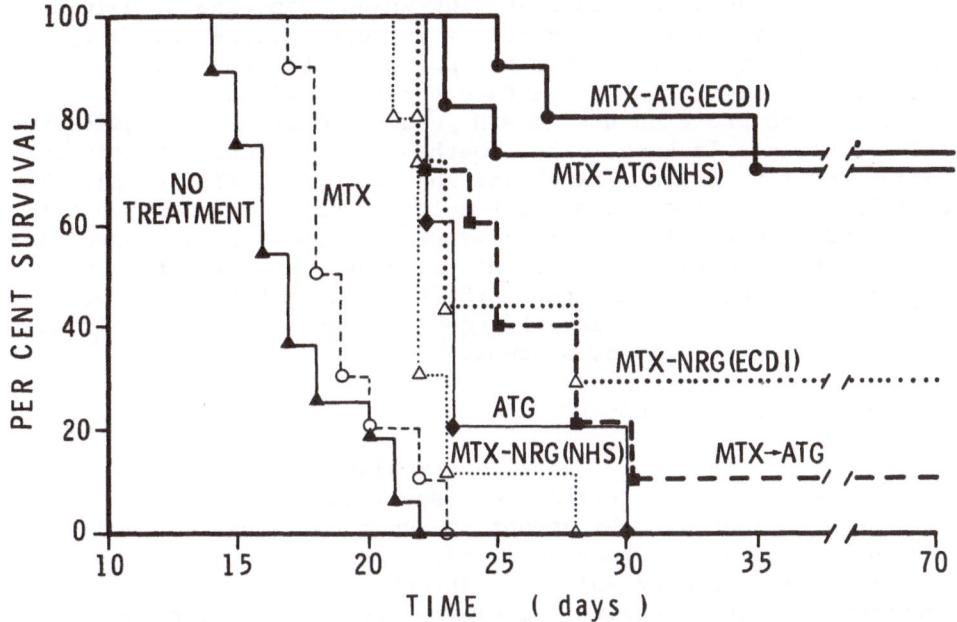

Fig. 1. Survival of EL4 tumor-bearing C57BL/6J mice injected with
methotrexate (MTX) antiEL4 antibody conjugates. Groups,
each containing at least 5 individuals, were inoculated
ip with 10⁴ EL4 cells per mouse. Starting 24 hr later,
different groups received on days 1, 4 and 7 one of the
following ip: MTX alone (O), antitumor IgG (ATG) alone
(◆), MTX followed by ATG (■), MTX linked to ATG (●)
by NHS or ECDI or MTX linked to nontumor specific IgG
(NRG) (△), by NHS or ECDI. The dose per injection of
MTX, administered conjugated or free, was 4 mg per kg and
the amount of free ATG per injection was 100 mg per kg.
The survival of a group injected with MTX followed by NRG
(100 mg/kg) was not significantly different from that of
the control group. Conjugates incorporated approximately
13 moles of MTX per mole of ATG or NRG.

To explain such differential tumor inhibition it is necessary to
determine whether the conjugate is capable of being internalised and,
if so, whether it uses a transport mechanism different from that of
the free drug and whether conjugated drugs ultimately interact with
the same target molecules as the free drug. So far, no study has
been carried out on the in-vivo fate of a drug linked by even a
single bond type.

Recent studies on binding toxins (particularly their enzymatically active A chains) to carriers are of interest in relation to
linkage group role because toxic action has been reported to require

reductive splitting of a disulfide link which joins the A chain to
the second moiety. This second moiety in turn governs uptake by
target cells[22]. Several methods are now available that are designed
to link two proteins or peptides together by disulfide bridges either
when one or both proteins has an -SH group available or in cases where
the -SH groups are lacking. These methods have allowed preparation
of conjugates between toxic A chains and IgG or Fab (Table 1A). The
general finding has been that the resulting conjugates display toxicity toward target cells governed by the antibody carrier specificity. However, selective toxicity has also been observed for conjugates in which binding has been effected via a thioether[29] or
alkyl[25] linkage, demonstrating the need for further study of linkage
parameters of toxin-antibody systems.

Linkage via Intermediaries

In linking methods employing intermediaries such as polyamino
acids and dextran or its derivatives (see Table 1B), the chief objective has been to increase the amount of agent bound per antibody molecule without loss of antibody activity. Linkage of these intermediaries with multiple drug molecules attached should increase drug incorporation without extensively modifying residues in the IgG molecule, which could lead to loss of antigen binding capacity. A spacer
intermediary that incorporates drug-binding groups of appropriate
chain length might also overcome steric hindrance with drug and/or
antibody activity. Special properties can also be exploited when drug-
intermediary-antibody conjugates are being designed; for example, polylysine may facilitate intracellular transport[40]. The optimal size
for an intermediary must be determined that is consistent with binding
effective amounts of drug without altering the size and charge of the
conjugate to produce diversion from the target tumor tissue. Finally,
the potential toxicity of spacers themselves must be considered.

TUMOR LOCALISATION OF ANTI-TAA ANTIBODIES

The rationale for the use of antibodies for targeting drugs or
radionuclides presupposes selective tumor localisation of systemically administered antibody. Investigation of localisation is
carried out by systemic administration of radiolabelled antibodies
followed by detection of localisation either by assay of radioactivity in tissues or by external photoscanning. This latter
technique involves the use of appropriate gamma emitting radionuclides and provides the basis of tumor imaging by antibody-linked
radionuclides (radioimmunodetection). Investigations on tumor
imaging stem from the observation of Pressman and Keighly in 1948
that labelled antibodies against normal tissues localize selectively
in the target organ[41]. A number of studies in experimental models
then demonstrated specific localisation of labelled antibodies in
tumors[37,42,43]. Our early studies showed that radioiodinated antibodies against cell-surface TAA bind to target tumor cells in vitro[44]

and selectively localise in tumors in vivo[45], permitting detection
of tumors by external protoscanning[5,42]. In an experiment designed
to establish the specificity of localisation, a specific xenoglobulin was raised against EL4 lymphoma cells; it did not react in
vitro with B16 melanoma cells[45]. In vivo, localisation occurred
only in the target EL4 tumor and not in a B16 melanoma in the same
mouse. We further showed that the extent of localisation of anti-
tumor immunoglobulin increases with the content of specific anti-TAA
molecules[5].

In a preliminary study, we observed tumor-specific localisation
of anti-TAA antibodies in metastases of renal cell carcinoma, squam-
ous cell carcinoma and malignant melanoma[42]. The presence of a TAA
common to human renal cell carcinoma was suggested by our early
observation that a precipitating antibody from a patient, who had
been subjected to immunotherapy with a renal cell carcinoma preparation, cross-reacted with homogenates of this carcinoma from other
patients but not with homogenates of normal renal tissues[46]. This
was confirmed using xenogeneic sera against human renal cell
carcinoma[47]. After intravenous administration of this xenoglobulin
labelled with ^{131}I, external photoscanning detected lesions in 13
out of 15 patients with primary tumors and 7 out of 8 patients with
metastases[5,48,49]. The tumor specificity of ^{131}I-labelled antitumor
xenoglobulins as imaging agents was supported in this study by several findings: 1) normal rabbit globulin and ^{99m}Tc-sulfur colloid
failed to image tumors; 2) there was immunofluorescent and autoradiographic evidence that i.v. administered ^{131}I-anti renal cell
carcinoma globulin localised in, and bound firmly to, tumor tissue
but did not do so in adjacent renal tissues; and 3) the tumor which
did not bind ^{131}I-anti renal cell carcinoma globulin could not be
visualised[5]. However, studies at this time were limited by the
lack of well-defined tumor markers or pure antibody. Goldenberg's
demonstration of the localisation of an affinity-purified antibody
against the well-defined oncofetal antigens, CEA, in xenografts of
human colonic carcinoma in hamsters was a major step in demonstrating the potential clinical usefulness of this technique[50]. Several
recent developments should make detection more precise and also aid
investigation of the dynamics and mechanism of antibody localisation:
1) identification of a wide range of human TAA and tumor markers for
antibody-mediated targeting[2]
2) availability of monoclonal and affinity-purified antibodies
against TAA and tumor markers (for example see reference 22,23,51)
3) breeding of nude mice which accept xenografts of human tumors as
experimental models.
As Pressman stated last year:"The stage has been set for the immuno-
logist, experimental oncologist and clinical oncologist to address
common objectives and problems in the improved detection and possible
therapy of neoplasms with specific antitumor antibodies...."[43].

Human TAA and Tumor Markers as Targets

The wide variety of human TAA markers that can be used for targeting has been recently discussed by McIntire[2]. To achieve adequate localisation of a targeting antibody, appropriate amounts of the antigens must be available for binding in the tumor, preferably on the cell surface. The number of TAA on the surface of experimental mouse lymphomas has been reported to vary from 5×10^4 to 6.9×10^6 per cell[52]. These numbers appear to be more than adequate for delivering lethal amounts of toxic agents. Targeting of a single molecule of a toxin such as diphtheria toxin, abrin or ricin, for example, is capable of killing a cell[53]. Results presented in Table 1A demonstrate that it is also possible to deliver cytocidyl amounts of cancer chemotherapeutic agents of various modes of anti-tumor action bound to anti-TAA antibodies. When a radionuclide such as ^{131}I is used for therapy (if one assumes the binding of 2 atoms of iodine per molecule of anti-TAA antibody) only a small fraction of the total antigenic sites need to be occupied by a radio-antibody in order to deliver 500 rads to the cell during one half-life[43]. If, for example, 100% of administered radiolabelled antibody bound to tumor cells and no biological loss of radioactivity occurred during its half-life, only 19.4 μg of anti-TAA antibody (with a specific activity of 362 μCi/μg) would be required per ml of blood from leukemic patients to kill 10^3 leukemia cells contained in that volume of blood[54]. At this dose level the total dose from γ - radiation to the soft tissue of the body would be less than 21 rads. It should be possible to kill almost all leukemic cells in the blood (or other circulating tumor cells) even at maximal clinically observed levels of these cells in the peripheral blood[54].

Concerning boron targeting for later activation by neutron capture, Bale et al.[55] have calculated that about 17 boron atoms need to be delivered to a cell to achieve a cytocidyl effect. Since a small tumor has comparatively few binding sites for the targeting antibody, localisation of bound agents can be increased by incorporating the maximal amount per antibody molecule. The only limitation is retention of antibody activity. Special considerations apply to the targeting of radionuclides. For a given amount of antibody bound in a tumor, the radiation emitted from the tumor area is directly proportional to the amount of isotope incorporated in the antibody. Therefore, the greater the specific radioactivity of the radionuclide and the greater the affinity of the carrier antibody for target TAA, the smaller is the tumor mass that can be detected.

TAA that become unavailable for binding because of modification of the cell surface after exposure to antibody are not suitable for targeting drugs or radionuclides. Antigens that elicit antibodies with low affinity are also not likely to be effective for targeting. Isso et al.[56] observed that even though more than 30% of administered antibody to a histocompatability antigen localised in an amount of tumor tissue equal to 1% of the total body weight of a rat, the antibody was lost rapidly from the tumor[56]. TAA that are shared by a given histologic type of tumor rather than associated with an individual type of tumor (e.g. as in renal cell carcinomas and melanomas) are likely to be particuarly useful for targeting. Even the less specific tumor markers, such as CEA, PAP or the B fragments of hCG, can be exploited for targeting against tumors which are detected to produce or contain such markers by assay of body fluids and/or tumor tissue. Most of these markers are available in pure form, facilitating production and affinity purification of antibodies against them. Antigens that are shared by the tumor and its normal tissue of origin, such as the prostate-specific antigen, can also be useful for targeting for diagnostic purposes to detect metastases and the recurrence of tumor after removal of the tumor-containing organ. Antibodies to such antigens can even be used for targeting cytotoxic agents if the antigen-containing organ is not vital (e.g. prostate) or if its function can be replaced (e.g. endocrines). TAA that induce production of large amounts of antibody and/or antibodies of high affinity in the tumor host seem to be undesirable for targeting. However, tumor markers such as oncofetal antigen or extopic hormones such as hCG have been reported not to be immunogenic in the host.

TAA that are shed from the tumor cell surface into the circulation also appear to be unsuitable for targeting. However, careful studies both by Goldenberg et al[57] and March et al[58] revealed that even very high levels of circulating CEA or hCG do not significantly interfere with the injected antibodies reaching the tumor. Whether this is true for other TAA remains to be investigated. This lack of interference is important because cell surface associated TAA are likely to be shed into the circulation.

AntiTAA Antibodies for Targeting

The ideal qualities of an anti-TAA antibody for targeting include high specificity, high affinity, characteristics appropriate for access to TAA on tumor cells leading to tumor localisation of a high proportion of administered antibody, availability in a state of high purity, low immunogenicity in the tumor host, and resistance to denaturation during conjugation procedures. Pressman[43] has pointed out that if the antigen-containing part of the tumor cell is freely exposed to circulating blood (e.g. intravascular invasion of a renal cell carcinoma or a choriocarcinoma) localisation is then determined primarily by the fraction of the cardiac output that reaches the tumor, which is usually small. However, if the antibody has to reach the tumor cell via the extravascular fluid then the extent of its binding to TAA depends upon the rate of diffusion of the labelled antibody, the metabolism of the blood antibody by endocytosis or shedding, and the number and rate of regeneration of TAA sites on the cell surface.

Fragments of anti-TAA antibodies. The transcapillary passage
and diffusion of the targeting antibody are likely to be improved by
using reactive fragments like Fab_2 and Fab. Removal of the Fc moiety
also renders immunoglobulins less antigenic and less suceptible to
binding to, and subsequent catabolism by, cells having Fc receptors,
for example, phagocytes.

Fab_2 and Fab fragments are cleared through the kidneys at a
much faster rate than intact IgG. While using fragments for imaging,
we and other investigators have observed that the detectability of
tumors and the improvement in the contrast of images by external
photoscanning correlates with the rate of clearance of radioactivity
from the system[32]. Rapid plasma clearance of labelled Fab_2 or Fab
fragments that are not bound to the tumor is one explanation for
the earlier visualisation of tumors when such reactive fragments are
used for radionuclide targeting. Reduction in the background
activity is also likely to allow resolution of smaller tumors and/or
tumors with low uptake of targeted radionuclide.

More recently, we have demonstrated that tumors in the central
nervous system (CNS) can be easily localised by external photoscanning after intravenous administration of ^{131}I-labelled Fab_2 fragments of anti-TAA IgG antibody[32]. At 120 hours after intravenous
administration of labelled agents, the Fab_2 fragment of the anti-TAA
IgG led to tumor:normal brain and tumor:blood ratios of ^{131}I activity of 17.9 and 3.3 respectively, whereas the corresponding figures
for intact IgG were 4.78 and 0.38. Thus the "blood brain barrier"
to circulating immunoglobulin in the CNS does not preclude the
application of this method of targeting of radionuclides and drugs.

There may be several disadvantages associated with the use of
these fragments for targeting of drugs. It is possible that labelled monovalent Fab will be less susceptible to endocytosis or shedding after binding to a tumor cell surface because it does not cap.
Although this property may improve imaging quality and aid the action
of conjugated cell surface active agents, it might render targeting
ineffectual for agents that interact with intracellular targets.
It has also been demonstrated that the cytotoxic effect of cancer
chemotherapeutic agents can be synergistic with complement-mediated
damage triggered by intact anti-TAA antibodies[8,10,11]. This
mechanism might contribute to superior tumor inhibition by drug-
linked antibodies and so would only be realised when the Fc moiety
is present.

Monoclonal antibodies. Theoretically, the high purity and
homogeneity of monoclonal antibodies against TAA should make them
superior to conventional polyclonal antibodies for targeting. However, only preliminary studies have been carried out on targeting of
drugs (see Table 1A) and radionuclides. Successful imaging by radiolabelled IgG, appropriately absorbed or affinity-purified, prompted

Ballou et al. to use a ^{131}I-labelled monoclonal anti-mouse terato-
carcinoma antibody to image that tumor in mice[59]. High tumor:normal
tissue ratios of radioactivity were obtained. A monoclonal IgG2a
against mouse Thy 1,1 antigen was studied by Houston et al.[60]
They demonstrated still higher ratios of localisation in target to
nontarget tissue when Fab$_2$ fragments rather than the intact IgG
were administered.

In our laboratory, we have used a hybridoma-produced monoclonal
IgG antibody against a human melanoma to image xenografts of human
melanoma in nude mice and metastases of melanoma in several patients.
This antibody was supplied by Dr. S. Ferrone who reported recently
on its specificity characteristics[51]. Intravenous injection of 50
μCi of ^{131}I-labelled antibody, followed by external scanning every
24 hours, distinctly visualised the tumor at 48 hours (Figure 2).
Tumor delineation was less distinct in mice given ^{131}I-labelled
conventional goat anti-melanoma IgG and tumors could not be localised
in mice given ^{131}I-labelled normal mouse globulin. The results of
assay of radioactivity in tissues of mice killed 6 days after injection of [131]-labelled anti-melanoma IgG or ^{131}I-labelled normal mouse
IgG are given in Table 2.

We also carried out a "paired label" experiment in which groups
of two melanoma-bearing mice were given a mixture of ^{131}I-labelled
monoclonal antimelanoma IgG and ^{125}I-labelled normal mouse globulin.
Tumor:blood ratios of activity were 0.32 for ^{131}I and 0.28 for [125]I-
24 hours after injection; at 48 hours, the respective ratios were
1.2 and 0.3. These results confirm that tumor imaging is not due
to such non-specific factors as increased tumor vascularity (producing an increase in blood volume in relation to surrounding tissues)
and increased permeability of tumor vasculature, but depends upon
the specific antibody content of the labelled antitumor globulin
preparations used for imaging. In a preliminary study, we also
confirmed the potential clinical usefulness of monoclonal antibodies
against human melanoma-associated antigens for radioimmunodetection
of human melanoma[4].

Selection of polyclonal or monoclonal antibodies for targeting
applications. A wide variety of conventional polyclonal and monoclonal antibodies against TAA and tumor markers are becoming increasingly available. Even TAA common to tumors of a given histologic type are known to be antigenically heterogeneous. Therefore,
the choice of TAA or markers and the appropriate antibody should
consider immunofluorescence or a radioimmunoassay-based comparison
of the binding of antibodies. If antibodies against more than one
marker or TAA in a given tumor are demonstrated to bind well to a
given tumor cell, then targeting with a cocktail of such antibodies
should increase the total binding and hence the amount of conjugated
agent delivered. An initial screening analysis of serum and other
appropriate body fluid may be useful in choosing antibodies for

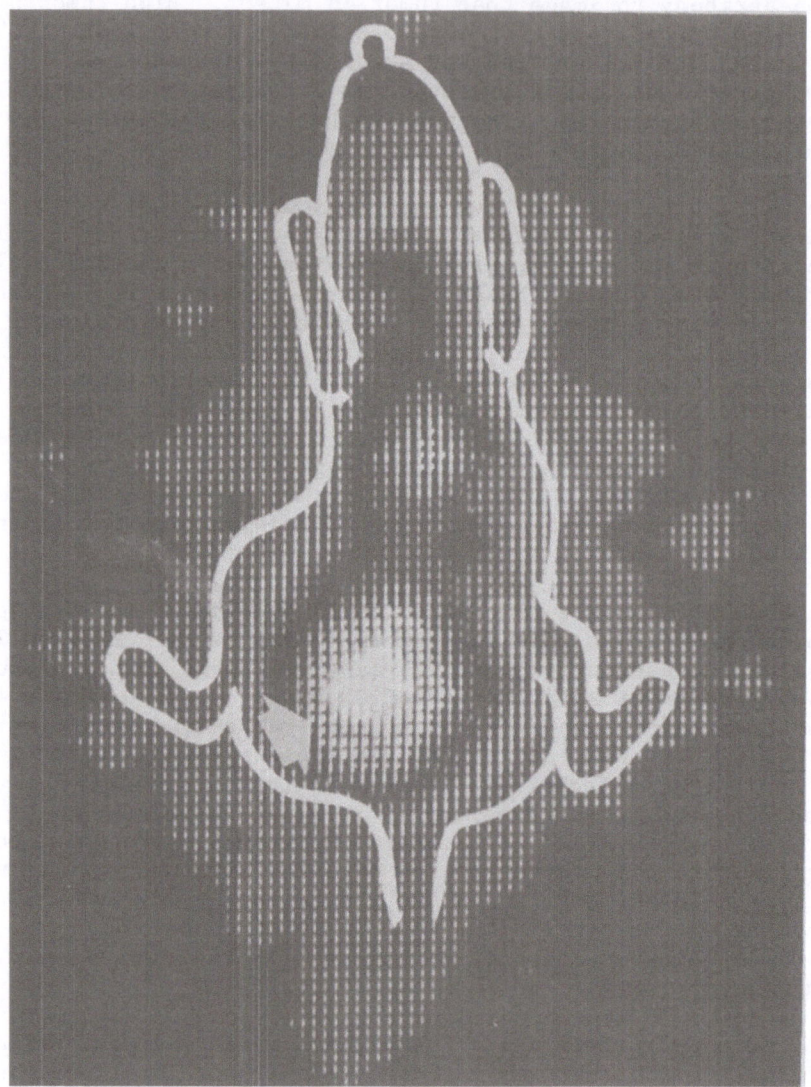

Fig. 2.   Scintiscan of an athymic mouse with a human melanoma
          xenograft 48 hours after intravenous injection of 50 μCi
          of ^{131}I bound to approximately 150 μg of hybridoma-
          produced antihuman melanoma IgG. The scan of ^{131}I
          distribution was obtained at 364 KeV with a 20 per cent
          window. Localisation of radioactivity in excess of the
          background can be seen in the melanoma which is indicated
          by an arrow.

Table 2. Tumor to Tissue Ratios of Radioactivity in Athymic
BALB/c Mice Bearing Xenografts of Human Melanomas[a]

| Tissue | Ratio of radioactivity in mice injected with: | |
	Mouse Monoclonal Antimelanoma IgG	Normal Mouse IgG
Normal muscle adjacent to tumor	7.20	4.27
Heart muscle	13.54	3.89
Kidney	4.10	1.70
Lungs	16.04	8.69
Spleen	4.21	2.37
Bone marrow	8.48	3.59
Liver	2.63	0.48
Blood	6.55	0.35

[a]Mice were injected intravenously with 50 μCi of ^{131}I bound
to about 150 μg of hybridoma-produced antihuman melanoma IgG
or normal mouse IgG and then killed 6 days after receiving
the labeled IgG. Blood was flushed out of organs by injecting
50 ml of warm saline into the heart after severing axillary
vessels.

targeting. For example, raised levels of serum CEA in association
with epithelial tumors indicate the use of antiCEA antibody. However, as already discussed, increased serum levels of other markers
might interfere with localisation of antibodies against them.

Induction of antibodies against targeting IgG (or fragments).
Our results as well as those from Goldenberg's laboratory demonstrate
that after injections of aggregate-free labelled xenoglobulins,
circulating antibody against them could not be detected even after
repeated injections of the xenoglobulin[34,57]. As already discussed,
removal of the F_c fragment of carrier immunoglobulins is also likely
to reduce their antigenicity. The experience obtained with monoclonal antibodies of mouse origin should provide useful guidelines
for later exploitation of monoclonal antibodies derived from human
myeloma lines. Use of TAA-sensitized B cells from lymph nodes
draining a tumor plus human myeloma cell lines to produce hybridomas might provide antibodies similar to autologous immunoglobulins.

Pharmacokinetics of labelled antibodies. Even very mild
treatment of antibodies during labelling may alter the handling of
the labelled antibody in vivo. For example, the half-life of
circulating antibodies has been observed to be considerably
shortened after ^{131}I labelling[42,45]. Though this short half-life
might be useful in tumor imaging by inducing rapid elimination of

heavily labelled denatured antibodies, rapid uptake and breakdown of
labelled specific antibody molecules by phagocytic cells could contribute to nonspecific localisation, thus increasing background
activity during imaging or reducing targeted drug delivery.

TARGETING OF RADIONUCLIDES FOR IMAGING

The design of an ideal imaging agent must consider the physical
decay scheme of the radionuclide and the effect of antibody linkage
on its biological behavior. The main attraction for binding radioisotopes of iodine to antibodies has been the availability of established methods that retain antibody reactivity. In fact, among
all the readily available gamma-emitting radionuclides, those of
iodine have the greatest synthetic versatility. The isotopes that
have been employed are ^{123}I, ^{125}I and ^{131}I. The very short half-life
of ^{123}I renders it impractical for imaging if it cannot be produced
locally. On the other hand, the relatively long half-life of
^{125}I causes unnecessary radiation exposure. ^{131}I has been the
most extensively-used isotope for binding to antibodies because it
has a gamma emission of appropriate energy and a more suitable
half-life of approximately 8 days. However, even this half-life
is unnecessarily long and its γ emission produces unnecessary tissue
exposure. Also, the high energy emission peaks of ^{131}I at 637 and
722 KeV pose problems in collimation. With all radioisotopes of
iodine, uptake by the thyroid must be blocked to prevent damage.
The excretion of iodine through the kidney also limits the usefulness
of radioiodine-labelled antibodies for detection of tumors in the
urinary tract[45].

One main reason for recent interest in the use of ^{111}In and
^{99m}Tc is that they have short half-lives compared to ^{131}I. This
should reduce exposure to the patient. ^{111}In, with its half-life
of 67.5 hours, should be appropriate for linkage to either IgG or
Fab$_2$ and Fab. ^{99m}Tc, with its half-life of about 6 hours, appears
to be appropriate if optimal ratios of tumor to normal tissue localisation are achieved early, as with fragments instead of intact IgG.
Another attractive feature of these two isotopes is that their gamma
emissions are particularly suited to external photoscanning. As in
any antibody-mediated targeting, the binding method should allow
these radionuclides to remain attached to the carrier molecule until
the carrier reaches its optimal concentration in target tissue. The
risk of premature dissociation in the blood is especially high when
a radionuclide is linked to the carrier molecule using noncovalent
bonds, for example, ^{111}In bound by chelation.[61] However, it has been
reported that ^{111}In chelated to antimyosin antibodies has remained
bound in vivo[62].

TARGETING OF RADIONUCLIDES FOR TUMOR THERAPY

Apart from their diagnostic use, nuclides linked to antibodies to TAA also have therapeutic potential as pointed out earlier. We have demonstrated in several mouse tumor models that tumoricidal amounts of ^{131}I can be delivered by anti-TAA antibodies both in vitro and in vivo[37,44,63]. As with chemotherapeutic drugs and toxins, targeting of radionuclides with anti-TAA antibodies depends upon retention of adquate antibody activity.

^{131}I is thus far the only radionuclide used for immunoradio-therapy. Using mild conditions (i.e. lactoperoxidase), Nord and Weisman demonstrated that five-sixths of the antigen binding capacity of anti-Moloney lymphoma ATG was retained when 2 moles of iodine were incorporated per mole of IgG[52]. At molar incorporation levels of 21 moles of iodine per mol IgG, about one-third of the antigen binding capacity was still retained by this antilymphoma antibody[52]. Employing the chloramine T method (i.e., the method usually used now for the radiodination of antibodies), Pressman had demonstrated earlier that incorporation of 2 atoms of I per molecule of IgG did not affect the activity of prototypes of tissue localising anti-bodies[42]. At an incorporation ratio of 19 atoms per molecule of IgG 30% to 50% of the original tissue localising activity of antibodies could be retained. However, incorporation of 25 iodine atoms per molecule of IgG led to complete loss of precipitating activity of antibodies. This loss of activity during radioiodination of anti-bodies could be prevented by protecting the binding site of the antibody with antigen[42].

About 500 rads delivered by β particles (tissue absorption of radiation is much less[54]) is tumoricidal for 100% of exposed HeLa and murine leukemia cells. We have found that between 1000 to 1750 rads of γ-irradiation (from ^{60}Co or ^{137}Cs beams) prevent in vivo proliferation of 100% of cells from several mouse tumors, such as Ehrlich ascites tumor, EL4 lymphoma and L2 lymphoma[63].

As Bale et al. reported, one advantage of using ^{131}I for immun-otherapy is that the effective β radiation from this iodine radio-isotope has a range in tissue corresponding to several times the diameter of a cell[55]. Thus, it is not imperative that the distribu-tion of ^{131}I in the tissue be asbolutely uniform since tumoricidal amounts of radiation can reach cells several diameters away from the site of bound radioactivity. However, this would lead to radiation damage to adjacent normal tissues. Furthermore, non-uniform distribution of radioactivity may fail to deliver lethal amounts of radiation to micrometastases or to small foci of cells even in large tumors with necrotic changes.

More precise and uniform targeting of radioactivity that spares adjacent normal tissues can be achieved by using radioisotopes that emit soft β rays, Auger electrons from ^{125}I, or alpha emitters. Because the effective range of these radiations does not exceed that of a single cell diameter, targeting antibody must reach every

tumor stem cell. Emission of a dense shower of low energy Auger
electrons leads to high electron density in the immediate vicinity
of the disintegrating radionuclide, which can irreversibly damage
sensitive intracellular target molecules[64]. Though some very
preliminary results on the therapeutic application of the Auger
cascade in cancer therapy merit a systematic investigation, Auger
emitters do not appear to be potentially useful for antibody-
directed targeting if nuclear DNA is assumed to be the site of action
of this type of radiation. Such DNA is likely to be out of reach of
Auger electrons from cell surface anti-TAA antibodies.

In another approach to radioimmunotherapy of cancer, ^{10}B was
incorporated into antibody against cell surface associated histocompatibility antigens[65,66]. It was postulated that localisation
of boron-containing compounds in the tumor tissue would render them
susceptible to destruction by slow neutron radiation because the
^{10}B nucleus would capture thermal neutrons with subsequent liberation of 2.79 MeV of energy. In this type of treatment, radiation
damage would be confined to the area exposed to the neutron beam
and effectiveness would depend upon the extent of antibody mediated
selective localisation of ^{10}B in tumor tissue. However, thermal
neutrons penetrate tissues poorly. Furthermore, whether the presence of ^{10}B does indeed enhance the relative biological effectiveness (RBE) of neutron beams appears to be controversial [67,68].

Tumor inhibition by ionizing radiations and cytotoxic agents
can be aided by the synergistic action of antibodies directed
against TAA[69]. This factor may contribute to the success of tumor
suppression by antibody-linked radionuclides. Tumor cell populations also vary in their sensitivity to ionizing radiations. Thus,
results from our laboratory show that though 500 μCi bound to
rabbit antiEL4 IgG produced long-term cure of most C57BL mice prein-
oculated with 10^4 EL4 lymphoma cells[44,63], only prolongation of
survival (but no long-term cure) could be obtained in AKR mice pre-
inoculated with L2 lymphoma cells after $\geqslant 1200$ μCi of ^{131}I-linked
to rabbit anti-TAA globulin was administered (unpublished observations). This amount of ^{131}I activity was lethal to about 10% of
the injected mice. Furthermore, no inhibition of subcutaneous
transplants of EL4 lymphoma could be detected when immunoradio-
therapy was instituted intravenously 3 days after tumor inoculation.
This approach to cancer therapy using conventional polyclonal antibodies thus appears to have little clinical potential. This conclusion appears to be supported by results reported in cancer
patients by Order et al[70]. Studies of tumor localisation of anti-
TAA antibodies have revealed that only a small fraction of the
administered labelled conventional anti-TAA antibody localises in
target solid tumor[55,58]. This is a major problem in therapy of
cancer with antibody-targeted agents but the use of reactive
fragments of monoclonal or affinity purified antibodies may
improve the extent of tumor localisation of targeted agents.

CONCLUSION

Initial indications that anti-TAA antibodies could be used for targeting drugs and radionuclides to diagnose and treat cancer were based on the use of relatively impure conventional polyclonal antibody preparations and methods of linkage whose appropriateness for the purpose had not been evaluated. Use of monoclonal antibodies (and fragments) against defined TAA and tumor markers, agents which have more potent cytotoxicity and improved binding methods, should produce conjugates that display increased tumor localisation, faster plasma clearance and reduced nonspecific localisation and toxicity. For imaging purposes, lower background activity and shorter intervals between administration and optimal imaging should be possible. However, an understanding of the mechanisms underlying the superior antitumor action of antibody-linked cytotoxic agents is needed before chemical linkages can be designed that will facilitate optimal interaction of the conjugate or an active catabolite with sensitive target molecules in vivo. Such knowledge should be of great help in the clinical application of antibody-targeted agents in the diagnosis and treatment of cancer.

ACKNOWLEDGEMENT

The investigations in our laboratory were supported by grants from the Medical Research Council of Canada, the National Cancer Institute of Canada, the Nova Scotia Division of the Canadian Cancer Society, and the Kidney Foundation of Canada. We are grateful to Mrs. B. Baird, Ms. D. Harvey and Mrs. H. Maxner for editorial and secretarial assistance.

REFERENCES

1. T. Ghose and A.H. Blair, Antibody-linked cytotoxic agents in the treatment of cancer: current status and future prospects, JNCI 61: 657 (1978).
2. K.R. McIntire, Tumor markers for radioimmunodetection of cancer, Cancer Res. 40: 3083 (1980).
3. T. Ghose, A.H. Blair, K. Vaughan, and P. Kulkarni, Antibody-directed drug targeting in cancer, in: "Targeted Drugs Polymers in Biology and Medicin," Vol. 2, E. Goldberg, L. Donaruma and O. Vogl, eds., John Wiley and Sons, Inc., New York (in press).
4.   T. Ghose, A.H. Blair, R.H. Martin, S.T. Norvell, S. Ramakrishnan, and P. Belitsky, Tumor imaging by antitumor antibody-linked radionuclides, in: "Tumor Imaging: the Radiochemical Detection of Cancer," S. Burchiel and B.A. Rhodes, eds., Masson Publishing U.S.A., Inc., New York (in press).
5. T. Ghose, S.T. Norvell, J. Aquino, P. Belitsky, J. Tai, A. Guclu, and A.H. Blair, Localization of ^{131}I-labeled antibodies in human renal cell carcinomas and a mouse hepatoma and corre-

lation with tumor detection by photoscanning, Cancer Res.
40: 3018 (1980).

6. T. Ghose and S.P. Nigam, Antibody as carrier of chlorambucil,
    Cancer 29: 1398 (1972).

7. T. Ghose, S.T. Norvell, A. Guclu, D. Cameron, A. Bodurtha, and
    A.S. MacDonald, Immunochemotherapy of cancer with chloram-
    bucil-carrying antibody, Brit. Med. J., 3: 495 (1972).

8. T. Ghose, A. Guclu, and J. Tai, Suppression of an AKR lymphoma
    by antibody and chlorambucil, JNCI 55: 1353 (1975).

9. J. Tai, A.H. Blair, and T. Ghose, Tumor inhibition by chlorambucil
    covalently linked to antitumor globulin, Eur. J. Cancer, 15:
    1357 (1979).

10. D.A.L. Davies and G.J. O'Neill, In-vivo and in-vitro effects of
    tumor specific antibodies with chlorambucil, Brit. J. Cancer
    1: 285 (1973).

11. R.D. Rubens and R. Dulbecco, Augmentation of cytotoxic drug
    action by antibodies directed at cell surface, Nature, 248:
    81 (1974).

12. H.F. Dullens, R.A. DeWeger, C. Vennegoor, and W. DenOtter, Anti-
    tumor effect of chlorambucil-antibody complexes in a murine
    melanoma system, Eur. J. Cancer, 15: 69 (1979).

13. F.L. Moolten, S.R. Cooperband, Selective destruction of target
    cells by diphtheria toxin conjugated to antibody directed
    against antigens on the cells, Science, 169: 68 (1970).

14. P.N. Kulkarni, A.H. Blair, and T. Ghose, Covalent binding of
    methotrexate to immunoglobulins and its effect on drug and
    antibody activities, Federation Proc. 40: 642 (1981).

15. P.N. Kulkarni, A.H. Blair, and T. Ghose, Covalent binding of
    methotrexate to immunoglobulins and the effect of antibody-
    linked drug on tumor growth in vivo, Cancer Res., (in press).

16. S. Burstein and R. Knapp, Chemotherapy of murine ovarian carcinoma
    by methotrexate-antibody conjugates, J. Med. Chem. 20: 950
    (1977).

17. Z.A. Latif, B.B. Lozzio, C.J. Wust, S. Krauss, M.C. Aggio, and
    C.B. Lozzio, Evaluation of drug-antibody conjugates in the
    treatment of human myelosarcomas transplanted in nude mice,
    Cancer, 45: 1326 (1980).

18. T. Ghose, J. Tai, A. Guclu, S.T. Norvell, A.H. Blair and J. Aquino,
    Use of cell surface localizing antihepatoma antibody for
    tumor imaging and therapy with drug-linked antibody, Trans-
    plant. Proc., 12: 192 (1980).

19. I. Kimura, T. Ohnoshi, T. Tsubota, Y. Sato, T. Kobayashi and
    S. Abe, Production of tumor antibody-neocarzinostatin (NCS)
    conjugate and its biological activites, Cancer Immunol.
    Immunother. 7: 235 (1980).

20. M. Belles-Isles and M. Page, In-vitro activity of daunomycin-
    anti-alphafoetoprotein conjugate on mouse hepatoma cells,
    Brit. J. Cancer, 41: 841 (1980).

21. F.H. Lee, I. Berczi, S. Fujimoto and A.H. Sehon, The use of anti-
    fibrin antibodies for the destruction of tumor cells.

III. Complete regression of MC-D sarcoma in guinea pigs by conjugates of daunomycin with antifibrin antibodies, Cancer Immunol. Immunother., 5: 201 (1978).

22. D.G. Gilliland, Z. Steplewski, R. Collier, K.F. Mitchell, T.H. Chang and H. Koprowski, Antibody-directed cytotoxic agents: Use of monoclonal antibody to direct the action of toxin A chains to colorectal carcinoma cells, Proc. Natl. Acad. Sci. USA, 77: 4539 (1980).

23. Y. Masuho, T. Hara, and T. Noguchi, Preparation of a hybrid of fragment Fab' of antibody and fragment A of diphtheria and its cytotoxicity. Biochem. Biophys. Res. Commun. 90: 320 (1979).

24. P.E. Thorpe, W.C.J. Ross, A.J. Cumber, C.A. Hinson, D.C. Edwards, and A.J.S. Davies, Toxicity of diphtheria toxin for lymphoblastoid cells is increased by conjugation to anti-lymphocytic globulin, Nature, 271: 752 (1978).

25. W.C.J. Ross, P.E. Thorpe, A.J. Cumber, D.C. Edwards, C.A. Hinson, and A.J.S. Davies, Increased toxicity of diphtheria toxin for human lymphoblastoid cells following covalent linkage to anti-(human lymphocyte) globulin or its $F(ab^1)_2$ fragment. Eur. J. Biochem. 104: 381 (1980).

26. K.A. Krolick, C. Villemez, P. Isakson, J.W. Uhr, and E.S. Vitetta, Selective killing of normal or neoplastic B cells by antibodies coupled to the A chain of ricin, Proc. Natl. Acad. Sci. USA, 77: 5419 (1980).

27. H.E. Blythman, P. Casellas, O. Gros, P. Gros, F.K. Jansen, F. Paolucci, B. Pau, and H. Vidal, Immunotoxins:hybrid molecules of monoclonal antibodies and a toxin subunit specifically kill tumor cells, Nature 290: 145 (1981).

28. F.K. Jansen, H.E. Blythman, D. Carriere, P. Casellas, J. Diaz, P. Gros, J.R. Hennequin, F. Apolucci, B. Pau, H. Poncelet, G. Richer, S.L. Salhi, H. Vidal, and G.A. Voisin, High specific cytotoxicity of antibody-toxin hybrid molecules (immunotoxins) for target cells Immunol. Lett. 2: 97 (1980).

29. R.J. Youle, and D.M. Neville, Jr., Anti-thy 1.2 monoclonal antibody linked to ricin is a potent cell-type-specific toxin Proc. Natl. Acad. Sci. USA, 77: 5483 (1980).

30. V. Raso, and T. Griffin, Specific cytotoxicity of a human immunoglobulin-directed Fab^1-ricin A chain conjugate J. Immunol. 125: 2610 (1980).

31. E. Hurwitz, R. Maron, A. Bernstein, M. Wilchek, M. Sela, and R. Arnon, The effect in vivo of chemotherapeutic drug - antibody conjugates in two murine experimental tumor systems, Int. J. Cancer, 21: 747 (1978).

32. T. Ghose, S. Ramakrishnan, P. Kulkarni, A.H. Blair, K. Vaughan, H. Nolido, S.T. Norvell and P. Belitsky, Use of antibodies against tumor-associated antigens for cancer diagnosis and treatment, Transplant. Proc., in press.

33. A. Guclu, T. Ghose, J. Tai and M. Mammen, Binding of chlorambucil with antitumor globulins and its effect on drug and antibody

activities, Eur. J. Cancer, 12: 95 (1976).

34. T. Ghose, S.T. Norvell, A. Guclu, A. Bodurtha, J. Tai, and
    A.S. MacDonald, Immunochemotherapy of malignant melanoma
    with chlorambucil-bound antimelanoma globulins: preliminary
    results in patients with disseminated disease, JNCI, 58:
    845 (1977).
35. T. Ghose, S.T. Norvell, A. Guclu and A.S. MacDonald, Immunochemo-
    therapy of human malignant melanoma with chlorambucil-
    carrying antibody, Eur. J. Cancer, 11: 321 (1975).
36. A. Guclu, J. Tai, and T. Ghose, Endocytosis of chlorambucil-bound
    antitumor globulin following "capping"in EL4 lymphoma cells,
    Immunol. Commun. 4: 229 (1975).
37. T. Ghose, J. Tai, A. Guclu, S.T. Norvell, A. Bodurtha, J. Aquino
    and A.S. MacDonald, Antibodies as carriers of radionuclides
    and cytotoxic drugs in the treatment and diagnosis of cancer,
    Ann. NY Acad. Sci., 277: 671 (1976).
38. D.G. Johns and J.R. Bertino, Folate antagonists, in: "Cancer
    Medicine," J.F. Holland and E. Frei, eds., Lea & Febiger,
    Philadelphia (1973).
39. E. Hurwitz, R. Levy, R. Maron, M. Wilcheck, R. Arnon and M. Sela,
    The covalent binding of daunomycin and adriamycin to anti-
    bodies, with retention of both drug and antibody activities,
    Cancer Res., 35: 1175 (1975).
40. W.C. Shen and H.J.P. Ryser, Conjugation of poly-L-lysine to
    albumin and horseradish peroxidase: a novel method of
    enhancing the cellular uptake of proteins, Proc. Natl. Acad.
    Sci. USA, 75: 1872 (1978).
41. D. Pressman, and G. Keighley, The zone of activity of antibodies
    as determined by the use of radioactive tracer; the zone of
    activity of nephrotoxic antikidney serum, J. Immunol., 59:
    141 (1948).
42. T. Ghose, A. Guclu, J. Tai, A.S. MacDonald, S.T. Norvell and J.
    Aquino, Antibody as carrier of ^{131}I in cancer diagnosis and
    treatment, Cancer, 36: 1646 (1975).
43. D. Pressman, The development and use of radiolabeled antitumor
    antibodies, Cancer Res., 40: 2960 (1980).
44. T. Ghose, M. Cerini, M. Carter and R.C. Nairn, Immunoradioactive
    agent against cancer, Brit. Med. J., 1: 90 (1967).
45. T. Ghose, J. Tai, J. Aquino, A. Guclu, S. Norvell and A.S.
    MacDonald, Tumor localization of ^{131}I-labeled antibodies by
    radionuclide imaging, Radiol., 116: 445 (1975).
46. R.C. Nairn, J. Philip, T. Ghose, I.B. Porteous, and J.E.
    Fothergill, Production of a precipitin against renal cancer,
    Brit. Med. J., 1: 1702 (1963).
47. T. Ghose, P. Belitsky, J. Tai, and D.T. Janigan, Production and
    characterization of xenogeneic antisera to a human renal cell
    carcinoma associated antigen, JNCI, 63: 301 (1979).
48. P. Belitsky, T. Ghose, J. Aquino, S.T. Norvell and A.H. Blair,
    Radionuclide imaging of primary renal-cell carcinoma by
    labeled antitumor antibody, J. Nucl. Med., 19: 427 (1978).

49. P. Belitzky, T. Ghose, J. Aquino, J. Tai, and A.S. MacDonald, Radionuclide imaging of metastases from renal-cell carcinoma patients by ^{131}I-labeled antitumor antibody, Radiol., 126: 515 (1978).

50. F.J. Primus, R. MacDonald, D.M. Goldenberg, H.J. Hansen, Localization of GW-39 human tumors in hamsters by affinity-purified antibody to carcinoembryonic antigen, Cancer Res., 37: 1544 (1977).

51. K. Imai, A.K. Ng, and S. Ferrone, Characterization of monoclonal antibodies to human melanoma-associated antigens, JNCI, 66: 489 (1981).

52. S. Nord, and I.L. Weissman, Radiolabeled antitumor antibodies. II. Quantitative analysis of Moloney tumor antigens on Moloney lymphoma cells (LSTRA), JNCI, 53: 125 (1974).

53. S. Olsnes, Directing toxins to cancer cells, Nature, 290: 84 (1981).

54. C. McGaughey, Feasibility of tumor immunoradiotherapy using radio-iodinated antibodies to tumor-specific cell membrane antigens with emphasis on leukemias and early metastases, Oncology, 29: 302 (1974).

55. W.F. Bale, M.A. Contreras, and E.P. Grady, Factors influencing localization of labeled antibodies in tumors, Cancer Res., 40: 2965 (1980).

56. M.J. Izzo, D.J. Buchsbaum and W.F. Bale, Localization of an ^{125}I-labeled rat transplantation antibody in tumors carrying the corresponding antigen, Proc. Soc. Exp. Biol. Med., 139: 1185 (1972).

57. D.M. Goldenberg, F. Deland, E. Kim, S. Bennett, F.J. Primus, J.R. Van Nagel, Jr., N. Estes, P. Desimone and P. Rayburn, Use of radiolabeled antibodies of carcinoembryonic antigen for the detection and localization of diverse cancers by external photoscanning, New Engl. J. Med., 298: 1384 (1978).

58. J.P. Mach, S. Carrel, M. Forni, J. Ritschard, A. Donath and P. Alberto, Tumor localization of radiolabeled antibodies against carcinoembryonic antigen in patients with carcinoma, New Engl. J. Med., 303: 5 (1980).

59. B. Ballou, G. Levine, T.R. Hakala and D. Solter, Tumor location detected with radioactively labeled monoclonal antibody and external scintigraphy, Science, 206: 844 (1979).

60. L.L. Houston, R.C. Nowinski and I.D. Bernstein, Specific in vivo localization of monoclonal antibodies directed against the Thy 1.1 antigen, J. Immunol., 125: 837 (1980).

61. G. Subramanian, B.A. Rhodes, J.F. Cooper, V.J. Sodd, eds., "Radiopharmaceuticals", Society of Nuclear Medicine, New York (1975).

62. B.A. Khau, J.T. Fallon, H.W. Strauss and E. Haber, Myocardial infarct imaging of antibodies to canine cardiac myosin with Indium-111-diethylenetriamine, Science, 209: 295 (1980).

63. T. Ghose, and A. Guclu, Cure of a mouse lymphoma with radio-iodinated antibody, Eur. J. Cancer, 10: 787 (1974).

64. K.G. Hofer, G. Keough and J.M. Smith, Biological toxicity of
    Auger emitters: molecular fragmentation versus electron
    irradiation, <u>Cur. Topics Radiation Res. Quarterly</u>, 12: 335
    (1977).
65. M.F. Hawthorne and R.J. Wiersema, Preparation of tumor specific
    boron compounds. 1. In-vitro studies using boron-labeled
    antibodies and elemental boron as neutron targets, <u>J. Med.
    Chem.</u> 15: 449 (1972).
66. A.G. Mallinger, E.L. Jozwiak, Jr., and J.C. Carter, Preparation
    of boron-containing bovine γ-globulin as a model compound
    for a new approach to slow neutron therapy of tumors,
    <u>Cancer Res.</u>, 32: 1947 (1972).
67. L.E. Farr and T. Koniwowski, Long range effects of neutron
    capture therapy of cancer in mice, <u>Int. J. Nucl. Med. Biol.</u>,
    3: 1 (1976).
68. T. Saigusa and Y. Veno, Calculated responses to a thermal neutron
    beam for hamster and HeLa cells containing Boron-10 at
    different concentrations, <u>Phys. Med. Biol.</u>, 23: 748 (1978).
69. T. Ghose and M. Cerini, Radiosensitization of Ehrlich ascites
    tumour cells by a specific antibody, <u>Nature</u>, 222: 993 (1969).
70. S.E. Order, J.L. Klein, D. Ettinger, P. Alderson, S. Siegelman,
    and P. Leichner, Use of isotopic immunoglobulin in therapy,
    <u>Cancer Res.</u>, 40: 3001 (1980).

ANTIBODY-TOXIN CONJUGATES AS POTENTIAL THERAPEUTIC AGENTS

D. Caird Edwards, Philip E. Thorpe and Anthony J.S.
Davies

Institute of Cancer Research: Royal Cancer Hospital
Chester Beatty Research Institute, Fulham Road
London, SW3 6JB, England

In his book 'Selective Toxicity', Adrian Albert[1] gave three
main principles upon which he averred drug selectivity to
depend. Defining the living matter to be injured as the
"uneconomic species", the principles were (1) accumulation by,
(2) injury to a chemical system important for, and (3) exclusive
reaction with cytological features of, the uneconomic species.
Commonly, more than one of these principles was to be seen in the
action of any selective agent. These rules provide a set of
guidelines to be followed in the design and testing of new
agents, the functional partition being particularly useful in the
present discussion of antibodies, toxins and their conjugates.
The role of antibody is to be accumulated, hopefully in an
exclusive fashion, by antigenic cytological features presented by
the target cells. This interaction itself need not be harmful
but fulfils two of Albert's three principles. For their part the
toxins, such as diphtheria toxin, abrin or ricin, are extremely
powerful cytotoxic agents but they lack the exquisite tissue
binding specificities which antibodies can be prepared to have.
By producing chemical conjugates of antibodies and toxins the
hope is to combine the desirable qualities of specificity of
binding and effectiveness in killing in order to generate a new
series of chemotherapeutic agents accumulated by and highly
injurious to the uneconomic species.

A useful aspect of the Albert principles is their emphasis
on the role of the target cell itself as the accumulator of the
agent. This active participation is in contrast to that of
passive victimisation implicit in models based on magic bullet or

similar concepts, and as will be seen is more realistic.

The function of the antibody in the conjugate

Antibodies are currently the most obvious and attractive
source of carrier molecules since the desired specificities can
be elicited by immunising appropriate hosts with the target
tissue itself. Their use is all the more plausible since the
recent introduction of the hybridoma technique[2] for producing
monoclonal antibodies in high yield and purity. Other molecules
such as hormones or lectins may in the future find use as
carriers and indeed pioneering studies with human placental
lactogen[3] and the β-subunit of human chorionic gonadotrophin[4]
have been undertaken already. Other moieties, such as mannose-6-
phosphate[5], epidermal growth factor[6] and insulin[7], have been
mainly used with the objective of exploring mechanisms of toxin
action rather than constructing chemotherapeutic agents.

The basic assumption made by all who utilize antibodies as
carriers is that antibodies display specificity and exclusivity
of reaction with the antigens to which they were raised, and
antibodies should thus fulfil the first and third of Albert's
criteria. Of these, exclusivity of reaction with the target
tissue, has been the easier to demonstrate. Indeed, such
reactions form the basis for the use of antisera in diagnosis of
bacterial and viral infections, for the determination of blood
groups and histocompatibility types, as well as in forensic and
other investigative sciences, specificity being authenticated by
strict observance of quality control measures.

Accumulation by an identified target tissue in a living
animal has not always been so convincingly shown. As this
problem has received particular attention in the cancer field
some discussion of the current position follows.

Although the very existence of specific tumour antigens has
been questioned[8] it is evident that certain specificities are
expressed on tumour cells which may be exploited with advantage.
Examples are the antigens said to have been found on chemically
or virally induced neoplasias, oncofoetal antigens and hormones,
and normal differentiation antigens sometimes expressed by tumour
cells[9]. In these last instances in which there is little or no
qualitative distinction between the malignant cell population and
the normal tissue from which it arose, it is envisaged that an
attack on the tumour could be made but only when a non-vital
organ or tissue is involved.

The ability of antibody to localise in target tissue _in vivo_
was the subject of a prolonged investigation of Pressman and his
colleagues. In their early work heterologous antibodies raised

against transplanted tumours were shown to be localised[10] but
later the same group found that much of this was due to the
previously unsuspected presence of antifibrinogen antibodies
which become extravascularised in areas where rapid cell growth
or inflammation were present[11]. In work subsequent to this
discovery they demonstrated convincing evidence for localisation
of rabbit antibodies to a hepatic tumour induced in rats with
N-2- fluoroamylacetamide. Antibodies to normal rat liver were
also taken up by the tumour but anti-fibrin antibodies as a rule
were not[12].

In 1971 Rief[13], using Pressman's paired-label method[14],
studied the localisation of rabbit antibody to a mouse myeloma
protein. In this case specific uptake by the melanoma was seen
in mice but not until 8 days after injection of antibody 4 days
after subcutaneous injection of 3×10^6 tumour cells. Despite
this positive evidence and some preferential localisation of
anti-lung, anti-kidney and anti-liver antibodies[15] the results
scarcely justified Ehrlich's optimistic view of antibodies as the
magic bullets of chemotherapy.

The discovery of onco-foetal antigens and in particular
carcinoembryonic antigen (CEA) gave fresh impetus to such
studies. For example, using affinity purified antibody and the
paired label technique, Primus et al.[16] found a four fold greater
accumulation of anti-CEA antibody than normal IgG by a human
tumour growing as a xenograft in the hamster. Later Mach et
al.[17] used an affinity purified anti-CEA previously shown to
localise in mice and injected it labelled with ^{131}I into
patients. ^{125}I normal IgG was also given and both isotopes
measured by scintillation counting in tumours and normal tissues
recovered after surgery. Although the total amount of antibody
accounted for in the tumour was only a small proportion of the
amount injected it was clear that it was the anti-CEA alone that
had localised in the tumour and that it had not accumulated in
the normal tissue. More recently Moshakis et al.[18] have studied
the ability of affinity purified goat anti-CEA to be accumulated
by human breast-carcinoma xenografts. Antibodies were shown to
become localised in tumour but not in normal tissues. The amount
trapped was correlated with the amount of tumour CEA but was
apparently unaffected by the levels of circulating CEA.

Houston et al.[19] have shown that lymph nodes from mice
expressing Thy 1.1 antigen injected intravenously with
radiolabelled monoclonal antibody contained 9 times more antibody
than lymph nodes from mice of a congenic strain expressing Thy
1.2 antigen. When $F(ab')_2$ was used the differential increased to
an impressive 144 times indicating that Fc binding is probably a
principal determinant of antibody localisation in the mammalian
body.

The improvements seen in the accumulation of antibodies by target tissue by the use of affinity purified and, more strikingly, monoclonal antibody justify some optimism that antibodies will fulfil the third of Albert's principles.

The function of the toxin in the conjugate

The choice of effector substance to injure the uneconomic species is in principle limitless and with specificity provided by the carrier moiety the criterion for choice becomes effectiveness. Many attempts have been made to attach clinically accepted drugs to antibodies using covalent and non-covalent bonds and some degree of success has been achieved (reviewed by Ghose & Blair[20] and O'Neill[21]).

Several groups of workers have preferred a more radical approach and have tried to harness the potential of the extremely potent naturally occurring cytotoxic agents like diphtheria toxin, abrin and ricin. The advantage of these substances over conventional drugs is that their action is catalytic and thus they are many times more effective than chemicals acting in a stoichiometric manner. This is seen as being particularly useful in situations where the target cell might have a paucity of antigens available for interaction with antibody either because of a low level of expression or by virtue of poor vascularity, or the inaccessibility of, for example luminal surfaces. This problem is likely to be exacerbated by the use of monoclonal antibodies reacting with single antigens which may further limit the number of antibody molecules able to attach to the cell surface. As far as the limited binding of monoclonal antibodies is concerned it may be possible to use a mixture.

The modes of action of the toxins have been thoroughly discussed in several recent articles[22,23] and this ground will not be covered here. It is sufficient merely to point out that each toxin in its active form comprises two polypeptide chains joined by a disulphide bridge. When separated, neither chain is cytotoxic. One subunit (the B chain) serves to effect primary interaction with a receptor molecule (usually a glycoprotein) on the cell surface. The second (the A chain) terminates protein synthesis in the cytosol compartment by a mechanism that is known to be enzymic in the case of diphtheria toxin and is likely to be so for abrin and ricin.

The disadvantage in the use of toxins lies in the role of the B chain in providing a point of interaction with the cell and thus a binding possibility in addition to that to be conferred on the conjugate by the antibody. As will be seen later various strategies have been devised in attempts to circumvent this problem.

The chemistry of conjugation

Most proteins have a number of free chemical groups available along the length of their polypeptide backbone which can be used in substitution reactions. Methyl, hydroxy, sulphy-dryl, amino and carboxyl are the most common, and that most used is the free ϵ-amino group of lysine.

To cross link two proteins in a defined manner is not a simple matter and various reagents have been used. Bifunctional reagents such as glutaraldehyde and di-isocyanates were among the first coupling agents to be exploited but suffer from some quite serious disadvantages. Having two identical reactive groups they are unselective and their use leads to the formation of homo-polymers of both protein species, and purification of the desired molecular combination can be difficult. Additionally with toxins non-reducible bonds between A and B chains may form which could prevent their dissociation and cause a loss of toxicity.

With these problems in mind, Thorpe et al.[24], devised a novel conjugation procedure based on the use of a derivative of chlorambucil, a nitrogen mustard used in the treatment of cancer. In the first studies the coupling agent was a mixed anhydride derivative of chlorambucil which was formed by reaction of the drug with butyl chloroformate. When this reagent was mixed with antibody at 4°C and allowed to react, primary amino groups on the protein interacted with the mixed anhydride radical to form an amide bond. At 4°C the chloroethylamino groups of the alkylating agent are relatively inactive. When toxin was added and the temperature raised to 25°C the chloroethyl amino groups were activated to react with free amino groups in the toxin (present in 4 fold molar excess), to form a piperazine ring. The conjugate so formed was readily purified by molecular sieve chromatography. This method of coupling had several merits. It prevented the formation of homopolymers of the second protein species (in this case toxin) and also did not cause intrachain bonds to be formed in the toxin. In an improved version of the method the N-hydroxysuccinimide ester of chlorambucil was employed[25]. This derivative had better solubility and gave more reproducible conjugation and somewhat higher yield.

Others have bound proteins together by the introduction of a disulphide link to mimic the bond naturally formed between the A and B chains of the toxins. In the most readily available method the 'SPDP' reagent, N-succinimidyl 3-(2-pyridyldithio) propionate, developed by Carlsson et al.[26], is used to introduce a disulphide group into one of the proteins to be coupled and a sulphydryl group into the other which then react together to form a conjugate with the two proteins linked by a disulphide bond. If the proteins to be modified possess a free sulphydryl group it

is of course only necessary to derivatise the other potential
partner. This is so when toxin A chains are used and disulphide
exchange reactions have commonly been employed for this purpose
(reviewed by Olsnes and Pihl[27]).

The art of conjugate formation has advanced rapidly and
reliable methods are now available for the introduction of both
reducible and non-reducible chemical bonds, with minimal damage
to either of the conjugate partners.

Experiments with antibody-toxin conjugates

The first attempts to employ antibody and toxin in chemical
combination were made by Moolten and Cooperband in 1970[28]. They
used diphtheria toxin conjugated to an anti-mumps virus antibody
to attack monkey kidney cells infected with mumps virus in tissue
culture. Later the same group[29] used affinity purified anti-
dinitro-phenyl antibodies attached to diphtheria toxin and
attempted to treat hamsters bearing subcutaneous implants of
dinitrophenylated sarcoma cells. Treatment with conjugate
delayed the appearance of tumours and prolonged life, and, when
small numbers of tumour cells were used (3×10^2), a reduction in
tumour incidence was seen. In 1975 they reported[30] that they had
coupled diphtheria toxin to immunopurified antibodies against
SV40-induced antigens and had produced conjugates more effective
at killing SV40 transformed cells than a conjugate in which
normal immunoglobulin (nIgG) was used in place of antibody.

Philpott et al.[31] using a similar approach conjugated rabbit
anti-trinitrophenyl antibody to diphtheria toxin and showed the
product to be toxic to TNP coated HeLa cells while sparing non-
substituted cells. They demonstrated the immunological
specificity of the effect by using the free hapten as a
competitive inhibitor of the conjugate.

Later Thorpe et al.[24] and Ross et al.[32] used the derivative
of chlorambucil already mentioned to attach diphtheria toxin to
horse anti-human lymphocyte globulin (AHLG) and to its F(ab')$_2$
fragment. The antibody in the conjugates was shown to have
retained its ability to bind specifically to the human lymphoblastoid cell lines, CLA 4 and Daudi, and using protein synthesis
inhibition as the marker, the antibody-toxin conjugate was found
to be more than one thousand times more toxic than free
diphtheria toxin in tissue culture. By contrast a conjugate made
using nIgG and toxin was between 50 and 100 times less potent
than the free toxin. The toxicity of the AHLG-toxin conjugate
could be blocked by pretreating the cells with excess free
AHLG and also by an anti-diphtheria toxin antibody. These
experiments gave clear evidence for primary and selective
binding of the conjugate and of injury to a vital chemical system

within the target cell.

The work also illustrated another aspect of the problem of
cell killing namely the ability of the injurious chemical to
penetrate into the cytosol. The human lymphoblastoid cells were
found to be surprisingly resistant to free diphtheria toxin.
Previously it had been thought that cells from a species
sensitive to the toxin would, with very few exceptions, be
equally sensitive. The increase in toxicity seen when the toxin
was attached to antibody was interpreted as indicating that the
cell presented many more sites for attachment of antibody than it
did for the toxin and that the resultant increase in
concentration of diphtheria toxin at the cell surface led to
greater internalisation of the toxin A chain.

The intact mouse is well known to be resistant to diphtheria
toxin and this is also true for mouse cells in tissue culture.
The cell free protein synthesising systems derived from mouse
cells are, however, fully sensitive to inhibition by the toxin A
chain. Using an anti-mouse lymphocyte globulin-diphtheria toxin
conjugate it was possible to ensure interaction with the cell
surface proteins of mouse splenic lymphocytes but the cells still
remained refractory to the toxin. It is evident from this
experiment that although primary binding to the cell surface is a
prerequisite of cytotoxicity it does not of itself guarantee it.
A mechanism for translocation of the toxic entity into or into
contact with the appropriate cellular compartment is necessary.

Anti-mouse lymphocyte globulin (AMLG) is a well known
immunosuppressive agent whose mode of action has been suggested
primarily to involve reaction with circulating lymphocytes[33].
Edwards et al.[34] attempted to impair the ability of the mouse to
react immunologically to an injection of sheep red blood cells by
treatment with a conjugate of AMLG and abrin. This conjugate was
about twice as effective as a control conjugate made with nIgG at
suppressing the formation of IgM antibody forming cells in the
spleen of the mouse. This two fold differential was about the
same as that seen when the same two conjugates were used against
mouse spleen cells in tissue culture.

In an extension of this work using the improved conjugation
method already mentioned and introducing a second gel filtration
step to purify the conjugate, the same group[25] obtained an
improved immunosuppressive differential of four-fold. In this
study the integrity of the A chain of the toxin in the conjugates
was formally demonstrated and thus differences in effectiveness
in vivo can be interpreted as indicative of the role of the
antibody binding sites in encouraging the binding of abrin to
cells engaged in the immune response.

The main objective of this work was to try to improve the
efficacy of AMLG by attachment of a highly active cytotoxic
moiety. The improvement in the ability of AMLG to immunosuppress
mice was in fact around 50,000 fold but this must be viewed
against the fact that the toxin itself proved to be highly
immunosuppressive. A bonus in this study was the fact that whole
body toxicity of abrin was greatly reduced on conjugation and
this along with the antibody carrier effect led to an increase in
therapeutic index from 2.8 for abrin to 19.0 for AMLG-abrin.

Ricin has been coupled to antibodies by several groups of
workers some of whom employed non-covalent linkages. Refsnes and
Munthe-Kass[35] used an anti-ricin B-chain antibody-ricin complex
to attack Kupffer cells and peritoneal macrophages in tissue
culture via interaction with their Fc-receptors. Raso and
Griffin[36] used a hybrid antibody of anti-ricin A chain and anti-
human IgG to encourage binding to and killing of human lymphoid
cells in tissue culture. A covalent conjugate containing a thio
ether linkage was prepared by Youle and Neville[37] from a
monoclonal anti-thy 1.2 antibody and ricin and was found to be as
toxic for EL4 cells as was ricin itself.

The toxic action of abrin and ricin upon tissue culture
cells seems to involve an interaction with terminal or
penultimate galactose residues presented by glycoproteins or
glycolipids on the surface of the cells. Thus this sugar, either
itself or as present in lactose, can be used as a competitive
inhibitor of the toxins in tissue culture. Youle and Neville[37]
showed that lactose antagonised the toxicity of their conjugate
to cells lacking Thy 1.2 antigen but that the toxic effect on EL4
cells was unimpaired. Similarly, Thorpe et al.[38] have
investigated the effect of excess free galactose on the toxicity
of abrin, AHLG- abrin and nIgG-abrin on Daudi cells and have
shown that in the presence of 100mM sugar only the antibody-abrin
toxicity is expressed.

The strategy most commonly employed to try to pre-empt the
cell binding properties of toxin moiety of conjugates is to use
isolated A chains or as in one case, to use a protein synthesis
inhibitor of plant origin equivalent to an A chain. In many such
instances the conjugates have been of rather low potency although
considerable selectivity has been demonstrated. The results can
be interpreted as showing that although exclusivity of interaction with specific sites on the cell surface occurs and
although the A chain provides the potential by which injury to
the vital apparatus of the cell may be effected, there is a
failure of accumulation within the required cytological compartment. It is encouraging nonetheless to find that Krolick et
al.[39] using an anti-idiotypic antibody conjugated to ricin A
chain could demonstrate selective toxicity against a murine

lymphoid tumour cell.   Similarly Gilliland et al.[40], with a
monoclonal antibody against colorectal carcinoma associated
antigen in conjugated form with either diphtheria toxin or ricin
A chains, could inhibit protein synthesis in, and growth of, two
different colorectal carcinoma cell lines and not of human
melanoma embryonal lung carcinoma cells or of normal lung
fibroblasts.

In two studies the production of extremely potent A-chain
conjugates have been reported.   In the first of these[41] immunopurified rabbit antibodies to dinitrophenyl-bovine gamma globulin
were linked to ricin A chain using a disulphide bridge and the
resulting conjugate found to be as active as native ricin when
used against DNP-coated cells in tissue culture.

Later, Thorpe et al.[42] coupled monoclonal anti-Thy 1.1 to
gelonin, a protein with A chain like properties first isolated by
Stirpe et al.[43], and produced a conjugate which inhibited T cells
from AKR mice with a potency equal to that of abrin.   This
conjugate was substantially without effect on B lymphocytes from
AKR mice or upon T lymphocytes from CBA mice which express the
Thy 1.2 allo antigen.

Current status and future prospects

The examples already cited illustrate the present state of
the art.   Of Albert's three principles, exclusivity of reaction
seems adequately to be satisfied.   The third, accumulation, has
been discussed earlier in terms of uptake of antibody by target
tissue in the living animal, where it was concluded that recent
work allows an optimistic view to be taken that this will not be
a major obstacle to future development.

There is a second aspect of accumulation that has been
touched on more briefly, this concerns the penetration of A chain
to the cytosol compartment where protein synthesis is taking
place.   This is as yet the unsolved problem; how to ensure
efficient translocation of A chain from the external to the
internal milieu (i.e. the cytosol) of the cell.

The means by which this is accomplished in the case of the
native toxins is still not clear.   There are basically two
theories, (1) the B chain contains regions or domains of high
lipophilicity which interact with the lipid bilayer of the plasma
membrane to form a pore through which the A chain can pass or is
passed into the cytosol, (2) the cell itself mediates in the
transport process perhaps by mistaken identification of the toxin
as a molecule required for cellular function.   One possibility is
that the glycoprotein toxins, abrin and ricin, penetrate cell
membranes by using a glycosyl activated translocation system,

perhaps similar to that described for the uptake in adsorptive pinocytosis[44]. The possible importance of carbohydrate molecules on ricin as a signal for the translocation mechanism was indicated in a recent study in which it has been shown that when ricin is demannosylated it is still capable of binding to the cell surface through its galactose acceptor site and its A chain still functions against isolated ribosomes but the toxin fails to kill cells[45]. As long as this aspect of the problem remains unsolved there is likely to be a restriction on the utility of A chain conjugates.

There are many circumstances in which the use of antibody-toxin conjugates could be advantageous. Cells of the lymphoid series exist in subsets defined both functionally and by the expression of surface antigens. These and the general existence of T cell specificity make possible not only prevention of delayed type hypersensitivity reactions and the abolition of antibody formation but also provide the means by which specific intervention might be achieved through destruction of helper or suppressor function, while the use of idiotypic specificity gives promise of induction of specific tolerance or elimination of clones responsible for autoimmune disease. The removal of unwanted cells from bone marrow grafts is seen as a likely early use for conjugates, since the conjugate is required only to recognise and kill the undesirable cells without cross-reacting with the haematopoietic stem cells. The ablation of T cells responsible for the development of graft-versus-host disease or of leukaemic cells and those of the neoplastic diseases such as neuroblastoma are seen as potential candidates with immediate possibilities of application.

The tissue localisation studies discussed earlier give rise to some optimism that antibodies displaying this ability may be used as carriers of toxins in attempts to treat tumours and in particular metastatic deposits. This view is reinforced by the recent development of a number of monoclonal antibodies reacting with tumour cells of human origin. Other possibilities for attack are inherent in the expression of idiotypic specificities by malignant lymphoid tissue and in the presence of normal differentiation antigens by tumour cells arising in expendable organs such as breast, ovary, prostate or testis.

Other potential targets for this modality of treatment and which have proved difficult to treat by conventional chemotherapy include protozoal and other parasitic infections. The stable expression of recognisable antigens by Trypanosoma cruzii make it a prime candidate along with the malaria parasite. In such circumstances the same rules already discussed will have to apply, i.e. localisation followed by internalisation and damage to a vital part of the parasites biochemical machinery.

Finally a non-destructive application that may be forseen is in the field of enzyme replacement therapy where delivery of a missing enzyme to a particular cell population followed by controlled uptake into an appropriate cell compartment would be required.

D.C.E. is an external staff member of the Wellcome Foundation Ltd.

REFERENCES
1. A. Albert, "Selective Toxicity," Chapman and Hall, London (1979).
2. G. Köhler, and C. Milstein, Derivation of specific antibody-producing tissue culture and tumour lines by cell fusion, Eur.J.Immunol. 6:511 (1976).
3. T-M. Chang, A. Dazord, and D.M. Neville, Jr., Artificial hybrid protein containing a toxic protein fragment and a cell membrane receptor-binding moiety in a disulphide conjugate, J.Biol.Chem. 252:1515 (1977).
4. T.N. Oeltmann, and C. Heath, A hybrid protein containing the toxic subunit of ricin and the cell specific subunit of human chorionic gonadotropin, J.Biol.Chem. 254:1028 (1979).
5. R.J. Youle, G.J. Murray, and D.M. Neville, Jr., Ricin linked to monophosphopentamannose binds to fibroblast lysosomal hydrolase receptors, resulting in a cell-type-specific toxin, Proc.Natl.Acad.Sci.USA 76:5559 (1979).
6. D.B. Cawley, H.R. Herschman, D.G. Gilliland, and R.J. Collier, Epidermal growth factor - toxin A chain conjugates, Cell 22:563 (1980).
7. W.K. Miskimins, and N. Shimizer, Synthesis of a cytotoxic insulin cross-linked to diphtheria toxin fragment A capable of recognizing insulin receptors, Biochem.Biophys. Res.Commun. 91:143 (1978).
8. H.B. Hewitt, E.R. Blake,and A.S.Wadler, A critique of the evidence for active host defence against cancer, Br.J. Cancer 33:241 (1976).
9. J.H. Coggin, Jr., and N.G. Anderson, Cancer, differentiation and embryonic antigens: some central problems, Adv.Cancer Res. 19:105 (1974).
10. L. Korngold, and D. Pressman, The localization of anti-lymphosarcoma antibodies in the Murphy lymphosarcoma of the rat, Cancer Res. 14:96 (1954).
11. E.D. Day, J.A. Planinsek, and D. Pressman, Localization in vivo of radioiodinated anti-rat-fibrin antibodies and radioiodinated rat fibrinogen in the Murphy rat lympho-sarcoma and in other transplantable rat tumours, J.Natl. Cancer Inst. 22:413 (1959).

12. E.D. Day, J.A. Planinsek, and D. Pressman, Localization of radioiodinated antibodies in rats bearing tumours induced by N-2-fluorenyl-acetamide, J.Natl.Cancer Inst. 25:787 (1960).
13. A.E. Rief, Studies on the localization of radiolabelled antibodies to a mouse myeloma protein, Cancer 27:1433 (1971).
14. D. Pressman, E.D. Day, and M.Blau, The use of paired labeling in the determination of tumor-localizing antibodies, Cancer Res. 17:845 (1957).
15. D. Pressman, and B.Sherman, The zone of localization of antibodies. XII Immunological specificities and cross reactions in the vascular beds of liver, kidney and lung. J.Immunol. 67:21 (1951).
16. F.J. Primus, R. MacDonald, D.M. Goldenberg, and H.J. Hansen, Localisation of GW-39 human tumours in hamsters by affinity-purified antibody·to carcinoembryonic antigen, Cancer Res. 37:1544 (1977).
17. J-P. Mach, S. Carrel, M. Forni, J. Ritschard, A. Donath, and P. Alberto, Tumor localization of radiolabelled antibodies against carcinoembryonic antigen in patients with carcinoma, New Eng.J.Med. 303:5 (1980).
18. V. Moshakis, M.J. Bailey, M.G. Ormerod, J.H. Westwood, and A.M. Neville, Localization of human breast-carcinoma xenografts using antibodies to carcinoembryonic antigen, Br.J.Cancer 43:575 (1981).
19. L.L. Houston, R.C. Nowinski, and D. Bernstein, Specific in vivo localization of monoclonal antibodies directed against the thy 1.1 antigen, J.Immunol. 125:837 (1980).
20. T. Ghose, and A.H. Blair, Antibody-linked cytotoxic agents in the treatment of cancer: current status and future progress, J.Natl.Cancer Inst. 61:657 (1978).
21. G.J. O'Neill, The use of antibodies as drug carriers, in: "Drug Carriers in Biology and Medicine," G. Gregoriadis, ed., Academic Press, London (1979).
22. R.J. Collier, Diphtheria toxin: mode of action and structure, Bact.Rev. 39:54 (1975).
23. S. Olsnes, and A. Pihl, Abrin, ricin and their associated agglutinins, in: "The Specificity and Action of Animal, Bacterial and Plant Toxins," P. Cuatrecasus, ed., Chapman and Hall, London (1977).
24. P.E. Thorpe, W.C.J. Ross, A.J. Cumber, C.A. Hinson, D.C. Edwards, and A.J.S. Davies, Toxicity of diphtheria toxin for lymphoblastoid cells is increased by conjugation to antilymphocytic globulin, Nature 272:752 (1978).
25. D.C. Edwards, A. Smith, W.C.J. Ross, A.J. Cumber, P.E. Thorpe, A.N.F. Brown and A.J.S. Davies, In vitro and in vivo effects of anti-mouse lymphocyte globulin abrin and their conjugates, Clin.exp.Immunol. submitted for publication.

26. J. Carlsson, H. Drevin, and R. Axén, Protein thiolation and
     reversible protein-protein conjugation, Biochem.J.
     173:723 (1978).
27. S. Olsnes, and A. Pihl, Chimaeric toxin, in: "Pharmacology
     of Bacterial Toxins," J. Drews and F. Dorner, eds.,
     Pergamon Press, London (1981).
28. F.L. Moolten, and S.R. Cooperband, Selective destruction of
     target cells by diphtheria toxin conjugated to antibody
     directed against antigens on the cells, Science 169:68
     (1970).
29. F.L. Moolten, N.J. Capparell, and S.R. Cooperband, Antitumor
     effects of antibody-diphtheria toxin conjugates: use of
     hapten-coated tumor cells as an antigenic target, J.Natl.
     Cancer Inst. 49: 1057 (1972).
30. F.L. Moolten, N.J. Capparell, S.H. Zajdel, and S.R.
     Cooperband, Antitumor effects of antibody-diphtheria toxin
     conjugates. II Immunotherapy with conjugates directed
     against tumor antigens induced by Simian virus 40, J.Natl.
     Cancer Inst. 55:473 (1975).
31. G.W. Philpott, R.J. Bower, and C.W. Parker, Improved
     selective cytotoxicity with an antibody-diphtheria toxin
     conjugate, Surgery 73:728 (1973).
32. W.C.J. Ross, P.E. Thorpe, A.J. Cumber, D.C. Edwards, C.A.
     Hinson, and A.J.S. Davies, Increased toxicity of
     diphtheria toxin for human lymphoblastoid cells following
     covalent linkage to anti-(human lymphocyte) globulin or
     its F(ab')$_2$ fragment, Eur.J.Biochem. 104:381 (1980).
33. A.M. Denman, and E.P. Frenkel, Mode of action of anti-
     lymphocyte globulin, Immunology 14:107 (1968).
34. D.C. Edwards, A. Smith, W.C.J. Ross, A.J. Cumber, P.E.
     Thorpe, and A.J.S. Davies, The effect of abrin, anti-
     lymphocytic globulin and their conjugates on the immune
     response of mice to sheep red blood cells, Experientia
     37:256 (1981).
35. K. Refsnes, and A.C. Munthe-Kass, Introduction of B-chain
     inactivated ricin into mouse macrophages and rat Kupffer
     cells via their membrane Fc receptors, J.Exp.Med. 143:1464
     (1976).
36. V. Raso, and T. Griffin, Delivery of ricin to immunoglobulin
     (Ig) bearing cells by hybrid antibodies, Proc.Amer.Assoc.
     Cancer Res. 20:207 (1979).
37. R.J. Youle, and D.M. Neville, Jr., Anti-thy 1.2 monoclonal
     antibody linked to ricin is a potent cell-type-specific
     toxin, Proc.Natl.Acad.Sci.USA 77:5483 (1980).
38. P.E. Thorpe, A.J. Cumber, N. Williams, D.C. Edwards, W.C.J.
     Ross, and A.J.S. Davies, Abrogation of the non-specific
     toxicity of abrin conjugated to anti-lymphocyte globulin,
     Clin.Exp.Immunol. 43:195 (1981).

39. K.A. Krolick, C. Villemey, P. Isakson, J.W. Uhr, and E.S. Vitetta, Selective killing of normal or neoplastic B cells by antibodies coupled to the A chain of ricin, Proc.Natl. Acad.Sci.USA 77:5419 (1980).

40. D.G. Gilliland, Z. Steplewski, R.J. Collier, K.F. Mitchell, T.H. Chang, and H.Koprowski, Antibody-directed cytotoxic agents: use of monoclonal antibody to direct the action of toxin A chains to colorectal carcinoma cells, Proc.Natl.Acad.Sci.USA 77:4539 (1980).

41. F.K. Jansen, H.E. Blythman, D. Carriere, P. Casellas, J. Diaz, P. Gros, J.R. Hennequin, E. Paolucci, B. Pau, P. Poncelet, G. Richer, S.L. Salhi, H. Vidal and G.A. Voisin, High specific cytotoxicity of antibody-toxin hybrid molecules (immunotoxins) for target cells, Immunol.Lett. 2:97 (1980).

42. P.E. Thorpe, A.N.F. Brown, W.C.J. Ross, A.J. Cumber, S.I. Detre, D.C. Edwards, A.J.S. Davies, and F. Stirpe, Cytotoxicity acquired by conjugation of an anti-thy 1.1 monoclonal antibody and the ribosome-inactivating protein, gelonin, Eur.J.Biochem. 116:447 (1981).

43. F. Stirpe, S. Olsnes, and A. Pihl, Gelonin, a new inhibitor of protein synthesis, non toxic to intact cells, J.Biol. Chem. 255:6947 (1980).

44. W.S. Sly, Saccharide traffic signals in receptor-mediated endocytosis and transport of acid hydrolases, in: "Structure and Function of the Gangliosides," L. Svennerholm, P. Mandel, H. Dreyfus, and P-F. Urban, eds., Plenum Publishing Corporation, New York (1980).

45. L.S. Simeral, W. Kapmeyer, W.P. MacConnell, and N.O. Kaplan, On the role of the covalent carbohydrate in the action of ricin, J.Biol.Chem. 255:11098 (1980).

SELECTIVITY IN CANCER CHEMOTHERAPY

T.A. Connors

MRC Toxicology Unit
Medical Research Council Laboratories
Woodmansterne Road, Carshalton, UK

Over the past thirty years a large number of chemicals of different structures have been found to inhibit the growth of animal tumours. A small number of these have subsequently been used with usually limited success in the treatment of a few types of human cancer. Anticancer agents have been discovered by 'screening' usually against transplanted rodent tumours, by a study of analogues of known active compounds or by the rational design of chemicals based on a knowledge of the biochemistry of a particular cancer.

A summary of the agents that have been used in the treatment of cancer and their mechanism of action is shown in Figure 1. The majority of the agents obviously have no particular specificity towards cancer cells and their detrimental effect on the growth of tumours is due to their action on cells in cycle. Most of the agents depicted in Figure 1 interfere more or less specifically with DNA, RNA or protein synthesis[1]. This causes an imbalanced growth of cycling cells and may result in cell death. A consequence of this mechanism of action is that normal host tissues which also proliferate rapidly (bone marrow, intestinal mucosa) are also sensitive to the cytotoxic effects of these normal tissues usually prevents the administration of a sufficient quantity of the drug to eradicate the tumour completely. The most common finding of chemotherapy is that tumours respond poorly or not at all to present day drugs. If they do show a significant regression, they often regrow once the drug has had to be discontinued because of excessive toxicity.

Since these drugs do have the ability to kill tumour cells they could be made considerably more effective if their selectivity was improved, that is, if some means were found by which the sensitive tissues of the host were protected from the action of the drug at

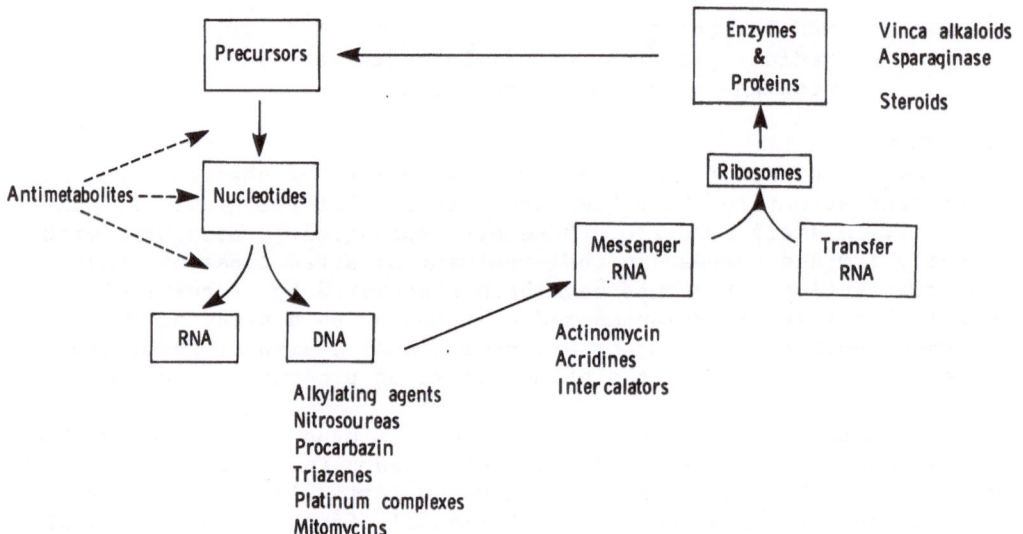

Figure 1.   Sites of Action of Anti Cancer Agents

the same time as the effect of the drug on the tumour was potentiated. While this could obviously be achieved by drug targeting implying the selective delivery of the drug to the tumour, there are other ways in which such an increase in selectivity can be achieved.

Improvements in chemotherapy have come from the discovery of new drugs, from better supportive care and from the rational use of this form of treatment integrated with surgery and radiotherapy. A major improvement has come from the use of drugs in combination. In the simplest case two drugs may have additive antitumour effects but major toxicity against different host tissues. By using a combination of the two drugs the total tumour cell kill may be increased at a tolerated level of toxicity.[2] Sometimes drug combinations are synergistic rather than just simply additive and their effects may be considerably enhanced by the concomitant use of agents to protect or rescue host tissues normally susceptible to the agents being used.

Using drugs based on a knowledge of cell kinetics has also greatly improved the results of chemotherapy. Some anticancer agents are cell cycle phase specific acting only at one stage of the cell cycle. It is clear that for such drugs there must be an optimum dose schedule which allows the minimum effective dose of the drug to be attained in the tumour environment for the period of time that it takes all the proliferating cells of the tumour to enter the sensitive phase of the cell cycle be it S, G_1, G_2, or M. For such drugs the method of administration can have a considerable effect on the antitumour effect observed. A simple example is shown in Table 1. Cytosine arabinoside is specific for cells in the S phase of the cell cycle and on injection is rapidly broken down to an inactive metabolite and excreted. Thus when given by a single injection every four days there is a considerable period of time between injections when it is not at a tumour effective concentration. During this period cells entering and passing through the S phase are unharmed. However, if the drug is given more frequently by several injections every four days, the tumour effective concentration is maintained for a much longer period of time and tumour cells are unable to escape the cytotoxic effects of the antimetabolite. In tests on tumour bearing animals the first dose schedule is ineffective and animals die at the same time as the controls and with the same number of tumour cells present. The second dose schedule, although more toxic, is curative. Since a smaller amount of drug has been used in the best schedule then the importance of dose scheduling is clear to see.[3]

These results must also be borne in mind when attempts are made to improve the selectivity of action of antitumour agents by targeting or by other means. Attaching cytosine arabinoside, for example, to a carrier will almost certainly alter its pharmacokinetic properties because it is no longer rapidly broken down. This in turn may result in a considerable improvement in its antitumour

Table 1

Effect of cytosine arabinoside on the L1210 leukaemia.[3]

Dose mg/kg	Time of injections	Total dose	No. of animals cured	Cancer cells at end of treatment
240	2,6,10,14	960	0/10	10^9
15	8 times daily or days 2,6, 10,14	480	10/10	None

properties even though selective concentration in the tumour or
targeting has not been achieved. Hence in measuring the effectiveness
of targeting one must compare the therapeutic index of the targeted
drug with the drug alone in both cases using optimum conditions for
administration of the drug. In the case of cytosine arabinoside the
optimum dose schedule would be continuous infusion for a defined
period of time while for targeted cytosine arabinoside the optimum
dose schedule might be daily injections. The therapeutic index is a
ratio of the dose which is toxic to the host and the dose which has
an antitumour effect. Conjugates of dextran with drugs have been
claimed to improve the therapeutic index of some anticancer agents.
Mytomycin C, for example, when covalently linked to a dextran of
70,000 molecular weight has a greater selectivity than the drug
alone. However this improvement may be due mainly to the improvement
of pharmacokinetic properties rather than an effect of drug targeting.[4]

Occasionally, for particular agents against particular tumours,
considerable selectivity of action may occur. This has been shown
to be due to concentration of the drug by active transport or by
some other property of the tumour, or by a specific activation in
the tumour of a prodrug. Proteins and other materials have also
been used with limited success as carriers of antitumour agents.

Some anticancer agents, such as the nitrogen mustards, melphalan
and HN2 may be taken up by some cells (including some tumour cells)
by proteins that are normally involved in the active transport of
other molecules. Thus melphalan is taken up against a concentration
gradient by active transport processes normally involved in amino
acid uptake and HN2 by a choline carrier.[5] Whether these carriers
might also take up selectively other toxic agents has not been
investigated in detail.

Selective concentration in tumour cells may also occur as a
result of some other specific property of the cell. It has been

reported for many years that tumours (both animal and human) tend to
be more acidic than normal cells. While newer techniques for measurement of intracellular pH have not confirmed this as a consistent
difference it is still possible that the overall 'tumour environment'
(tumour cells, stroma and extracellular fluid) is more acidic than
other tissues. Certainly sulphadiazine concentrates specifically
in many tumours, and it has been proposed that this is due to the
acidic environment of the tumour which leads to the precipitation
of sulphadiazine in its unionised and very insoluble form. Attempts
to exploit this effect by using sulphadiazene as a carrier for cytotoxic alkylating agents and N,N-dimethyl triazene groups were not
particularly successful.[6]

     Prodrugs are defined as chemicals which are not themselves
cytotoxic but which can be converted by enzymes or other means into
cytotoxic agents. Selectivity can be achieved by the use of prodrugs
if the activating enzyme is only present in the tumour cells. In one
recent study advantage is taken of the fact that malignant cells
(both animal and human) produce large amounts of plasminogen activator compared with normal tissues.[7] This results in a high level
of the protease plasmin being continually produced in the region of
the tumour by conversion of plasminogen. Any of the enzyme moving
away from the tumour is rapidly deactivated so that the net result
is a tumour environment particularly high in plasmin. Plasmin
hydrolyses poteins by 'recognising' certain amino acid sequences.
If one of these sequences or 'specifiers' is attached to a low molecular weight compound then it will be rapidly cleaved in the presence
of plasmin. Thus in the structure D-valine-leucine-lysine-aniline
the leucine-lysine sequence is recognised and aniline is cleaved
from the peptide. If aniline is replaced by a drug which is non-toxic
when linked to the peptide but highly toxic by itself then it should
be selective in tumours secreting large amounts of plasminogen activator. One suitable prodrug is shown in Figure 2 p-phenylene-diamine
mustard (Figure 2.II) is a very toxic alkylating agent, but derivatives made by substitution of the primary amine group have very much
less toxicity. If the substituting group is a specifier for plasmin
(Figure 2.I) then activation would take place specifically in the
tumour region. Preliminary results using cells in vitro have shown
that antitumour selectivity can be achieved by this method. This
idea could obviously be extended to the use of proteins as carriers
of cytotoxic agents. A protein might conceivably be used to carry
a large number of molecules of a cytotoxic agent. There would be
little toxicity if the protein did not enter cells. However, if the
cytotoxic molecules were linked to the protein through a plasmin
specifier sequence then the cytotoxic molecules would be released in
the region of the tumour. If the agent released was p-phenylenediamine mustard described above then considerable selectivity might
occur. It would be readily taken up by tumour cells and since it
is chemically very reactive much of the drug escaping from the
vascular bed of the tumour would hydrolyse to harmless products before

reaching sensitive tissues such as the bone marrow.

Other attempts at prodrug design include the use of the
O-glucuronide of aniline mustard (a metabolite of aniline mustard)
which is selctively converted in tumours high in β-glucuronidase to
the highly toxic p-hydroxyaniline mustard and azomustards which are
metabolised by azoreductase in liver tumours to cytotoxic amine
mustards.[8]

Another interesting recent example of prodrug design concerns
the enzyme γ-glutamyl transferase. This enzyme is sometimes an
early marker of developing malignant hepatocytes and is very high in
certain liver cancers. The enzyme removes γ-glutamyl moieties from
substrates coverting relatively non-toxic substrates such as
γ-glutamyl-p-phenylenediamine mustard into highly toxic products.
Preliminary in vitro studies have shown that γ-glutamyl-p-phenylene-
diamine mustard is a selective cytotoxic agent for hepatocytes high
in the transferase enzyme.[9]

In many tumours, especially rapidly growing ones, there is a
continuous stimulation of growth of new blood vessels at the periphery
and a breakdown of earlier formed ones towards the centre of the
tumour. As the tumour grows there can usually be observed a peripheral region containing viable cells, many of them in cycle, and a
central ischaemic region of necrotic tissue. Between these two
regions is a zone of cells which are viable but which are not well
vascularised and are relatively anoxic. It has been found that these
cells can reduce certain heterocyclic nitro derivatives to the
corresponding amino derivatives in the course of which cytotoxic
intermediates are generated. Some time after injection of labeled
drug, radioactivity is concentrated in the anoxic zone as a result
of specific activation of the drug in these areas, and covalent
binding of the reactive intermediates to macromolecules.[10]

· Some chemicals have an affinity for tumours for unknown reasons
and the suggestion has been made as with the case of sulphadiazene,
mentioned earlier, that these could be used as carriers of cytotoxic
agents. Some suggested tumour localisers are listed in Table 2.
Certain porphyrins for example selectively concentrate in tumours
and besides their use as carrier molecules they have been studied
experimentally as agents for phototherapy of suitable tumours of
skin and bladder.[11] The use of mitomycin C linked to dextrans has
already been discussed and while its therapeutic index can be
improved it has not yet been proven that dextrans do act as carrier
molecules concentrating agents specifically in tumours. A result
of particular interest has been obtained by conjugating methotrexate
to poly(L-lysine). In in vitro experiments an increased transport
of the antimetabolite in active form was obtained and it proved
possible to overcome the resistance to methotrexate of transport
resistant mammalian cells.[12]

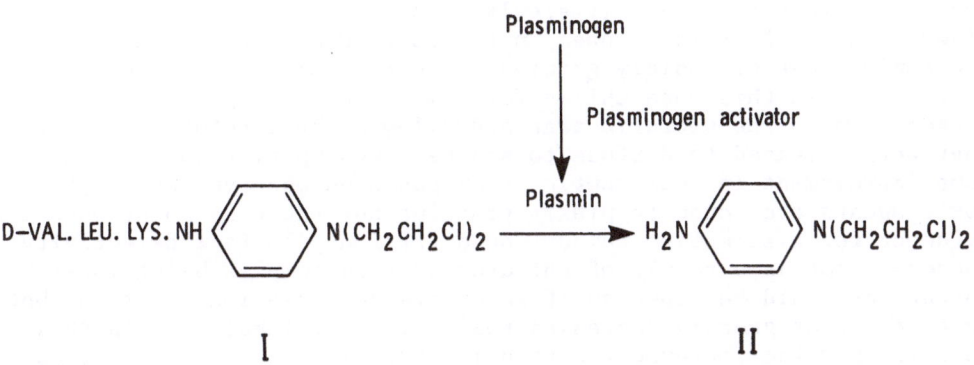

Figure 2. Activation by Plasmin

Table 2

Tumour Localisers

Porphyrins	γ-globulin
Sulphadiazene	Dextrans
Fibrinogen	Polylysine
Albumin	Con-A

The use of proteins to carry drugs selectively to tumours is not a new idea and has been based on observations that a number of proteins - particularly plasma proteins - appear to accumulate in solid tumours.[13] It is not clear whether there is in fact an artefact, the protein being only slowly cleared from the body as a result of which some of it is trapped in the increasing necrotic and ischaemic areas of rapidly growing tumours. Selectivity would not be achieved in this case unless for some reason the protein was broken down in the necrotic area and allowed the cytotoxic molecules that were released to diffuse to and be taken up by viable cells. Some improvement in therapeutic index has been observed when cytotoxic agents are bound to plasma proteins but there is no strong evidence for a selective tumour concentration. In fact selectivity increases not as a result of the drug-protein complex being more potent, as would be expected if selective accumulation occurred, but as a result of greatly decreased toxicity. The likelihood in this case is that the improved therapeutic index is due to a protection of host tissues for example, by the inability of the protein-drug complex to be taken up by bone marrow.

Attempts to direct drugs to tumours by attachment to monoclonal antibodies raised against a specific tumour receptor is a very much more logical approach[14] and would seem to be a rational method for the design of new anticancer agents. Many cell types contain specific receptors and unusual proteins are often expressed by certain tumours. Some of these are listed in Table 3 and could be a starting point for the manufacture of monoclonal antibodies. Some early experiments using monoclonal antibodies for cell targeting have shown that while binding is very specific it is at only a low concentration, because of the small numbers of receptors available for binding. This has meant that it might not be possible to achieve a lethal concentration of the carried cytotoxic drug at the cell surface. One suggestion has been to use a panel of monoclonal antibodies but some receptors would seem to be more suitable targets than others. γ-glutamyl transferase, for example, which has already been discussed is present in some malignant hepatocytes at extremely high concentration. Since the enzyme is in the cell membrane and facing outwards it would

Table 3

Specific   Receptors

Galacto-glycoproteins	Hepatocytes
Phosphomannose residues	Fibroblasts
N-Ac glucosamine/mannose	Kuppfer cells, macrophages
Polyaspartamate polymers	Kidney cells
Polypeptide receptors	Malignant cells
Pi 4.0 glycoprotein	Malignant cells
γ-glutamyl transferase	Malignant hepatocytes

appear to be a particularly suitable target for antibody-toxin
conjugates.

A related approach has been to utilise agents which localise in
particular tissues as carriers for drugs used in the treatment of
cancers arising from that tissue. This approach makes the doubtful
assumption that the malignant cells of a particular tissue possess
the same ability as the normal cells of that tissue to concentrate
the agent, presumably even when they have metastasised to a distant
site. Some agents which concentrate in particular organs or certain
cells of those organs are shown in Table 4. 4-ipoemanol is a particularly interesting example.[15] It is a naturally occurring furan
derivative causing characteristic lung lesions as a result of a
highly specific toxic action on one cell type, the non ciliated
bronchiolar or Clara cell. This cell can convert ipoemanol into a
toxic metabolite at a much greater rate than any other cell including
hepatocytes, which are usually by far the most efficient at carrying
out microsomally mediated reactions. Further studies on this chemical
would clearly add to the knowledge of the function of this cell type
and may be of importance in the design of drugs for the treatment of
cancers arising from Clara cells.

Following the report that high levels of dl-propanolol concentrate in the lung, the d-propanolol isomer which has no β-blocking
activity was suggested as a carrier of agents specific for the
treatment of lung cancer. Two propanolol nitrogen mustards have
been synthesised but have not been shown to have any particular
affinity for lung cancer in animal models.[16]

Table 4

Tissue Localisers

D-propanolol	Lung
Vitamin E	Lymphatic
Methoxsalen	Skin
Ipoemanol	Clara cell
Hydantoins	CNS

Besides the use of biopolymers such as protein and DNA as carrier molecules for drug targeting the possible value of a range of synthetic homo and co-polymers has been studied. Such models can be designed as a polymer backbone to which are attached by appropriately labile spacer groups not only cytotoxic agents but also solubilising and transport groups.[17] Although synthetic polymers are sometimes thought of as potentially toxic materials which are difficult to remove from the body there is no doubt that the technology is already advanced enough to overcome this problem and polymers can be designed which are susceptible to enzymatic hydrolysis and excretion.[18]

Thus, while very few highly selective agents are available for the treatment of cancers, as knowledge of the biochemistry of cancers increases - particularly using human tumour xenografts in rodents which may be more relevant 'biochemical' models of human cancer - so it will be possible to rationally design chemicals which are superior to the presently available drugs. Drug targeting will obviously play a major role in this approach in the future.

REFERENCES

1. T.A. Connors, Drugs used in the treatment of cancer, Febs Lett. 57: 223 (1975).
2. R.H. Blum and E. Frei, III. Comination chemotherapy, Methods in Cancer Research, XVII: 215 (1979).
3. H.E. Skipper, F.M. Schabel and W.S. Wilcox, Experimental evaluation of anticancer agents, Cancer Chemother. Rep. 51: 125 (1967).
4. T. Johima, M. Hashida, S. Muranishi and H. Sezaki, Mitomycin C-dextran conjugate: a novel high molecular weight prodrug of mitomycin C, J. Pharm. Pharmacol. 32: 30 (1980).
5. F.M. Sirotnak, P.L. Chellow and R.W. Brockman, Potential for exploitation of transport systems in anticancer drug design,

Methods in Cancer Research, XV1: 381 (1979).

6. G. Abel, T.A. Connors, W.C.J. Ross, Nguyen-Hoang-Nam, H. Hoellinger and L. Pichat, The selective concentration of sulphadiazine and related compounds in malignant tissue, Europ. J. Cancer 9: 49 (1973).

7. P.L. Carl, P.K. Chakravarty, J.A. Katzenellenbogen and M.J. Weber, Protease activated prodrugs for cancer chemotherapy, Proc. Nat. Acad. Sci. USA., 77: 2224 (1980).

8. T.A. Connors, Alkylating agents, Topics in Current Chemistry 52: 141 (1974).

9. M.M. Manson, R.F. Legg, J.V. Watson, J.A. Green and G.E. Neal, An examination of the relative resistances to aflatoxin B and susceptibilities to γ-glutamyl-p-phenylene diamine mustard of γ-glutamyl transferase negative and positive cell lines, Carcinogenesis 2: 661 (1981).

10. J.D. Chapman, A.J. Franko and J. Sharpun, A marker for hypoxic cells in tumours with potential clinical applicability, Br. J. Cancer 43: 546 (1981).

11. M. Tsutsui, C. Carrano and E.A. Tsutsui, Tumor localizers, porphyrins and related compounds (unusual metalloporphyrins XXIII), Ann. N.Y. Acad. Sci. 244: 674 (1975).

12. H.J.P. Ryser and W. Shen, Conjugation of methotrexate to poly (L-lysine) increases drug transport and overcomes drug resistance in cultured cells, Proc. Nat. Acad. Sci. USA., 75: 3867.

13. M. Szekerke, R. Wade and M.E. Whisson, The use of macromolecules as carriers of cytotoxic groups (Part 1), Conjugates of nitrogen mustard with proteins, polypeptidyl proteins and polypeptides, Neoplasma 19: 199 (1972).

14. D.G. Gilliland, Z. Steplewski, R.J. Collier, K.F. Mitchell, T.H. Chang and H. Koprowski, Antibody directed cytotoxic agents. Use of monoclonal antibodies to direct the action of toxin A chains to colorectal carcinoma cells, Proc. Nat. Acad. Sci. USA., 77: 4539 (1980).

15. M.R. Boyd, Evidence for the Clara cell as a site of cytochrome P450 dependent mixed function oxidase activity in lung, Nature (London) 269: 713 (1977).

16. L.V. Feyns, J.A. Beisler, J.S. Driscoll and R.A. Adamson, Synthesis of propranolol mustard as a possible lung specific agent, J. Pharm. Sci. 69: 190 (1980).

17. D.S. Zaharko, M. Przybylski and V.T. Oliverio, Binding of anti-cancer drugs to carrier molecules, Methods in Cancer Research XVI: 347 (1979).

18. N.B. Graham, Polymeric inserts and implants for the controlled release of drugs, British Polymer Journal, 10: 260 (1978).

DRUG CONJUGATES OF POLYMERIC MICROSPHERES AS TOOLS IN

CELL BIOLOGY

I. Pecht, N. Mazurek, A. Petrank and S. Margel

Departments of Chemical Immunology and Plastic Research
The Weizmann Institute of Science
Rehovot 76100, Israel

Visualisation and identification of specific sites on cell
surfaces is of great importance for understanding various biological
phenomena, such as cell—cell recognition in development, cell communication and differences between normal and tumor cell surfaces.
Mapping of antigens and carbohydrate residues on the surface of
cells has been studied intensively by various techniques, for
example, using fluorescent, or radioactive antibodies or lectins[1-3]
or by binding biological macromolecules as markers, e.g. ferritin[4],
hemocyanin[5], viruses[6] and peroxidase[7] to antibodies or lectins.
The latter macromolecules were used as markers for transmission
electron microscopy or for scanning electron microscopy (SEM).
Synthetic markers would naturally have several important advantages
over the available biological reagents. Prominent amongst these
advantages are control over a wide range of sizes of the microspheres,
the modification of their chemical and mechanical properties and the
possibility of introducing fluorescent or magnetic compounds into
them. The latter compounds serve an essential role in the visualisation of the beads bound to the cells by their fluorescence in
the microscope or their opacity in the electron microscope. Furthermore they allow for sorting and separation of components in cell
populations. Synthetic polymer microspheres were also used as
markers for cell labelling. Thus conjugates of polystyrene latex
particles have been utilised as immunological markers in the SEM
techniques[8]. However, the applications of polystyrene microspheres are limited by the hydrophobic properties of these particles
which cause them to adhere non-specifically to the surface of many
cells. Several types of hydrophilic polymeric microspheres based
on acrylic monomers were also synthesized and used for labelling of
cell surface receptors[9]. These microspheres carried a variety of
functional groups, such as carboxylates, hydroxyl, amide and/or

pyridine groups on their surfaces. These functional groups were
used for covalently binding proteins to the microspheres by means
of a series of reactions[10]. The last step of the microsphere derivatization technique, prior to antibody binding, consisted of a
reaction with glutaraldehyde designed to introduce reactive aldehyde groups on the beads surface.

In order to simplify the derivatization procedure, polyglutaraldehyde (PGL) microspheres were synthesized. These new microspheres also carry reactive aldehyde groups on their surface through
which covalent binding of a variety of ligands like peptides,
proteins or drugs, under physiological pH, can be achieved. The
binding to the microspheres is based on the reaction between the
aldehyde groups and primary amino groups on the ligands to yield
Schiff base product:

$$R_1 - \overset{C}{\underset{H}{C}} + R_2NH_C \rightleftharpoons R_1CH \quad NHR_2 + H_2O$$

Reduction of the Schiff base will then add to the stability of the
conjugates. PGL microspheres were prepared[11-13] by polymerizing
glutaraldehyde under alkaline conditions in presence of an appropriate surfactant. Under these conditions glutaraldehyde was poly-
merized through the aldol condensation mechanism and resulted in
the formation of a polymer containing aldehyde, hydroxyl and
carboxylate groups.

The presence of primary hydroxyl and carboxylate groups is due
to the Cannizzaro reaction which occurs between two aldehyde groups
under aqueous basic conditions. PGL microspheres meet the essential
requirements necessary for specific labelling of cell surface membrane sites: hydrophylicity and presence of negatively charged
carboxylate groups which prevent microspheres from aggregation and
thereby reduce nonspecific interactions between cells and microspheres. Homodisperse, fluorescent PGL microspheres were synthesized in sizes ranging from 0.1 micron to about 1.0 micron. Fluorescent PGL microspheres were prepared by carrying out the glutaraldehyde polymerization in presence of the appropriate fluorescent
labelling compounds, e.g., fluorescein isothiocyanate, propidium
iodide, 9-amino acrydine or tetramethyl rhodamine isothiocyanate.
Since a large number of fluorescent molecules can be covalently
entrapped in these microspheres, the fluorescence intensity of
cells labelled by these fluorescent microspheres can be enhanced.

Different subpopulations of cells were resolved according to
their different surface antigens by labelling the cells with immunomicrospheres, i.e., microspheres to which a specific antibody
lectin antigen is covalently bound. Figure 1 illustrates the
procedure employed in direct and indirect labelling. In the direct

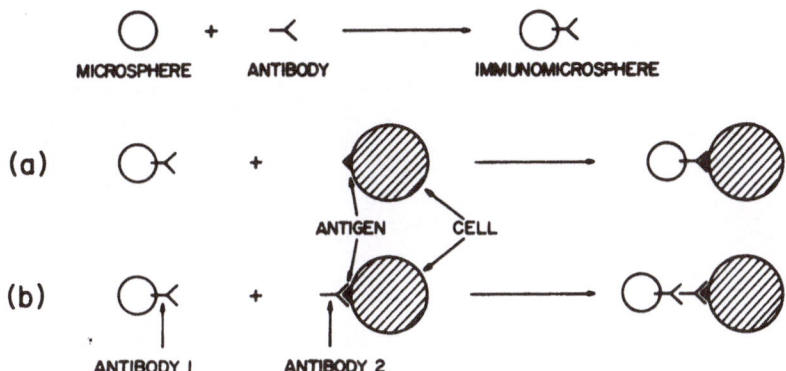

Fig. 1.   Schematic representation of direct(a) and indirect(b)
          labelling of cells by means of immunomicrospheres.

procedure an immunomicrosphere selects out its target site and
binds to it (Fig. 1a) and in the indirect method (Fig. 1b) an
intermediate antibody is employed.

    The labelling of cell surface receptors by means of fluorescent
or non-fluorescent PGL microspheres was found to be simple and
efficient as evidenced by numerous tests using human red blood cells
(RBC). The specificity of the labelling was ascertained by using
mixtures of RBC sensitized with rabbit anti-human RBC and unsensitized cells. The sensitized cells were labelled with fluorescent PGL
microspheres-goat anti-rabbit conjugate[12]. The labelled cells were
followed by fluorescence microscopy or by SEM. Fig. 3 shows SEM
photomicrographs of human RBC labelled with non-fluorescent PGL
microspheres. The control experiments (Fig 3a vs. 3c) show that
practically no labelling of unsensitized RBC by microsphere antibody conjugates takes place. Polyglutaraldehyde microspheres in
size of 0.7 micron bound to human immunoglobulin were also used
successfully for labelling Fc receptors on human lymphocytes. The
results are shown in Table 1.

    In our efforts to improve the non-specific interaction between
cell surfaces and microspheres a novel method for preparation of a
new polyaldehyde microspheres "polyacrolein" was developed recently
[14]. These microspheres can be formed in sizes ranging from 0.06
micron to 40 micron. They are hydrophylic and negatively charged.
Most clearly, high specficity was observed when using these microspheres for labelling of human red blood cells (Fig. 3), or for
specific labelling of human red blood cells in a mixture of human

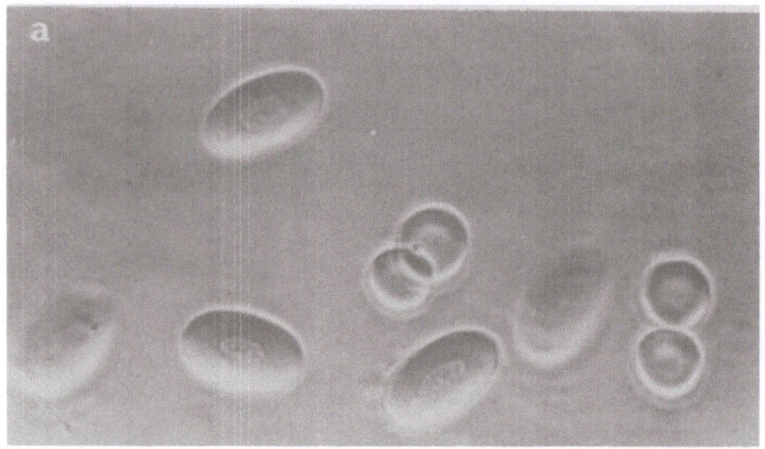

Fig. 2.   Fluorescence and phase micrographs of labelled human red
          blood cells in a mixture containing human and turkey red
          blood cells. a) Phase mode, b) Fluorescence mode.

and turkey red blood cells. Further research related to the
potential use of polyacrolein microspheres as a specific marker
for mapping of cell surface receptors is under investigation.
The non-specifically labelled cells in control experiments had a
maximum of only 4 beads on the cell surface. The appearance of
specifically labelled cells is shown in Fig. 2.

A very informative application of the microsphere beads has
been to the investigation of the action mechanism of certain membrane receptors of mast cells and basophils. Thus the anti-allergic
drug disodium cromoglycate (disodium salt of 1,3-bis-(2-carboxy

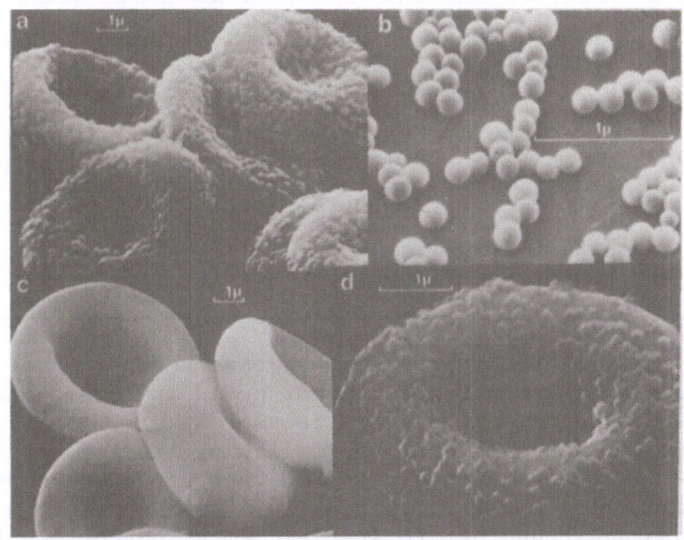

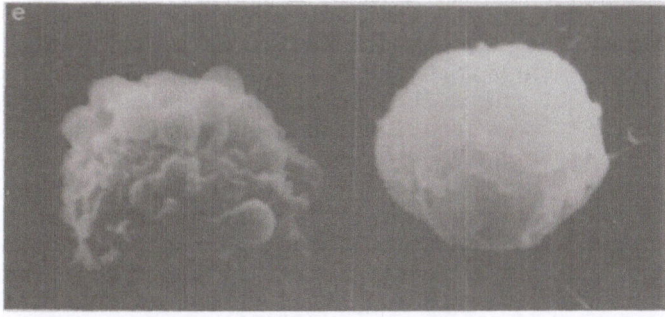

Fig. 3. SEM photographs of human red blood cells treated with PGL
microspheres carrying specific and human RBC on their surface. a) and d) cells labelled and magnified 10000 and
20000 fold, respectively. b) the PGL microspheres.
c) non labelled control RBC. e) SEM of human lymphocytes
labelled with PGL microspheres carrying human IgG on their
surface. f) SEM of unlabelled control.

Table 1

Experiment	Type of microspheres	Antibody (mg)	% Labelled cells
1	IgG Conjugate	0.19	8.8
	Unreacted microspheres (control)	–	0
2	IgG conjugate	0.29	20.7
	Unreacted microspheres (control)	–	6.7
3	IgG conjugate	0.45	17.9
	Unreacted microspheres (control)	–	4.6
4	IgG conjugate	1.9	17.2
	Unreacted microspheres (control)	–	2.9

chromon-5-yloxy)-2-hydroxypropane) has been shown to have specific binding sites on the membranes of mast cells and basophils through which its pharmacological activity is expressed[15]. These conclusions have been reached through the following line of work: several agents can induce the degranulation and secretion of anaphylactic mediators from mast cells and basophils: immune reaction between the cell membrane bound IgE to specific allergens or the binding of neurotransmitter peptides like substance P or neurotensin as well as compounds of unknown action mechanism like compound 48/80 and dextran. The next defined event ensuing after the interaction of one of the above agents with the cells, is a marked increase in the Ca^{2+} permeability of the membranes of these cells. This increase in intracellular Ca^{2+} concentration has been proposed to lead to the degranulation and secretion steps[16-18].

DSCG has been found to act by inhibiting the degranulation and secretion process of the mast cells and basophils and therefore found wide application in the treatment of allergic bronchial asthma [19,20]. Accumulated evidence suggested that this inhibition takes place by blocking the calcium influx[15,21]. The chemical nature of the drug led us to examine its potential Ca^{2+} chelation properties. Indeed such a drug - Ca^{2+} complex is formed with a fair affinity and specificity[22]. This finding led us to formulate a working hypothesis according to which the drug acts by forming a ternary complex-drug-Ca^{2+}-receptor. We have further postulated that this receptor is related to the membrane Ca^{2+} gates, probably constituting part of it[15]. The formation of such a ternary complex which involves specific interactions between the membrane's drug receptor and both Ca^{2+} ions and the drug perturbs the Ca^{2+} influx and hence the degranulation-secretion events are inhibited. To examine this hypothesis we first have looked for the site of binding and action of

Table 2. Examination of the specificity of binding of DSCG to basophils and to mast cells as monitored by the fluorescence activated cell sorter (FACS).

Cell Types	Type of microspheres	Staining Procedure	Percent cells stained
RBL-2H3	−	None	7
"	Non-conjugated micro-spheres	Regular	20
"	DBC	"	97
"	"	Preincubation with DSCG	32
"	"	Ca^{2+} free medium	40
RPMC	−	Regular	5
"	Non-conjugated micro-spheres	"	8
"	DBC	Competition by:	71
"	DBC	1) Preincubation with DSCG $(5-10^{-3}M)$	33
"	DBC	2) Co-inhibition with DSCG $(10^{-2}M)$	19
"	DBC	Ca^{2+} free medium	6
"	DBC	Preincubation with trypsin	30
"	Microspheres conjugated to glutamate	Regular	20
Lympho-cytes	−	"	14
"	Free beads	"	18
"	DBC	"	14
P-815	−	"	4
"	Free beads	"	4
"	DBC	"	4

The procedure of sample preparation for the FACS analysis involved incubation of 10^6 cells, with the appropriate staining agents in Tyrode solution for 30 min at room temperature and mild mixing. Regularly $10^7 - 10^8$ microspheres/ml were added to the mixture

cont. next page.*

Table 3.The inhibition effect of DSCG conjugated to PGL micro-
         spheres on the histamine secretion from antigen challenged
         rat   peritoneal mast cells.

DSCG	Non conjugated microspheres	DBC	% release
–	–	–	3 *
–	–	–	35
200 μM	–	–	6
–	$10^7 - 10^8$ B/ml	–	34
–	–	$10^7 - 10^8$ B/ml **	8

Inhibition of histamine release after pre-incubation of sensitized
mast cells with DSCG, or DBC, before antigen challenge. Results
are the mean of 2 experiments in which each is a duplicate.
*   Spontaneous release
** Drug/DBC, $10^6 - 10^{10}$ molecules/bead.

the drug. This has been done by covalently conjugating DSCG to
fluorescent microsphere beads (made of polyacrylamide or polyglutaraldehyde, 0.7 or 0.2 μm in diamter respectively and containing
either fluorescein or rhodamine as fluorophores). The conjugation
was made so as not to impair the activity of the drug and the beads
served both to visualize the loci of the drug binding as well as
preventing it from penetration through the membrane[15].

A specific, Ca^{2+} dependent binding of the DSCG-beads conjugates
(DBC) to rat peritoneal mast cell (RPMC) and basophil (RBL-2H3)
membrane was found[15]. This was monitored by fluorescence microscopy
and also analysed quantitatively by the automated fluorescence cell
sorter (FACS II). An example of the visualization and localization
of DSCG binding sites on basophils using the image itensified
fluorescence microscopy is shown in Fig 4, while the representative
fluorescence histograms obtained by the FACS analysis of cells
stained with DBC are shown in Fig. 5. When rat basophilic leukemia
cells (2H3) are incubated with DBC, areas of bright fluorescence
spread all over the cell surface are clearly observed (Fig. 4), and
97% of the cells are stained (Fig. 5, Table 2). Specificity of
DBC binding to the cells has been critically examined from two points
of view (Table 2): That of the binding and its Ca^{2+} dependence and

---

*DBC = Drug conjugated beads. RBL= Rat basophilic leukemia cells.
Trypsinization of the cells was carried out with a 0.25% trypsin
solution for 30 min at 37ºC. Controls for target cells were BW-
5147AKR/J thymoma cells and P-815 BALB/c mastocytoma. Competition
with free DSCG was carried out by preincubation at room temperature.

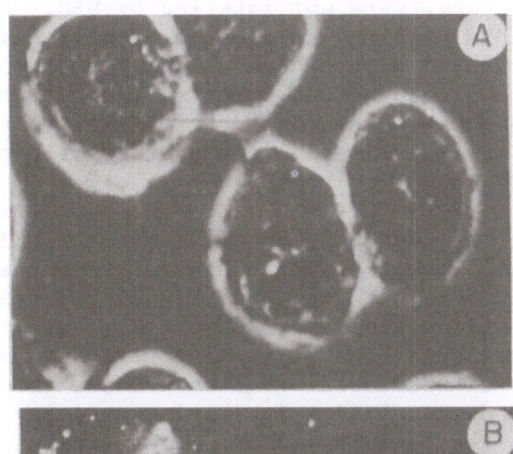

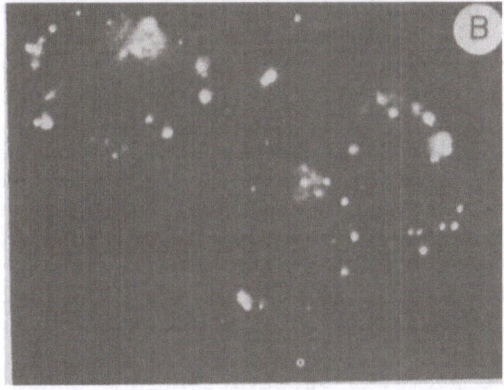

Fig. 4. Fluorescence and phase micrographs of basophils labelled
         by fluorescein containing PGL microspheres. The pictures
         were taken from a TV screen onto which an intensified
         image of the cells is projected. Rat basophilic leukemia
         cells (RBL-2H3) were incubated with the DSCG conjugated
         microspheres in Tyrode solution (137 mM NaCl, 2.7 mM KCl,
         0.4 mM NaH_2PO_4, 10 mM HEPES, 5 mM glucose, 1.8 mM $CaCl_2$,
         1.0 mM $MgCl_2$ and 2% BSA) at 25°C for 30 min. a) phase
         mode b) fluorescence mode.

that towards the target cells. One group of controls was concerned
with excluding non-specific binding of the beads (with or without
the drug). Free DSCG was found to competitively inhibit the binding
of the bead-conjugated drug (Fig 5, Table 2). Non specific staining
due to the extra electrostatic charges of the drug's carboxylates was
also tested using beads to which glutamate has been covalently conjugated. Trypsinization of mast cells (resulting in removal of
membrane proteins) reduced significantly the binding of the conjugated beads. Another group of controls was concerned with the
target cells binding specificity of DBC: BW5147 AKR/J thymoma
cells and P-815 BALB/c mastocytoma cell line, which are known to be

histamine non-secretory, were not labelled by DBC. Finally, the Ca^{2+} dependence of the DBC binding was clearly established when RPMC or RBL cells were incubated with DBC in a Ca^{2+} free medium and a drastic reduction of staining was observed (Fig. 5, Table 2). Also addition of a strong Ca^{2+} chelating agent (EDTA) to the staining mixture caused an effectively full attenuation of the labelling of the cells by the DBC.

All the above observations, notably the strict dependence on the presence of Ca^{2+} ions, led us to suggest that the cromoglycate-Ca^{2+} binary complex form a ternary complex with a specific site on the cell membrane of mast cells and basophils. The main question emerging was whether this binding is also relevant to the pharma-cological activity of DSCG. In order to provide an answer to this question, the degranulation inhibiting activity of the DBC has been examined. On the basis of molar concentration of DSCG, the activity of the drug conjugated to the beads was found to be main-tained and even somewhat amplified (Table 3). Hence the binding sites identified on these cells' membrane are also the sites of the drug's action. As pointed out before, these binding sites may be related to the Ca^{2+} gates or perhaps be part of these interesting membrane components. In extending this line of thought one should bear in mind that for the formulation of the specific ternary complex formed between DSCG, Ca^{2+} and the receptor, both the cromone nucleus of the drug as well as its Ca^{2+} chelating capacity are considered to be essential.

In view of the previous observations and conclusions, we have addressed ourselves to examining possible relationship between the DSCG binding sites on the mast cells and basophil membranes and the IgE binding sites. In this endeavour, the fluorescent beads have also been very useful reagents. One type of experiment in-volved examination of interrelation between the capping process of membrane bound IgE and the state of aggregation of the DSCG binding sites on the same cell membrane. The aggregation and capping of the IgE were induced by reacting anti-IgE antibodies with monoclonal, rhodamine labelled IgE residing in their specific Fc receptors on membranes of rat basophil leukemia cells (2H3). The drug-bead conjugates are polyvalent and will therefore undergo patching and capping at room temperature and at 37°C, respectively without requiring further crosslinking agent (Fig. 6).

The distributions of the differently labelled agents (IgE and DBC) have been examined at different stages of the distribution process on the cells membrane by fluorescence microscopy (on in-dividual cells) and by fluorescence activated cell sorting (on whole populations). An indicator for the state of aggregation of the cell membrane receptors is the fluorescence intensity signal as detected by the fluorescence activated cell sorter (FACS II). Thus, pronounced differences of fluorescence were found for patched

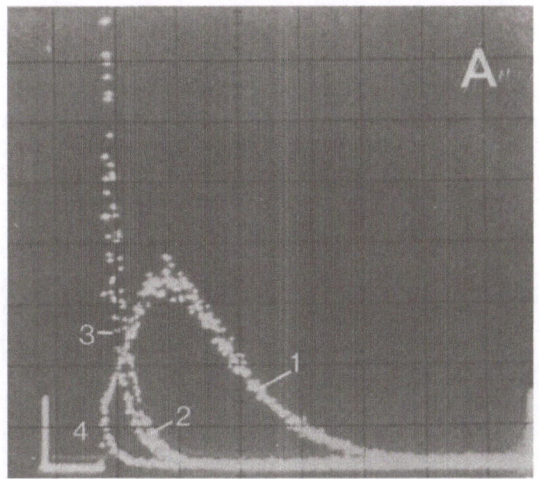

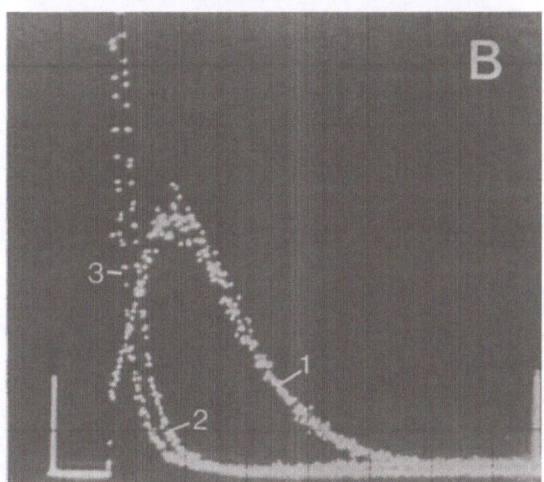

Fig. 5. Fluorescence histograms of rat basophilic leukemia cells
(RBL-2H3) labelled with polyglutaraldehyde microspheres conjugated with DSCG and containing tetramethyl rhodamine were
obtained by a fluorescence-activated cell sorter (FACS-II,
Becton-Dickinson). the 400 mW, 514.5 nm line from an argon
ion laser (Model 164, Spectra-Physics) intersects the stream
just below the nozzle so that the cells are illuminated
while they are in the fluid jet. The 580-nm large-pass
filter (Dictric Optics) and the 590-nm large-pass filter
(No. 2-73 Corning Glass Works) improved the red colour separation. Only living cells in the size range of 14 μm were
analysed, that is, FACS was size-gated to exclude small
cells (as lymphocytes) and smaller-appearing dead cells.
The cells were treated as for fluor- (Cont. next page)

escence microscopy. A. Four histograms are shown: 1, specific binding of DBC; 2, cells with DBC in a Ca^2-free medium;
3, cells in the presence of drug-free beads; 4, autofluorescence of the cells. B. Competitive inhibition exerted by
the addition of free DSCG (see Table 2) causes a shift towards low fluorescence which resembles that due to the non-
specific staining (2), compared with the specific binding
curve (1).

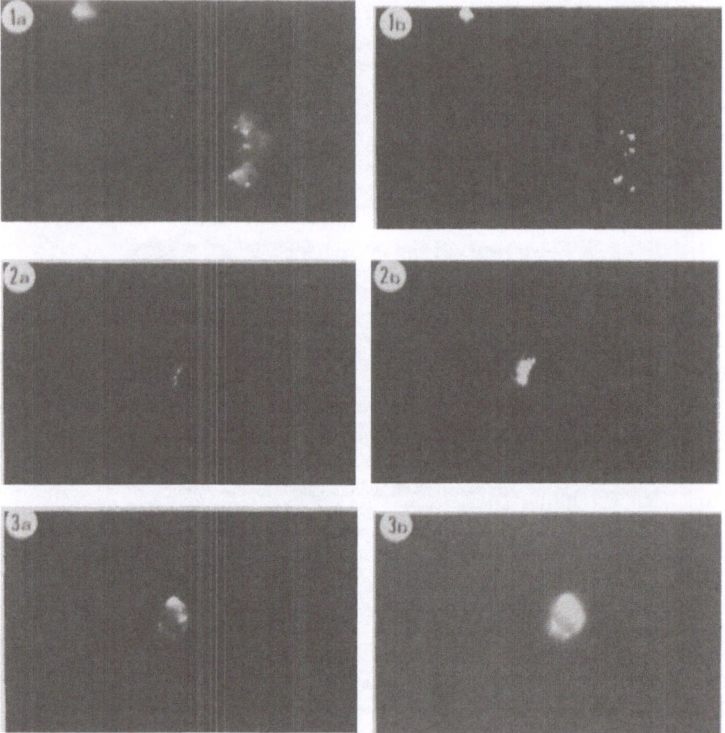

Fig. 6.   Examples of co-capping experiments on RBL-2H3 cells using
          double labelling with fluoresceinated monoclonal IgE and DSCG
          conjugated on fluorescent (tetramethyl rhodamine) PGL micro-
          spheres (DBC). Three different procedures were employed in
          order to examine the occurrence of co-capping: 1. The cells
          were reacted with the fluorescein labelled IgE at 4°C yield-
          ing a diffuse pattern of staining. After several washings,
          anti-IgE antibodies were added and the temperature raised to
          37°C leading to the formation of fluorescent IgE caps (1a).
          Then the cells were fixed by paraformaldehyde and reacted
          with the rhodaminated DBC at 4°C resulting in the superim-
          position of DBC with the IgE cap (1b). 2. The cells were
          stained with both DBC and IgE at 4°C yielding a diffuse
          pattern. Then they were transferred   (Cont. next page)

and capping cells as expressed in the broadening and shifting of the maxima in the histograms while monitoring the same probe (Fig. 7). From the results of these measurements we have learned that a certain extent of correlation between the DSCG and IgE binding sites indeed does exist. Thus, while there was hindrance (probably steric) to the binding of the drug-bead conjugates on cells where cross-linked aggregates of IgE have already been formed, the binding of DBC limited to a certain degree the clustering of the IgE molecules. Furthermore, we found that clustering of the beads causes coclustering and eventual cocapping of the membrane bound IgE molecules[23]. These experiments provided us with the first hints concerning possible interactions between the IgE and DSCG receptors on basophils and on mast cells. By the same token these experiments are also illustrative of the usefulness and wide application range of these beads as visualising agents and probes.

CONCLUSION

We have tried to summarise in this report our experience gained in employing synthetic polymer microspheres in biochemical studies of cells. These microspheres have been found very useful markers, visualising the bind of ligands to receptors on cell membranes. They serve also an important role of preventing low molecular weight ligands, like drugs or hormones, from penetrating into the cells. Hence resolution between binding sites present <u>on</u> the cell surface and <u>within</u> them may be attained. The control can be exerted in the synthesis of microspheres in terms of fluorescence, opacity, magnetic properties, size and mechanical characteristics makes microspheres very useful tools. The application of the DSCG conjugated PGL microspheres to the study of specific receptors for that drug and its mode of activity constitutes one detailed illustration for that case.

---

to 37°C and co-capping of both IgE (2a) and DBC (2b) was observed. (DBC is multivalent with respect to DSCG and therefore is capable of inducing aggregation.) 3. The cells were capped with DBC at 37°C (3b), then fixed with paraformaldehyde and reacted with fluoresceinated IgE at 4°C (3a). Once again an overlap of the fluoresceinated IgE and the rhodaminated DBC was observed. The intensity of the fluoresceinated IgE at the cap is relatively weak. This is probably due to steric hindrance caused by the microspheres of the DBC.

Fig. 7.

Three dimensional presentation of
the histograms obtained by the
FACS II for the co-capping experiments. RBL-2H3 cells were double
labelled with flouresceinated IgE
(F-IgE) and rhodamine containing
DBC(R-DBC) as outlined above
(Legend to Fig. 6). The top picture represents diffuse staining
with both the F-IgE and the R-DBC.
The double staining appears on the
same cell population. Transferring the cells to 25°C caused
co-patching of both labels, as
indicated by the shift of the peak
towards a higher fluorescence intensity zone and its broadening
(middle picture). Further increase of the temperature to
37°C caused co-capping of both
F-IgE and R-DBC as presented at
the bottom histogram, which shows
further shifts towards higher
fluorescence intensity and even
further broadening of the peak.

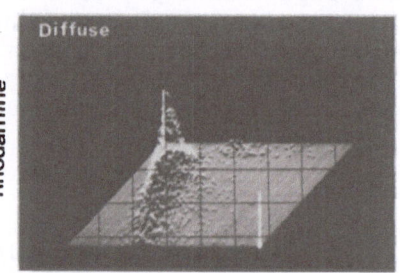

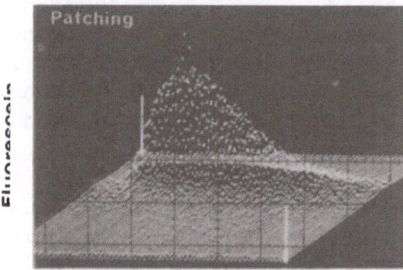

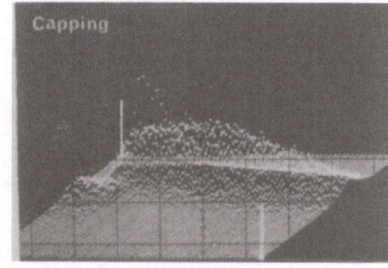

REFERENCES

1. E.R. Unanue, W.D. Perkins, and M.J. Karnovsky, Ligand induced
    movement of lymphocyte membrane macromolecules, J. Exp. Med.
    136: 885 (1972).
2. I. Yahara, and G.M. Edelman, Restriction of the mobility of
    lymphocyte immunoglobulin receptors by Concanavalin A,
    Proc. Natl. Acad. Sci. USA 69: 608 (1972).
3. B. Pernis, L. Forni, and L. Amante, Immunoglobulin spots on the
    surface of rabbit lymphocytes, J. Exp. Med. 132: 1001 (1970).
4. S. Depetris, and M.C. Raff, Movement of lymphocyte surface
    antigens and receptors: the fluid nature of the lymphocyte
    plasma membrane and its immunological significance, Nature,
    241: 257 (1973).
5. S.B. Smith, and J.P. Ravel, Mapping of concanavalin A binding
    sites on the surface of several cell types, Dev. Biol. 27:
    234 (1972).
6. T. Aoki, E. Boyse, L. Old, E. De harven, U. Hammerling, and
    M. Wood, G (Gross) and H-2 cell-surface antigens: location
    on gross leukemia cells by electron microscopy with visually
    labelled antibody, Proc. Natl. Acad. Sci. USA 65: 569 (1970).
7. S. Avrameas, Immunoenzyme techniques: enzymes as markers for
    the localization of antigens and antibodies, Int. Rev. Cytol.
    27: 349, (1970).
8. D.S. Linthicum, and S. Fell, Topography of lymphocyte surface
    immunoglobulin using scanning immunoelectron microscopy,
    J. Ultrastr. Res. 51: 55 (1975).
9. A. Rembaum, and S. Margel, Design of polymeric immunomicro-
    spheres for cell labelling and cell separation, Brit.
    Polymer J. 10: 275 (1978).
10. R.S. Molday, W.J. Dreyer, A. Rembaum, and S.P.S. Yen, New
    immunolatex spheres: visual markers of antigens on lympho-
    cytes for scanning electron microscopy, J. Cell Biol. 64:
    75 (1975).
11. A. Rembaum, S. Margel, and J. Levy, Polyglutaraldehyde: a new
    reagent for coupling proteins to microspheres and for
    labelling cell surface receptors, J. Immunol. Meth. 24:
    239 (1978).
12. S. Margel, S. Zisblatt, and A. Rembaum, Polyglutaraldehyde: a
    new reagent for coupling proteins to microspheres and for
    labelling cell surface receptors. Simplified labelling
    method by means of non-magnetic and magnetic polyglut-
    araldehyde microspheres, J. Immunol. Meth. 28: 341 (1979).
13. S. Margel, and A. Rembaum, Synthesis and characterization of
    polyglutaraldehyde, potential reagent for protein immobili-
    zation and cell separation, Macromolecules 13: 19 (1980).
14. S. Margel, U. Beitler, and M. Offarim, A novel method for
    preparation of polyacrolein microspheres and their biological
    applications, Fourth Internatl. Conf. on Surface and
    Colloid Science, IUPAC, Jerusalem, Israel, p. 14 (1981).

15. N. Mazurek, G. Berger and I. Pecht, A binding site on mast cells
     and basophils for the anti-allergic drug cromolyn, Nature 286:
     722 (1980).

16. J.C. Foreman, M.B. Hallet, and J.L. Mongar, The relationship
     between histamine secretion and ^{45}calcium uptake by mast
     cells, J. Physiol. 271: 193 (1977).

17. J.C. Foreman, and J.L. Mongar, Desensitization in the process of
     histamine secretion induced by antigen and dextran,
     J. Physiol. 239: 381 (1974).

18. J.C. Foreman, J.L. Mongar, and B.D. Gomperts, Calcium ionophores
     and movement of calcium ions following the physiological
     stimulus to a secretory process, Nature 245: 249 (1973).

19. J.S.G. Cox, Disodium cromoglycate (FPL 670) (Intal): a specific
     inhibitor of reaginic antibody-antigen mechanisms, Nature
     216: 1328 (1976).

20. R.E.C. Altounyan, Review of clinical activity and mode of action
     of sodium cromoglycate, Clin. Allergy 10: 481 (1980).

21. J.C. Foreman, and L.G. Garland, Cromoglycate and other anti-
     allergic drugs: a possible mechanism of action, Br. Med. J.
     1: 820 (1976).

22. N. Mazurek, C. Geller-Bernstein, and I. Pecht, Affinity of
     calcium ions to the anti-allergic drug, dicromoglycate,
     FEBS Lett. III: 194 (1980).

23. N. Mazurek, G. Berger, and I. Pecht, Co-capping of fluorescently
     labeled IgE-receptor complexes and cromolyn-beads conjugates
     on clutured rat basophilic cells, submitted.

RECONSTITUTED SENDAI VIRUS ENVELOPES AS A VEHICLE FOR THE INTRO-
DUCTION OF SOLUBLE MACROMOLECULES AND MEMBRANE COMPONENTS INTO
ANIMAL CELLS

M. Beigel, G. Eytan* and A. Loyter

Department of Biological Chemistry
The Hebrew University of Jerusalem
Institute of Life Sciences
Jerusalem, Israel
*Department of Biology
Technion, Israel Institute of Technology
Haifa, Israel

INTRODUCTION

During the past few years attempts have been made by different
groups to develop methods for the introduction of macromolecules into
living cells[1-3]. Such technology can serve as an excellent tool for
the study of various problems in modern cell biology and medicine,
which otherwise could not have been studied.

Many of the intracellular processes in the living cell are
complex and cannot be reproduced in a cell-free system. Regulation
and control of gene expression, transformation of cells by oncogenic
viruses (or by carcinogens), or protein turnover are just a few
examples of multi-step biological processes, the investigation of
which necessitates the use of the intact cell.

Similarly, membrane associated phenomena such as the function
of polypeptide hormones, virus-cell interaction, or transport of ions
or macromolecules can properly be studied only by following the
structure and function of the components involved within the intact
biological membrane. It appears, therefore, that in cell biology and
in medical research we are approaching a stage where the intact
eucaryotic cell (whether it be a mammalian or a plant cell) will be
used as a test tube in order to study the relationship between the
structure and function of various macromolecules of biological
interest. Evidently, such an approach will be feasible only with

125

the development of methods for the microinjection of macromolecules
into the intracellular space or the insertion of membrane components
into membranes of the living cell.

Resealed membranous vesicles can be used as carriers for the
introduction of macromolecules into living cells. In principle,
three kinds of vesicles have been developed: (i) Resealed erythrocyte
ghosts in which macromolecules, especially proteins, can be enclosed
if added during the hemolysis process which is utilized to prepare
the erythrocyte ghosts[2,4]. Loaded erythrocyte ghosts can be fused,
by the aid of various fusogenic agents, with living cells in culture.
[2,4-7]   (ii) Vesicles made of pure phospholipids[1,8]. Different
methods have been used to trap macromolecules within phospholipid
liposomes[8]. When loaded liposomes are incubated with living cells
in culture, most of them are being phagocytosed, thereby introducing
the trapped material into secondary lysosomes[8]. However, the possibility that a few of the cell-attached liposomes are fused with the
cell plasma membrane and thus inject their content directly into the
cytoplasm, cannot be excluded[8]. (iii) Reconstituted envelopes of
fusogenic animal viruses such as Sendai virus[9-11]. The infection of
cells by enveloped viruses, especially those belonging to the para-
myxovirus group, is composed of two main steps: (a) binding of the
virus to the cell surface, and (b) fusion of the viral envelope with
the plasma membrane of the recipient cell, with the concomitant
injection of the viral nucleocapsid into the cell interior.

Soluble macromolecules or purified membrane components can be
trapped either within the "intraviral" space or inserted into the
viral envelope, especially when added during reconstitution of the
viral envelope[9-11]. Since such reconstituted envelopes are able to
fuse with plasma membranes of living cells, as do intact virus
particles[9-11], it is conceivable that any material enclosed within
the virus envelope would be injected into the cytoplasm of the recipient cell, while any component inserted into the viral envelope will
be transplanted via the fusion process into the plasma membrane of
the living cell[12,13]. Using reconstituted Sendai virus envelopes
(or envelopes made of some other fusogenic virus) as a carrier to
introduce biological material into living cells in culture, may be
efficient, simple and reproducible, since no external fusogenic
agent is required to promote fusion between the virus envelopes and
cell membranes.

INTRODUCTION OF MACROMOLECULES (PROTEINS AND DNA) INTO THE CYTOPLASM
OF LIVING CELLS BY THE USE OF RECONSTITUTED SENDAI VIRUS ENVELOPES
(RSVE) AS A CARRIER

In our laboratory in Jerusalem we have used the detergent
Triton X-100 for solubilization of intact Sendai virus particles[10].
Removal of the detergent from the supernatant obtained after centri-
fugation of the detergent-insoluble nucleocapsid, resulted in the

formation of membranous vesicles containing the two viral envelope glycoproteins and the viral phospholipids[10]. Hosaka and his colleagues in Japan have used the detergent NP-40 for solubilization of Sendai virus particles[14].

In our experiments we have shown that when a soluble enzyme such as cytochrome-C (cyt-C) is added to the detergent solubilized viral glycoproteins, it is trapped within the vesicle formed after removal of the detergent[15]. Incubation of the loaded fusogenic reconstituted viral envelopes with Friend erythroleukemic cells (FELC) resulted in the direct injection of the trapped cyt-C into the cytoplasm of the FELC with relatively high efficiency[15]. Uchida et al.[9,16] demonstrated the successful application of RSVE for the introduction of the non-toxic mutant protein, CRM-45 related to diphtheria toxin, or of Fragment A of diphtheria toxin into mouse cells. This can be done either by sonication of the virus particles in the presence of Fragment A or by a similar method to the one used in our laboratory[15], namely, to add Fragment A to the reconstitution system[16]. In these experiments about 0.2 to 0.3% and 7% of the total Fragment A added were enclosed in the viral envelopes formed by sonication or after solubilization with detergents, respectively[9,16].

Electron microscopic techniques have been used by us to follow the enclosure of ferritin particles within RSVE. It has been observed that when ferritin particles are added to the reconstitution system, they are trapped and occupy the entire "intraviral" space of the RSVE[17]. Using ^{125}I-IgG as a marker, we have found that about 4 to 6% of the added IgG can be trapped within 3 mg of RSVE. Incubation of IgG-loaded RSVE with FELC, resulted in the injection of about 3 to 4 x 10^4 IgG molecules into each FELC[17]. Trapped IgG molecules were resistant to digestion by trypsin, whereas externally absorbed IgG molecules were readily removed by incubation of RSVE with trypsin [17].

Recently, we have demonstrated that also ^{3}H-DNA molecules can be enclosed within RSVE when added to the viral envelope reconstitution system[17,18]. Autoradiographic techniques have been employed to demonstrate trapping of ^{3}H-labeled PMB-9 plasmid in viral envelopes, and the introduction of the plasmid into FELC via fusion-mediated microinjection. Lately, we have used RSVE as a vehicle to introduce naked SV_{40}-DNA into various cell lines[18]. RSVE loaded with SV_{40}-DNA transferred the latter to SV_{40}-susceptible and resistant cell lines[18]. Our experiments indicated that the DNA molecules were not affected by the reconstitution process and remained biologically active. Between 5 to 20% of the cells (such as African green monkey cells) incubated with SV_{40}-DNA-loaded RSVE exhibited synthesis of SV_{40} specific T-antigen [18]. DNA-loaded RSVE can also serve as a vehicle for the introduction of SV_{40}-DNA into cells that are not infected by intact SV_{40}. T-Antigen synthesis was induced in F1 1'-4 cells (an established rat cell line) after fusion-mediated injection of SV_{40}-DNA[18].

Thus, it seems to us that the delivery of DNA molecules through the use of fusogenic membrane vesicles may have an enormous potential in several areas of cell biology and of medicine. With some laboratory manipulations, this technology might be used for genetic engineering purposes on the level of cell culture and, eventually, for the delivery of DNA molecules into tissues of living organisms.

THE FORMATION OF "HYBRID" SENDAI VIRUS ENVELOPES: INSERTION OF FOREIGN PROTEINS INTO RECONSTITUTED VIRUS VESICLES

As already mentioned above, when an isolated membrane protein (or even a crude preparation of membrane components) is added to the Sendai virus (SV) reconstitution system, it is inserted into the virus envelope formed after removal of the detergent[12,13]. This results in the formation of "hybrid" vesicles containing both the viral envelope glycoprotein and the foreign component inside one vesicle[12,13]. In order to study and to demonstrate the formation of "hybrid" vesicles, we have used the human erythrocyte band 3 poly-peptide as a model system[12,13]. The human erythrocyte band 3 is well defined transmembrane protein of 100,000 daltons, whose function is to exchange anions across the erythrocyte membrane[19]. In addition, the band 3 polypeptide can be isolated and purified by methods which do not affect its function[19]. In our experiments we have shown that, indeed, the purified detergent-soluble polypeptide can be inserted into SV envelopes. Several experimental approaches have been used by us to demonstrate the formation of "hybrid" vesicles, containing the viral glycoproteins and the human erythrocyte band 3 polypeptide [12,13]. Band 3 can be covalently and stoichiometrically labeled with the radioactive agent 4,4'-diisothiocyano-2,2'-ditriostilbene disulfonic acid ($^3H_2$-DIDS) which also inhibits anion exchange activity[19]. We have shown that after $^3H_2$-DIDS-labeled band 3 was inserted into the virus envelopes, anti-viral antibodies were able to precipitate the labeled human erythrocyte polypeptide[12,13]. Precipitation of inserted $^3H_2$-DIDS labeled band 3 was highly dependent upon the concentration of the anti-viral antibody (Fig. 1A). High concentrations of antibodies were able to precipitate up to about 85% of the total band 3 protein present in the virus envelopes. In the absence of anti-viral antibodies no precipitation of $^3H_2$-DIDS-labeled band 3 was observed (not shown).

Anti-viral antibodies were used by us also as a tool to study the question of how many band 3 molecules could maximally be inserted into the viral reconstituted envelopes without impairing their fusogenic activity.

Figure 1B shows that the antiviral antibody is able to precipitate as many as 9.5×10^{14} molecules of $^3H_2$-DIDS-labeled inserted band 3 polypeptide/mg viral proteins. In all cases about 80 to 85% of the total band 3 polypeptides present in the "hybrid" vesicles were precipitated by the anti-viral antibody. At higher ratios of

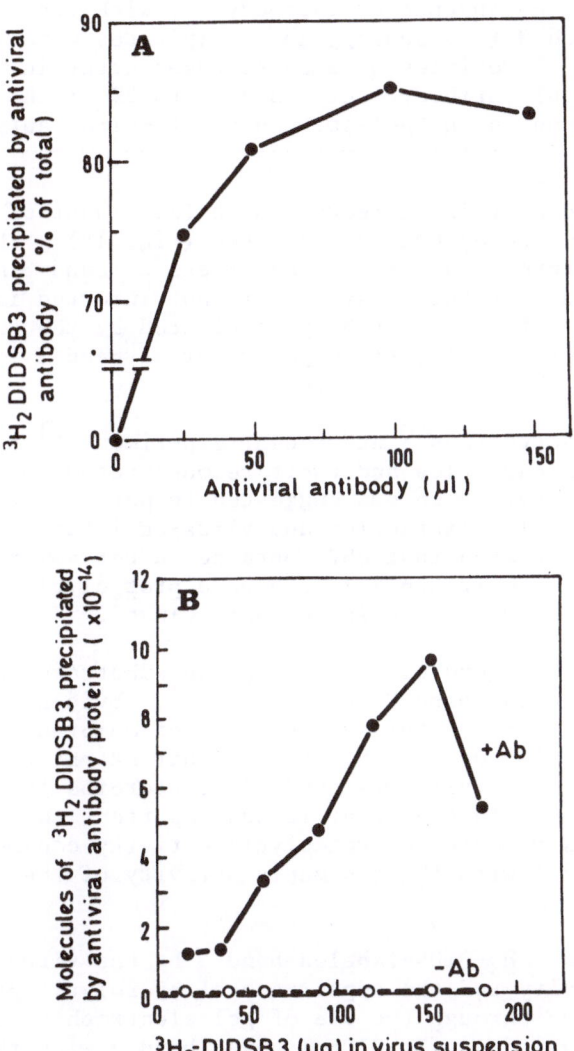

Fig. 1.   Precipitation of viral associated band 3 by anti-Sendai
          virus antibodies. A, Precipitate of $^3H_2$-DIDS-labeled
          band 3 by increasing concentrations of anti-viral antibody.
                                    (Continued on next page)

B, Precipitation of increasing amounts of viral associated $^3H_2$-DIDS band 3 by anti-viral antibody. Band 3 was labeled with $^3H_2$-DIDS, inserted into viral envelopes and precipitated by anti-viral antibodies as described before[12]. Note that in the absence of antibody, or with vesicles containing only band 3 (not shown), no precipitates were formed. When the band 3 vesicles were centrifuged after incubation with anti-viral antibody, only about 1 to 2% of the total counts were found in the pellet. Ab = anti-viral antibody.

---

band 3/viral glycoprotein, a reduction in the amount of the precipitable $^3H_2$-DIDS-labeled band 3 was noted (Fig. 1B). This observation can be interpreted as either the excess of band 3 molecules, present in the reconstitution system, is not inserted into the viral envelopes and therefore cannot be precipitated by the anti-viral antibody, or alternatively, the high amount of band 3 interferes with the formation of the "hybrid" vesicles.

Previous observations[20] and recent experiments[21] have shown that Sendai virus particles and their reconstituted envelopes exhibit proteolytic activity, which was suggested to participate in the process of virus-cell interaction and virus-cell fusion. Furthermore, it has been demonstrated that RSVE obtained after solubilization of intact particles with Triton X-100, have a proteolytic activity of higher specific activity than intact particles[21].

RSVE are able to hydrolyze polypeptide substrates such as ^{125}I-β-insulin, histone and band 3 polypeptides[21]. Evidently, in order to use the RSVE as a carrier for implantation of membrane proteins, it was important to find out whether and to what extent the virus associated proteolytic activity will hydrolyze proteins inserted into the virus envelope. In addition, it was important to study whether and how the virus associated proteolytic activity can be blocked without interfering with the fusogenic activity of the "hybrid" vesicles.

Hydrolysis of $^3H_2$-DIDS-labeled band 3 by the virus associated proteolytic activity and the appearance of hydrolytic products has been studied by us through the use of gel electrophoresis. Figure 2 shows that incubation of $^3H_2$-DIDS-labeled band 3 with the virus envelope glycoproteins in a solution containing Triton X-100 (2%), resulted in a marked hydrolysis of band 3 and led to the appearance of proteolytic products (compare Fig. 2,1 with Fig. 2,2).

Pretreatment of the viral glycoproteins and of band 3 polypeptides with 1 mM phenylmethylsulfonyl fluoride (PMSF) prevented proteolysis of band 3 (Fig. 2,6). When the viral glycoproteins were pretreated with 1 mM PMSF but the band 3 polypeptides with only 0.1 mM PMSF, digestion of band 3 was still observed (Fig. 2,5) most

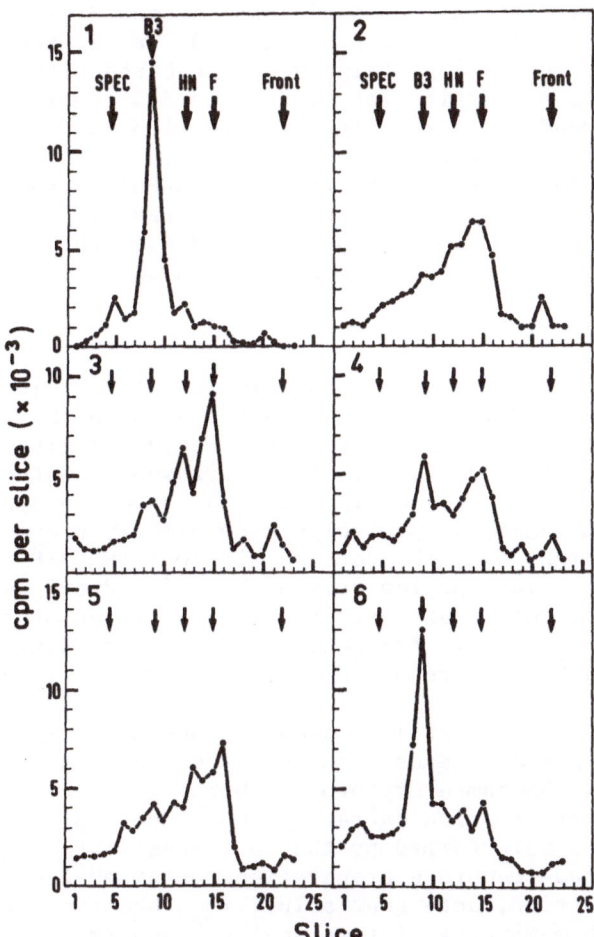

Fig. 2. Proteolysis of $^3H_2$-DIDS-labeled band 3 polypeptides during co-reconstitution with SV glycoproteins. $^3H_2$-DIDS-labeled

(Continued on next page)

band 3 was co-reconstituted with Sendai virus glycoproteins as described before[12]. After the co-reconstitution
process, the "hybrid" vesicles formed were washed in
isotonic buffer and subjected to SDS-acrylamide gel
electrophoresis (7.5% acrylamide). The gels were studied
and analysed for radioactivity as described before[12].
1. Control $^3H_2$-DIDS-labeled band 3 polypeptides. 2.
Analysis of the $^3H_2$-DIDS-labeled band 3 after co-reconstitution with SV glycoproteins. 3. as 2, but band 3 and
the virus glycoproteins were incubated with 10^{-4} M PMSF
before reconstitution[12]. 4. Band 3 treated with 10^{-3} M
PMSF and the viral glycoprotein with 10^{-4} M PMSF. 5.
Viral glycoproteins treated with 10^{-3} M PMSF and band 3
with 10^{-4} M PMSF. 6. Both the $^3H_2$-DIDS-labeled band 3 and
the viral glycoproteins were treated with 10^{-3} M PMSF.
Spect = erythrocyte spectrin; B3 = erythrocyte band 3;
HN = viral hemagglutinin neuraminidase; F = viral fusion
protein.

---

probably due to the presence of proteolytic activity in the band 3
preparation[22]. Proteolysis was also observed when the band 3 polypeptides were treated with 1 mM PMSF but the viral glycoproteins with
only 0.1 mM PMSF (Fig. 2,4), due to the virus-associated proteolytic
activity. Only when both the viral and the band 3 polypeptides were
treated with 1 mM PMSF was proteolysis completely blocked (Fig. 2,6).
Obviously, treatment of both proteins with 0.1 mM PMSF (Fig. 2,3) was
not sufficient to block proteolysis of band 3. Previous experiments[20]
clearly indicated that treatment of virus particles or RSVE with 1 mM
PMSF does not affect their fusogenic activity. Much higher concentrations of PMSF (5 mM) are required to block virus-cell fusion.

"Hybrid" membrane vesicles can be formed not only by co-reconstitution of SV glycoproteins with isolated and pure membrane
proteins such as the human erythrocyte band 3, but also with crude
membrane preparations or an extract of whole cell plasma membranes.
"Hybrid" vesicles were formed by the co-reconstitution of SV glycoproteins with crude membrane preparations obtained from mouse lymphocytes[23]. In addition, detergent solubilized membrane fragments from
H-2 antigen-rich membranes of tumor cells[24] and from SV_{40}[18] or
Epstein-Barr virus receptor-rich[25] membranes were co-reconstituted
with the SV envelope glycoproteins.

THE USE OF RSVE FOR IMPLANTATION OF MEMBRANE PROTEINS INTO PLASMA
MEMBRANES OF LIVING CELLS

Since fusion of SV with living cells leads to the implantation
of the viral envelope glycoproteins into the plasma membranes of the
recipient cell, it is conceivable that this will be the fate of any
protein that is inserted into the viral envelope.

In our experiments we have fused "hybrid" vesicles containing the band 3 polypeptides with various cell lines in order to study their fate and function in the new environment. Fusion of these "hybrid" vesicles with FELC resulted in implantation of band 3 into the plasma membrane, as was demonstrated by electron microscopic techniques as well as by other methods[11-13]. Ferritin conjugated anti-erythrocyte antibodies stained the plasma membranes of FELC after fusion-mediated implantation of band 3[12]. Furthermore, our experiments clearly demonstrated that the band 3 polypeptides remained active in their new environment[12,13]. Quantitative determinations using "hybrid" vesicles with $^3H_2$-DIDS-labeled band 3 showed that an average of 5×10^5 band 3 polypeptides were transferred into the membranes of each FELC[12].

Table 1 compares the amount of band 3 polypeptide molecules that were transferred — using RSVE as a vehicle — into membranes of FELC, L-cells and hepatoma tissue cultured cells (HTC cells). The results summarized in Table I indicate that many more band 3 polypeptides can be transferred into L-cells than into FELC or HTC cells.

Table 1. Binding and Implantation of Band 3 Polypeptides into Various Cell Lines by the Use of RSVE as Vehicles

Cell line	Temperature:	4°C		37°C
Time of incubation (min)		15	20	180
FELC		1.2×10^6	8.0×10^5	6.0×10^5
L-Cell		2.6×10^6	2.0×10^6	1.6×10^6
HTC cell		9.2×10^5	7.0×10^5	5.7×10^5

No. of band 3 molecules/cell

Band 3 polypeptides were labeled with $^3H_2$-DIDS and inserted into SV envelope glycoproteins, as previously described[12]. "Hybrid" vesicles were incubated with the different cells at 4°C and at 37°C, and the number of $^3H_2$-DIDS-labeled band 3 bound to the cell surface (4°C) and inserted into these membranes (37°C) was calculated as previously described[12].

A rough calculation revealed that as many as 1 to 3×10^6 molecules of band 3 can be incorporated into each L-cell as compared with about 5 to 8×10^5 molecules transferred to FELC. It is conceivable that a certain amount of the "hybrid" vesicles which

interact with L-cells are incorporated into these cells by phagocytosis and not necessarily via the membrane fusion process. L-Cells,
as opposed to FELC or HTC cells, are characterized by high phagocytic
and endocytic activities[26].

The same electron microscopic methods used by us to study the
fate of RSVE and band 3 after insertion into FELC[12], were applied to
follow the fate and localization of these proteins after incubation
of the "hybrid" vesicles with L-cells. Ferritin-conjugated anti-
viral antibodies stained plasma membranes of L-cells containing SV
glycoproteins (Fig. 3). A close examination of the plasma membranes
seen in Fig. 3,B reveals the presence of numerous ferritin particles,
indicating implantation of viral glycoproteins into these membranes.
This situation arises only by fusion of "hybrid" vesicles with the
L-cells. However, the electron micrograph seen in Fig. 3,C shows
that L-cells are probably also able to phagocytose the "hybrid"
vesicles. A few "hybrid" vesicles (arrows in Fig. 3,C) can be seen
in the process of being phagocytosed. Phagocytosis of either RSVE
or "hybrid" vesicles was not observed when these membrane vesicles
were incubated with either human erythrocytes or with FELC.

DISCUSSION AND CONCLUSIONS

        Since the pioneering work of Okada and his colleagues in Japan
[27,28], it became evident that Sendai virus particles are able to
interact with cells in culture and to promote cell-cell fusion. This
results in the formation of either homo- or heteropolykaryons[27].
From studies performed in Okada's laboratory[28] as well as in others[29]
it became clear that the first step in inducing cell-cell fusion is
the fusion between the viral envelope and the recipient cell plasma
membrane. Cell-cell fusion and virus-cell fusion are two distinct
steps which, under specific experimental conditions or with certain
cell lines, can be separated from one another[28,29]. Virus-cell fusion
will take place in the presence of high concentrations of mono- or
di-saccharides[28] or with erythrocyte ghosts[29], but not so cell-cell
fusion. However, under these conditions, single cells containing
the viral nucleocapsid are formed[28,29].

        These observations led us as well as others to make attempts to
develop methods in which Sendai virus envelopes will be used as a
carrier for the introduction of macromolecules into animal cells. The
fact that Sendai virus particles fuse with cell membranes, thereby
injecting their content directly into the cytoplasm of the recipient
cells, makes them a very powerful syringe. The results of the present
work show that Sendai virus envelopes can serve also as an efficient
vehicle of membrane components. As many as 1 to 2 x 10^6 molecules of
band 3 can be transferred into membranes of L-cells by using RSVE as
a carrier. We suggest that, in addition to the process of virus-cell
fusion, a process of phagocytosis takes place. The possibility that
a certain amount of the SV population is taken into the cell by

phagocytosis, cannot be eliminated. Phagocytosis was suggested to be
the main route by which Semliki Forest viruses are being taken by and
infecting cells[30]. Nevertheless, phagocytosis of Semliki Forest particles occurs only at neutral pH[30]. When these virus particles are
incubated with cells at low pH (pH < 6.0), they fuse with the cell
plasma membrane, thus delivering their cell content directly into
the cell cytoplasm and not into the lysosomes[31]. From these studies
it appears that, similar to the phospholipid liposomes[8], enveloped
animal viruses can either fuse with or be phagocytosed by cells in
culture (see scheme in Fig. 4). It should be emphasized, however,
that when liposomes interact with cells in culture, most of them are
being phagocytosed and only a very small percentage fuse with the
cell plasma membranes[1,8]. With enveloped animal viruses such as
Semliki Forest virus or Sendai virus, the picture is more complex.
It appears that the quantitative relationship between the process of
virus-cell fusion and phagocytosis is probably dependent on the cell
type, the pH of the medium, and the biological activities of the
virus.

    In spite of recent extensive research, it is still unclear how
viral envelope components such as the F-protein of Sendai virus
promote fusion between the viral envelope and the cell plasma membrane. It is conceivable that in the absence of the viral F-protein
(or when it is inactive) the interaction between the viral particles
and cell plasma membrane will result in phagocytosis, as occurs with
any other particles which come into close association with plasma
membranes of living cells (see Fig. 4). Evidently, the fusogenic
viruses possess a membrane factor, such as the F-protein of Sendai
virus envelopes, which probably promotes a quick and direct contact
between the viral envelope and cell plasma membrane phospholipids.
Such a tight contact will lead to the formation of membranous tetra-
layer structures which are probably unstable and will spontaneously
collapse. Disruption of these contact areas between the virus envelope and the cell plasma membrane, will obviously result in virus-
cell fusion. We suggested[20] that such contact may be possible after
specific and local hydrolysis of the dense layer of the cell surface
glycoproteins by a viral-associated proteolytic activity. Alternatively, it has been suggested[32] that the SV fusion factor is an
hydrophobic protein which is able to cross the cell surface glycoprotein layer and to penetrate through the phospholipid bilayer.

    Based on these considerations and various observations, it can
be assumed that the quantitative relationship between the processes
of virus-cell fusion and phagocytosis of virus particles will be
dependent upon the following factors: 1. the cell type with which
the virus particles interact, and 2. the activities of the viral F-
protein and/or the virus-associated proteolytic enzymes.

    Cell lines, such as the mouse L-cell line, which are character-
ized by a highly phagocytic activity, will take up enveloped viruses
by both processes: virus-cell fusion and phagocytosis (Fig. 4, process

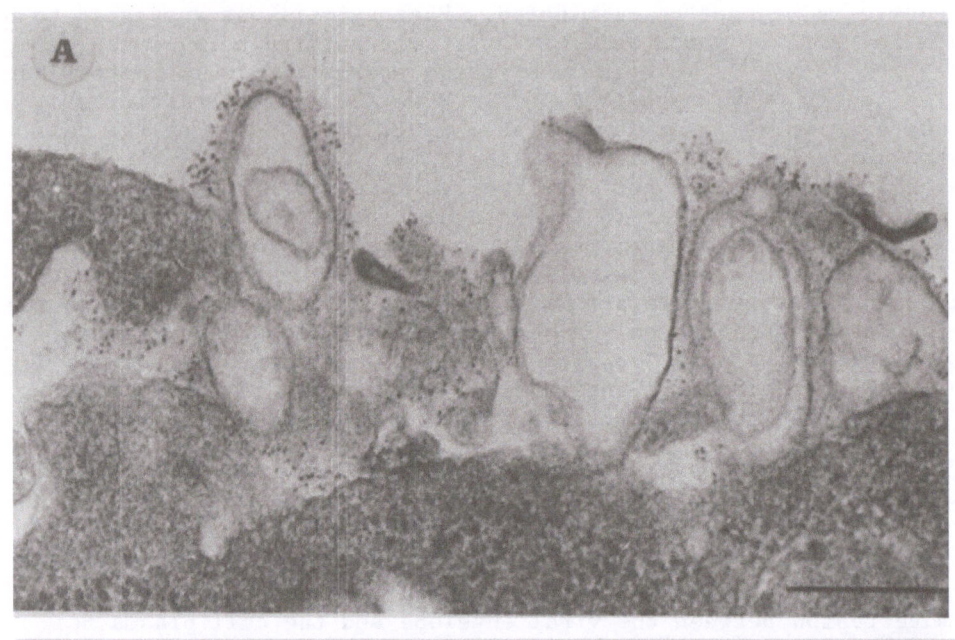

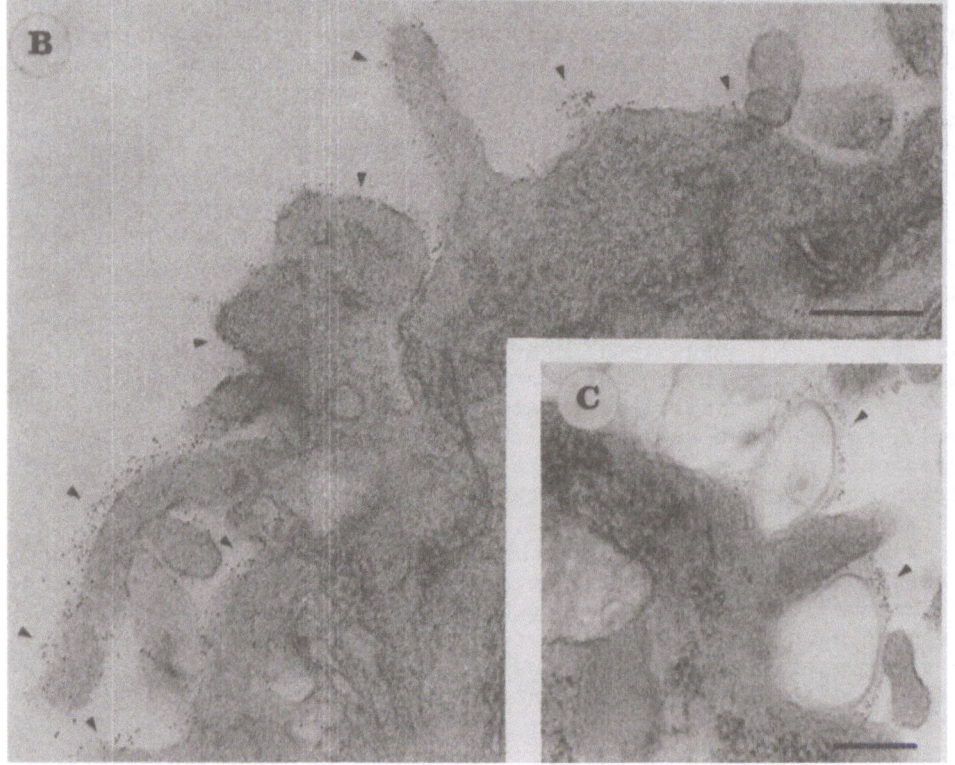

2). This will lead to incorporation of viral associated material to
the cell cytoplasm and to the lysosomal system. On the other hand,
animal cells such as FELC or red blood cells which show very little
or no phagocytic activity, will be subjected — after binding of virus
particles at 4°C — only to the process of virus-cell fusion (Fig. 4,
process 1). In these cells viral associated material will be inserted
exclusively into the plasma membrane and microinjected directly into
the cell cytoplasm.

Fig. 3.   Interaction of RSVE with L-mouse cells. SV envelopes were
          reconstituted and incubated with L-cells as previously
          described for FELC[12]. The cell suspension was fixed with
          2.5% glutaraldehyde and stained with ferritin-conjugated
          anti-viral antibodies as described before[12]. Samples were
          prepared for electron microscopic observation, as before
          [33,34]. A, RSVE were incubated with L-cells at 4°C. Nume-
          rous membrane vesicles surrounded by ferritin particles are
          seen attached to the cell plasma membrane. B, Cells were
          fixed and prepared for electron microscopic observation after
          3 hours of incubation at 37°C with RSVE. No intact RSVE
          (vesicles) can be seen. Numerous ferritin particles (arrows)
          are seen attached to the cell plasma membrane, indicating
          RSVE-cell fusion. C, Cells were prepared for electron micro-
          scopic observation after 30 minutes of incubation at 37°C.
          It appears (arrows) that a few RSVE are being phagocytosed
          by the cells (arrow). Bar = 0.25μ.

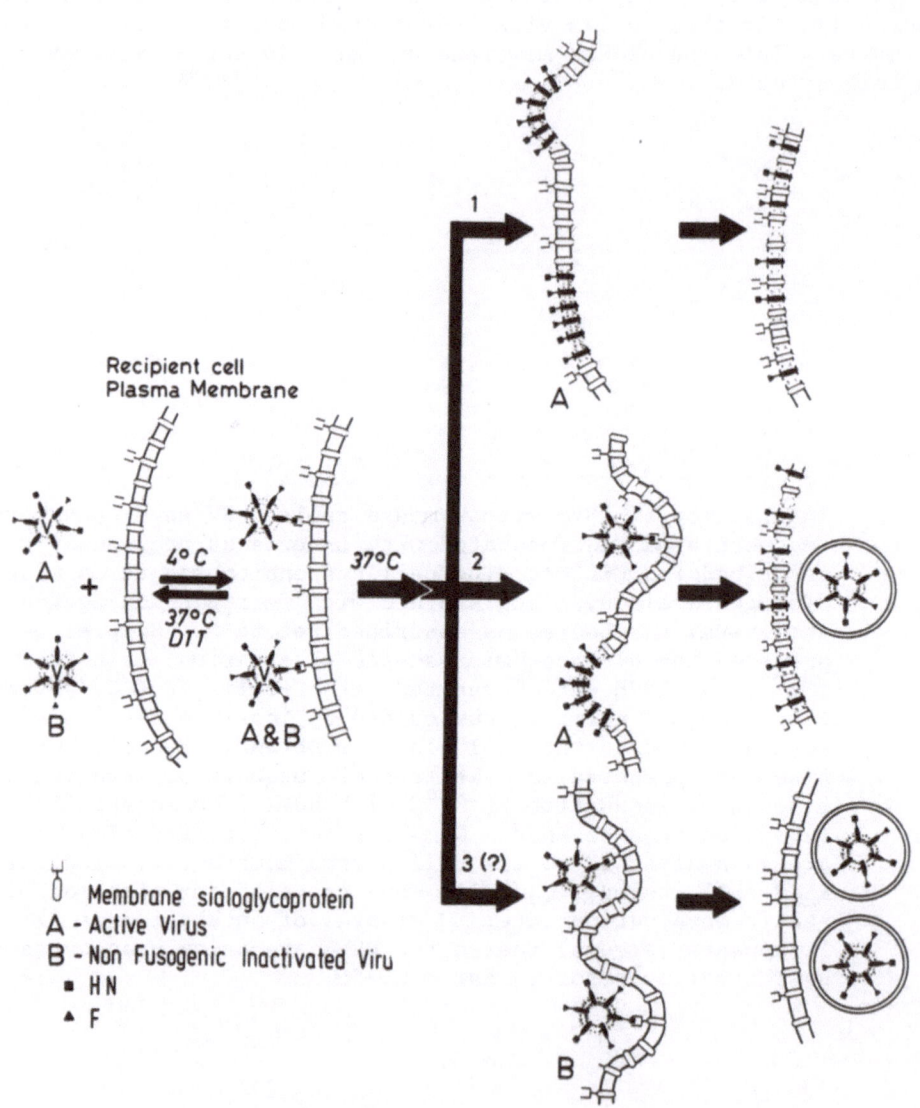

Recipient cell
Plasma Membrane

ͷ Membrane sialoglycoprotein
A - Active Virus
B - Non Fusogenic Inactivated Viru
 ▪ HN
 ▲ F

Fig. 4.   Schematic outline showing fusion and phagocytosis of SV
          particles. Interaction of SV particles with living cells
          at 4°C results in binding of the virus particles to cell
          surface sialoglycoproteins via the viral envelope hemag-
          glutinin/neuraminidase (HN) protein. Both active virions
          (A) and non-fusogenic virions (B) are able to interact
          with membrane sialoglycoproteins. At 37°C the virions are
          either released from the cell surface after hydrolysis of
          the membrane sialoglycoproteins by the viral neuraminidase
          or fused (processes 1 and 2) and/or being phagocytosed
          (processes 2 and 3). When the virus particles interact with
          cells that do not show any phagocytic activity, such as red
          blood cells, only process 1 will take place; namely, the
          virus particles will fuse with the cell plasma membrane.
          On the other hand, when the virus interacts with cells of
          high phagocytic activity such as the mouse L-cells, both
          fusion and phagocytosis will occur (process 2). The SV
          fusion protein can be inactivated by high temperatures (56°C,
          3 min) or by treatment with reagents such as PMSF or DTT.
          Such a non-fusogenic virus (B) is still able to interact at
          4°C with cell plasma membranes. However, at 37°C the non-
          fusogenic virions are unable to fuse with the cell membrane
          and probably will only be phagocytosed by cells with high
          phagocytic activity (process 3). V = virus; HN = hemag-
          glutinin/neuraminidase viral glycoprotein; F = fusion
          protein.

It is conceivable that inhibition of Sendai virus-associated proteolytic activity[20] or inactivation of its fusion protein (by high temperature or by reducing agents such as DL-dithiothreitol (DTT) will result in the formation of virus particles which cannot fuse with cell plasma membranes but which probably will be taken by phagocytosis (Fig. 4, process 3). Preliminary results in our laboratory showed that Sendai virus particles treated with the inhibitor of proteoyltic enzymes, PMSF, do not fuse with mouse L-cells. The question whether PMSF-treated Sendai virus particles are taken into L-cells by phagocytosis is currently being studied in our laboratory.

We believe that a better knowledge of the factors which control virus-cell fusion versus phagocytosis of virus particles, as well as a better understanding of the quantitative relationship between these two processes will lead to the possibility of constructing a specific and powerful "biological syringe". Incorporation of the Sendai virus F-protein into phospholipid vesicles, together with the viral proteolytic enzyme, may result in the formation of a fusogenic vesicle. It might be suggested that the quantitative ratio between the viral F-protein and the phospholipids in such vesicles may control the efficiency by which these vesicles will be fused or phagocytosed by living cells.

ACKNOWLEDGMENT

This work was supported by a grant, No. 015-7349 (to A.L.) from the United States-Israel Binational Science Foundation, Jerusalem.

REFERENCES

1. G. Poste, and D. Papahadjopoulos, Lipid vesicles as carriers for introduction of biologically active materials, in: "Methods in Cell Biology," Vol. 4, D.M. Prescott, ed., Academic Press, New York (1976).
2. R.G. Kulka and A. Loyter, The use of fusion methods for the microinjection of animal cells, in: "Current Topics in Membranes and Transport," Vol. 12, F. Bronner and A. Kleinzeller, eds., Academic Press, New York (1979).
3. M. Furusawa, M. Yamaizumi, T. Nishimura, T. Uchida and Y. Okada, Use of erythrocyte ghosts for injection of substances into animal cells by cell fusion, in: "Methods in Cell Biology", Vol. 14, D.M. Prescott, ed., Academic Press, New York (1976).
4. M. Wasserman, N. Zakai, A. Loyter and R.G. Kulka, A quantitative study of ultramicroinjection of macromolecules into animal cells, Cell, 7: 551 (1976).
5. A. Loyter, N. Zakai and R.G. Kulka, "Ultramicroinjection" of macromolecules or small particles into animal cells,

J. Cell Biol., 66: 292 (1975).

6. M. Furusawa, T. Nishimura, M. Yamaizumi and Y. Okada, Injection
    of foreign substances into single cells by cell fusion,
    Nature, 249: 449 (1974).

7. A.B. Schlegel, and C.M. Rechsteiner, Microinjection of thymidine
    kinase and bovine serum albumin into mammalian cells by
    fusion with red blood cells, Cell, 5: 371 (1975).

8. R.E. Pagano and J.N. Weinstein, Interactions of liposomes with
    mammalian cells, Annu. Rev. Biophys. Bioeng., 7: 435
    (1978).

9. T. Uchida, M. Yamaizumi, E. Mekada and Y. Okada, Methods using
    HVJ (Sendai virus) for introducing substances into viable
    cells, in: "Introduction of Macromolecules into Mammalian
    Cells," Alan B. Liss, Inc. (1980).

10. D.J. Volsky and A. Loyter, An efficient method f_or reassembly
    of fusogenic Sendai virus envelopes after solubilization of
    intact virions with Triton X-100, FEBS Lett., 92: 190
    (1978).

11. A. Loyter, and D.J. Volsky, The use of reconstituted Sendai virus
    envelopes as carriers for the introduction of biological
    material into animal cells, in: "Cell Surface Reviews,"
    G. Poste and G.L. Nicolson, eds., North Holland Publishing
    Co., Amsterdam (in press).

12. D.J. Volsky, Z.I. Cabantchik, M. Beigel and A. Loyter, Implanta-
    tion of the isolated human erythrocyte anion channel into
    plasma membranes of Friend erythroleukemic cells by use of
    Sendai virus envelopes, Proc. Natl. Acad. Sci. USA, 76: 5440
    (1979).

13. Z.I. Cabantchik, D.J. Volsky, H. Ginsburg and A. Loyter, Reconsti-
    tution of the erythrocyte anion transport system: In vitro
    and in vivo approaches, in: "Annals of the New York Academy
    of Science", Vol. 341 (1980).

14. Y. Hosaka and K.Y. Shimizu, Artificial assembly of envelope
    particles of HVJ (Sendai virus). I. Assembly of hemolytic
    and fusion factors from envelopes solubilized by Nonidet
    P-40, Virology 49: 627 (1972).

15. A. Loyter and D.J. Volsky, The use of reconstituted Sendai virus
    envelopes for microinjection of macromolecules or for
    transfering of membrane components into animal cells, in:
    "Membrane Bioenergetics," C.P. Lee, G. Schatz and L. Ernster,
    eds., Addison-Wesley Publ. Co., Massachusetts (1979).

16. T. Uchida, M. Yamaizumi and Y. Okada, Reassembled HVJ (Sendai
    virus) envelopes containing non-toxic mutant proteins of
    diphtheria toxin show toxicity to mouse L-cells, Nature,
    266: 839 (1977).

17. A. Vainstein, J. Atidia and A. Loyter, Reconstituted Sendai virus
    envelopes as a biological carrier for microinjection of
    proteins and DNA molecules into animal cells, in "Liposomes
    in the Study of Drug Activity and Immunocompentent Cell
    Function," A. Paraf and C. Nicolau, eds., Academic Press,

London, New York (1981).

18. A. Loyter, A. Vainstein, M. Graessmann and A. Graessmann, Fusion
    mediated injection of SV_{40}-DNA: Introduction of SV_{40}-DNA
    into tissue culture cells by the use of DNA loaded recon-
    stituted Sendai virus envelopes, Proc. Natl. Acad. Sci. USA
    (submitted for publication).

19. Z.I. Cabantchik, A. Knauf and A. Rothstein, The anion transport
    system of the red blood cell: The role of membrane protein
    evaluated by the use of "probes", Biochim. Biophys. Acta,
    515: 239 (1978).

20. A. Loyter, D. Ginsberg, D.J. Volsky, N. Zakai and Y. Laster,
    Association between enveloped viruses and host cell membrane:
    A specific case of ligand receptor interaction, in: "Recep-
    tors for Neurotransmitters and Peptide Hormones," G. Pepeu,
    M.J. Kuhar and S. Enna, eds., Raven Press, New York (1980).

21. S. Israel, N. Zakai, D. Ginsberg, Y. Laster, Z.I. Cabantchik,
    J. Gordon and A. Loyter, Proteolysis and its possible role
    in virus-cell fusion, in: "13th FEBS Meeting," Jerusalem
    (1980) (Abstract).

22. G. Tarone, N. Hamasaki, M. Fukuda and U.T. Marchesi, Proteolytic
    degradation of human erythrocyte band 3 by membrane associ-
    ated protease activity, J. Memb. Biol. 48: 1 (1979).

23. A. Prujansky-Jakobowitz, D.J. Volsky, A. Loyter and N. Sharon,
    Alteration of lymphocyte surface properties by insertion of
    foreign functional components of plasma membranes, Proc.
    Natl. Acad. Sci. USA, 77: 7247 (1980).

24. D.J. Volsky, A.L. Richter, T. Dalianis and G. Klein, Implantation
    of mouse histocompatibility antigensinto membranes of cul-
    tured tumoral cells, Eur. J. Immunol. (in press).

25. D.J. Volsky, M.I. Shapiro and G. Klein, Transfer of Epstein-Barr
    virus receptors to receptor negative cells permits virus
    penetration and antigen expression, Proc. Natl. Acad. Sci.
    USA, 77: 5453 (1980).

26. M.R. Steinman, E. Brodie and A.Z. Cohn, Membrane flow during
    pinocytosis: A sterologic analysis, J. Cell Biol., 68: 665
    (1976).

27. Y. Okada, Factors in fusion of cells by HVJ, in: "Current Topics
    in Microbiology and Immunology," Vol. 48, W. Arber and A.
    Braun, eds., Springer-Verlag, Berlin (1969).

28. Y. Maeda, J. Kim, I. Koseki, E. Mekada, Y. Shiokawa and Y. Okada,
    Modification of cell membranes with viral envelopes during
    fusion of cells with HVJ (Sendai virus), Exp. Cell. Res.,
    108: 95 (1977).

29. A. Lalazar and A. Loyter, Involvement of spectrin in membrane
    fusion: Induction of fusion in human erythrocyte ghosts by
    proteolytic enzymes and its inhibition by antispectrin anti-
    body, Proc. Natl. Acad. Sci. USA, 76: 318 (1979).

30. A. Helenius, J. Kartenbeck, K. Simons and E. Fries, On the entry
    of Semliki Forest virus into BHK-21 cells, J. Cell Biol.
    84: 404 (1980).

31. J. White, J. Kartenbeck and A. Helenius, Fusion of Semliki Forest
    virus with the plasma membrane can be induced by low pH,
    J. Cell Biol., 87: 264 (1980).
32. M.C. Hsu, A. Scheid and W.P. Choppin, Activation of the Sendai
    virus fusion protein (F) involves a conformational change
    with exposure of a new hydrophobic region, J. Biol. Chem.
    256: 3557 (1981).
33. G.D. Eytan, Liposome cell interaction: Adsorption of ferritin
    loaded liposomes. Introduction of ferritin in cytoplasm of
    Ehrlich ascites tumor cells, J. Cell Biol., (submitted for
    publication).
34. A.E. Gad, R. Broza and G.S. Eytan, Fusion of cells and proteo-
    liposomes: Incorporation of beef heart cytochrome oxidase
    into rabbit erythrocytes, FEBS Lett., 102: 230 (1979).

ERYTHROCYTES AS CARRIERS FOR RECOMBINANT CLONED DNA

Garret M. Ihler

Texas A&M College of Medicine
College Station, Texas 77843, USA.

INTRODUCTION

The concept of carriers in pharmacology has evolved because various problems complicate the objective of delivering pharmacologically-active substances to the appropriate target in appropriate amounts. One objective achieved by carriers is protection. Small molecular weight drugs for example can be protected from serum enzymes and binding proteins by a carrier. Enzymes and proteins can be protected from circulating antibodies and it is possible that they can be sequestered from the immune system so that an immune response is not initiated. A second objective is carrier-mediated delivery to specific target sites. For example several groups (Alving et al., 1978; Black et al., 1977; New et al., 1978) have shown that liposomes containing antimonial drugs are more effective than the free drug for the treatment of leishmaniasis, presumably because liposomes are specifically taken up by the same reticulo-endothelial cells that are infected by the intracellular parasite.

Our work has primarily focused on the use of resealed erythrocytes as carriers. During hypotonic hemolysis, rather large holes or pores open reversibly in the membrane through which substances as large as macromolecules can pass. The holes close when the original osmotic conditions are restored, trapping substances added to the external medium within erythrocytes. A variety of possible applications for these resealed erythrocytes have been proposed (Ihler, 1979). Damaged carrier erythrocytes are taken up quickly by the reticuloendothelial system, like liposomes, and could be used in the treatment of leishmaniasis or to introduce lysosomal enzymes such as glucocerebrosidase into erythrophagocytic cells of patients with lysosomal storage diseases such as Gaucher's disease (DeLoach

145

et al., 1977). Carrier erythrocytes which continue to circulate
for substantial periods of time could be used as slow-release capsules for drugs or could contain enzymes which could function in
patients with diseases such as phenylketonuria to degrade unwanted
substrate molecules such as phenylalanine which can be transported
into the erythrocytes. Even the resealed erythrocyte itself could
become a therapeutic agent. Erythrocytes loaded with magnetic iron
could be halted within capillaries of solid tumors by a magnetic
field so that they might reversibly occlude the blood supply to the
tumor, in addition to potential applications as magnetically-con-
trolled delivery vehicles for anti-tumor compounds as previously
proposed for magnetic microspheres (Widder et al., 1979).

METHODS OF GENE TRANSFER

        Current developments in molecular biology have now made it
likely that DNA soon will be employed therapeutically for the treatment of certain diseases just as drugs are used today. This is
especially true for treatment of genetically inherited diseases.
The thalassemias, for example, might be controlled by addition of
DNA containing the normal allele to appropriate hematopoietic cells
of the bone marrow. The implications of this new technology in
areas such as plant or animal science are even more important than
they are to medicine since it appears likely that entirely new
species of living creatures with properties important to man can be
developed.

        These developments have depended on two factors, development
of the necessary techniques for isolating and studying defined segments of DNA in vitro and development of procedures for reintrodu-
cing these segments back into living cells. Isolation of defined
segments of DNA and cloning of those segments on viral or plasmid
DNA has become remarkably simple since the discovery and development of restriction enzymes. In addition, cloned DNA can now be
readily sequenced. Specific base substitutions or deletions in the
nucleotide sequence of a gene can be accomplished if desired.

        This DNA can be reintroduced in vitro into eucaryotic or pro-
caryotic cells so that viable cells with altered genetic information
result. Procedures for the introduction of DNA basically fall into
four categories - those which depend on cell or membrane fusion,
those which use a virus-like vector, those which involve direct
injection and those which depend on uptake of either chromosomes
or chromatin or of free DNA by the recipient cells. For many types
of studies it is most desirable to use only defined and hence
fairly small fragments of DNA consisting of one or more genes and
thus procedures which permit the uptake and expression of defined
fragments of DNA are very desirable.

        One procedure utilizes transformation by free DNA. The

efficiency of this procedure is enhanced if the DNA is precipitated with calcium phosphate. Despite this improvement, the probability that a particular cell will be transformed is very low, so that a selective technique is necessary to identify the transformants. Wigler et al. (1979) have demonstrated that cells which have taken up a selectable marker have a much higher probability of being transformed for other, nonselectable markers, apparently due to physical linkage of the incorporated DNA (Perucho et al., 1980). This procedure may represent at least a partial answer to the efficiency problem. Capecchi (1980) has partially circumvented the efficiency problem by direct microinjection into the nucleus, which initially results in nearly 100% expression of the injected DNA. However stable transformants can be rare, a complicating factor since only a limited number of cells can be manually microinjected.

Thus it seems that a procedure may be needed in which a sufficiently large population of cells is transformed to allow selection of rare stable integrants, in which multiple copies per recipient cell of the DNA are transferred, and in which a high percentage of recipient cells receive the DNA to allow isolation of transformants at high efficiency.

ENTRAPMENT OF VIRUS PARTICLES IN ERYTHROCYTES

We have recently found conditions suitable for the entrapment in erythrocytes of viruses which are being used as vectors for cloned DNA (Humphreys et al., 1981). Although we had found in 1973 that low levels of the small bacteriophage ϕX174 could be encapsulated using the dilution procedure (Thorpe and Ihler, unpublished results) the levels of entrapment were very low compared to enzymes or small molecules. Similar results for the encapsulation of virus T2 were reported by Loyter et al. (1975).

There have been no reports concerning the successful incorporation of free DNA into erythrocytes. Free double-stranded DNA might not be readily loaded into erythrocytes because of its length and negative charge, but it seemed likely to us that DNA would enter if it were condensed and neutralized, for example with polylysine or histones, or precipitated, perhaps with calcium phosphate. However the condensed form of DNA obtained most conveniently is the virus particle and so we decided to reinvestigate the encapsulation of virus particles prior to attempting to encapsulate other forms of condensed DNA or free DNA.

We have now determined conditions that not only allow the encapsulation of small and medium sized virus particles in erythrocytes but also achieve a high level of equilibration. Using the dialysis procedure for loading (DeLoach and Ihler, 1977) at a hematocrit of 10-20%, the intracellular and extracellular

concentrations of bacteriophage ϕX174 come nearly to equilibrium.
ϕX174 is one of the smallest viruses known, being an icosahedron of
diameter 25nm and containing 5386 nucleotides of single stranded
DNA. Its diameter is only about four times the diameter of a hemo-
globin molecule and so it is not too surprising that this virus
can be efficiency encapsulated. ϕX174 however is not especially
useful as a carrier of cloned DNA.

LAMBDA AS A CLONING VEHICLE

Bacteriophage lambda has several properties which have led to
its extensive use as a cloning vehicle. Lambda phage heads can
accomodate between 38 and 52 kb of DNA. Although lambda wild type
DNA contains about 49kb, several large DNA deletions are available,
including those in the b_2 region and nin 5, which do not include
essential genes. Lambda DNA containing appropriate deletions can
carry more than 20 kb of non-lambda DNA and still be packaged into
lambda phage heads.

A variety of cloning vectors are now available, allowing the
use of various restriction enzymes. Recently de Wet et al. (1980)
published restriction maps for twenty-one Charon vector phages,
allowing cloning with a single restriction enzyme or pair of
enzymes. Various selective procedures are available to ensure that
the phage carry recombinant DNA. Selection can be achieved by
using phage whose DNA, after cutting with the restriction enzyme
and resealing without incorporation of foreign DNA, would be too
small to be packaged (Thomas et al., 1974) or by use of the Dam
system (Sternberg et al., 1977). Libraries containing all sequences
of a eucaryotic genome present on lambda phage are readily constructed (Maniatis et al., 1978).

Viable phage particles can be produced from infectious lambda
DNA either by transfection of $CaCl_2$-treated cells (Mandel and Higa,
1970) or with helper phage (Kaiser and Hogness, 1960). However
the DNA can be more efficiently encapsulated in vitro in λ heads
to which can be joined the tails needed for absorption to the
bacterial cell surface (Hohn and Murray, 1977). Plasmids, called
cosmids, which contain the lambda cos site (cohesive ends of lambda)
can also be packaged into lambda heads (Collins and Bruning, 1978).
This permits the lambda cloning system to be utilized in conjunction
with plasmid cloning systems.

ENTRAPMENT OF LAMBDA IN ERYTHROCYTES

Bacteriophage lambda has a head diameter of 55 nm and a tail
150 nm in length. It can be entrapped in erythrocytes, but four to
ten-fold less efficiently than ϕX174. Presumably this decreased
efficiency reflects the increased size of the bacteriophage head
rather than the presence of the tail since lambda and T7 load with

equivalent efficiencies even though T7 has only a short tail of 15 nm in length.

The most efficient entrapment procedure which we have found so far is the dialysis procedure of DeLoach and Ihler (1977) modified by the use of a relatively low hematocrit (10-20%). Under these conditions ϕX174 equilibrates almost completely and lambda reaches about 7%-10% of complete equilibration. In some of these experiments lambda virus carrying cloned DNA were used. Using the higher hematocrits (80%) which permit retention of most of the intracellular proteins and enzymes of the erythrocyte, levels of equilibration of ϕX174 drop to about 2% and to about 0.5%-1% for lambda. Values similar to those obtained with 80% hematocrits were obtained by us using the preswell procedure devised by Schlegel and Rechsteiner (1975).

Although it is clearly useful to employ conditions which permit high levels of equilibration, this is less important than might be thought since the extracellular concentration of bacteriophage used can be very high. For example at a concentration of 6.1×10^{12} lambda phage/ml, an equilibration of only 1.5% nevertheless permitted the entrapment of nearly nine lambda phage per erythrocyte. Moreover the concentration of lambda used may be much higher than this if desired. At lower concentrations of virus at least, the number of virus encapsulated is proportional to the extracellular concentration.

FUSION OF CARRIER ERYTHROCYTES AND RECIPIENT CELLS

There are several fusion procedures available which have been used to fuse erythrocytes containing various substances, including proteins and tRNA, with recipient cells. Capecchi et al. (1977) demonstrated that tRNA introduced by fusion is functional Kaltoft and Celis (1978) have shown that enzymes introduced by fusion are functional. Consequently we do not anticipate difficulty in introducing DNA present as phage or virus particles into the cytoplasm of recipient cells. We do not know however the ultimate fate of these particles in the recipient. Viruses are exceptionally resistant to DNases and proteases and so it is possible that they might persist indefinitely as intact virus particles. Alternatively there might be some mechanism akin to "uncoating" which would release the DNA, either in the cytoplasm or in the nucleus.

However we have also found that release of the DNA within the carrier erythrocyte can be readily accomplished so that DNA can be introduced into recipient cells either as free DNA or within virus particles. Bacteriophage lambda binds to a specific outer membrane protein on the bacterial cell surface, the lam B protein, which is a component of the maltose transport system. This protein is a single polypeptide of 47,000 MW (Endermann et al., 1978) which tends to aggregate in the absence of detergent (Roa and Scandella, 1976), as do many membrane proteins. The receptor binds to the tail fiber of phage lambda but wild type phage do not release their DNA directly as a consequence of this binding. However the addition of chloroform or ethanol to the phage-receptor complex causes the DNA to be ejected from the phage head through the tail (Randall-Hazelbauer and Schwartz, 1973).

A variant of lambda, λh exists which has an extended host range so that it can infect E. coli B193 or CR63 to which λ wild type will not absorb. λh mutants are readily selected by simply plating on these strains (Appleyard et al., 1956). The h mutations map in gene J which specifies the tail protein to which antibodies that neutralize phage infectivity bind. Phage carrying the λh host range mutation are directly inactivated with release of their DNA after binding the E. coli receptor (Randall-Hazelbauer and Schwartz, 1973). Consequently addition of chloroform or ethanol to accomplish irreversible binding and DNA release is not necessary with h phage. The same is true for wild type lambda if receptor protein isolated from certain other bacterial species such as Shigella is used (Schwartz and LeMinor, 1975).

Binding of the receptor to the phage occurs at 4°C but release of the DNA does not take place unless the temperature is raised above 15°C (Mackay and Bode, 1976). This permits the receptor to be bound to the phage at 4°C and the complex to be loaded into erythrocytes at 4°C. Alternatively receptor and phage may simply be mixed and loaded separately. DNA release then can be readily accomplished at a later time, such as during cell fusion, simply by raising the temperature.

PROTECTION OF THE DNA FROM DEGRADATION BY NUCLEASES

There is no danger of enzymatic degradation of the DNA in the erythrocyte as long as it is contained in virus particles. Even free DNA in the erythrocyte is not likely to be degraded since erythrocytes do not contain lysosomes or major amounts of degradative enzymes. However nucleases contaminating the receptor preparation would enter the erythrocyte during loading and could potentially degrade the DNA. This problem should be minimized by preparing receptor protein from E. coli endo I$^-$ exo I$^-$ deficient bacteria. Even rather unpurified preparations of receptor protein isolated from this bacterial strain can be used to release DNA in the erythrocyte without significant degradation of the DNA. It may however be that inclusion of receptor protein to release the DNA is not actually required. The λh virus, as originally observed by Randall-Hazelbauer and Schwartz (1973) and as confirmed by ourselves, is rather unstable and can spontaneously release its DNA. In our experiments using λh phage, a small fraction of the λh DNA is released in the erythrocytes even when the lambda receptor

protein is not added. This indicates that inclusion of lambda
receptor may not actually be necessary for λh phage and its omission
may actually be desirable because of possible nuclease contamination
in the receptor preparation.

PROTEINS AND DNA CAN BE TRANSFERRED TO RECIPIENT CELLS

As discussed earlier, erythrocytes may have important advantages over other DNA entry procedures. However the most important
advantage of erythrocyte carriers may be the ability to transfer
both DNA and various proteins such as histones, RNA polymerase, or
regulatory proteins. Since histones partition predominantly into
the nucleus, it is possible that their inclusion with the DNA
might facilitate entry of the DNA into the nucleus. A wide variety
of studies on the functions of histones and other enzymes and proteins might be possible using this system.

SURVIVAL OF ENTRAPPED VIRUSES IN VITRO

The possibility of using erythrocyte carriers to introduce
DNA into cells in vivo seems rather remote, if only because erythrocytes are generally confined to the vascular system and do not come
into contact with most cell types, although it is conceivable that
some sort of targeting and fusion mechanism might be developed.
Bacteriophage however provide a sensitive assay to determine
whether erythrocytes carrying virus could survive in the circulation
for any appreciable time and to determine whether the viruses are
shielded from the immune system. Circulatory half-lives of ϕX174
loaded into erythrocytes were determined in either sensitive mice
or mice immunized against ϕX174 (Humphreys et al., 1981). We found
that free phage injected into sensitive mice had essentially
disappeared after one day and free phage injected into immunized
mice could not be detected at any time after injection. ϕX174
encapsulated into erythrocytes however had a half-life of 4-6 days
and continued to circulate up to 30 days at which time the
experiment was terminated. Identical half lives were observed
whether the erythrocytes were injected into sensitive or immunized
mice. Normal mouse erythrocytes have been reported to have a half
life of 20 days as measured by the ^{51}Cr procedure. This experiment
directly demonstrates that carrier erythrocytes are capable of
survival for extended periods and that their contents are protected
from circulating antibodies.

ACKNOWLEDGMENTS

This work was supported by grant 1-618 from the National
Foundation - March of Dimes and by grants GM 24432 and GM 27727
from the National Institutes of Health.

REFERENCES

Alving, C. R., Steck, E. A., Chapman, W. L., Waits, V. B., Hendricks,
    L. D., Swartz, G. M., and Hanson, W. L., 1978, Therapy of
    leishmaniasis: Superior efficacies of liposome-encapsulated
    drugs, Proc. Nat. Acad. Sci. U.S.A., 75:2959.
Appleyard, R. K., McGregor, J. F., and Baird, K. M., 1956, Mutation
    to extended host range and the occurrence of phenotypic mixing
    in the temperate coliphage lambda, Virology, 2:565.
Black, C. D. V., Watson, G. J. and Ward, R. J., 1977, The use of
    Pentostam liposomes in the chemotherapy of experimental
    leishmaniasis. Trans. Royal Soc. Trop. Med. Hyg., 71:550.
Capecchi, M. R., Vonder Haar, R. A., Capecchi, N.E., and Sveda,
    M. M., 1977, The isolation of a suppressible nonsense mutant
    in mammalian cells, Cell, 12:371.
Capecchi, M. R., 1980, High efficiency transformation by direct
    microinjection of DNA into cultured mammalian cells, Cell,
    22:479.
Collins, J., and Bruning, H.J., 1978, Plasmids useable as gene-
    cloning vectors in an in vitro packaging by coliphage λ:
    "Cosmids", Gene, 4:85.
DeLoach, J., and Ihler, G., 1977, A dialysis procedure for loading
    erythrocytes with enzymes and lipids, Biochim. Biophys. Acta
    496:136.
DeLoach, J., Peters, S., Pinkard, O., Glew, R., and Ihler, G.,
    1977, Effect of glutaraldehyde treatment on enzyme-loaded
    erythrocytes, Biochim. Biophys. Acta 496:507.
de Wet, J. R., Daniels, D. L., Schroeder, J. L., Williams, B. G.,
    Denniston-Thompson, K., Moore, D. D., Blattner, F. F., 1980,
    Restriction maps for twenty-one Charon vector phages, J. Virol.
    33:401.
Endermann, R., Hindennach, I., and Henning, U., 1978, Major proteins
    of the Escherichia coli outer cell envelope membrane, FEBS
    Let., 88:71.
Hohn, B., and Murray, K., 1977, Packaging recombinant DNA molecules
    into bacteriophage particles in vitro, Proc. Nat. Acad. Sci. USA,
    74:3259.
Humphreys, J., Edlind, T., and Ihler, G., 1981, Entrapment of viral
    vectors for recombinant DNA in erythrocytes, J. Appl. Biochem.,
    (in press).
Ihler, G., 1979, Potential use of erythrocytes as carriers for
    enzymes and drugs, in:"Drug Carriers in Biology and Medicine",
    Gregoriadis, G., ed., Academic Press, London.
Kaiser, A. D., and Hogness, D. S., 1960, The transformation of
    Escherichia coli with deoxyribonucleic acid from bacteriophage
    lambda - dg, J. Mol. Biol. 2:392.
Kaltoft, K., and Celis, J. E., 1978, Ghost mediated transfer of
    human hypoxanthine-guanine phosphoribosyl transferase into
    deficient Chinese hamster ovary cells by means of polyethylene
    glycol-induced fusion, Exptl.Cell. Res., 115:423.

Loyter, A., Zakai, N., and Kulka, R. G., 1975, "Ultramicroinjection" of macromolecules or small particles into animal cells, J. Cell Biol., 66:292.

Mackay, D. J., and Bode, V. C., 1976, Binding to isolated phage receptors and λDNA release in vitro, 72:167.

Mandel, M., and Higa, A., 1970, Calcium-dependent bacteriophage DNA infection, J. Mol. Biol., 53:159.

Maniatis, T., Hardison, R. C., Lacy, E., Lauer, J., O'Connel, C., and Qon. D., 1978, The isolation of structural genes from libraries of eucaryotic DNA, Cell, 15:687.

New, R. R. C., Chance, M. L., Thomas, S. C., and Peters, W., 1978, Antileishmanial activity of antimonials entrapped in liposomes, Nature, 272:55.

Perucho, M., Hanahan, D., and Wigler, M., 1980, Genetic and physical linkage of exogenous sequences in transformed cells, Cell, 22:309.

Randall-Hazelbauer, L., and Schwartz, M., 1973, Isolation of the bacteriophage Lambda receptor from Escherichia coli, J. Bacteriol., 116:1436.

Roa, M., and Scandella, D., 1976, Multiple steps during the interaction between coliphage lambda and its receptor protein in vitro, Virology, 72:182.

Schlegel, R., and Rechsteiner, M., 1975, Microinjection of thymidine kinase and bovine serum albumin into mammalian cells by fusion with red blood cells, Cell. 5:371.

Schwartz, M., and Le Minor, L., 1975 Occurrence of the bacteriophage lambda receptor in some enterobacteriaceae, J. Virology, 15:679.

Sternberg. N., Tiemeier, D., and Enquist, L., 1977 In vitro packaging of a λ Dam vector containing EcoRl DNA fragments of Escherichia coli and phage Pl, Gene, 1:255.

Thomas, M., Cameron, J.R., and Davis, R. W., 1974. Viable molecular hybrids of bacteriophage lambda and eukaryotic DNA, Proc. Nat. Acad. Sci. USA., 71:4579.

Widder, K., Flouret, G., and Senyei, A., 1979, Magnetic microspheres: synthesis of a novel parenteral drug carrier, J. Pharm. Sci., 68:79.

Wigler, M., Sweet, R., Sim, G. K., Wold, B., Pellicer, A., Lacy, E., Maniatis, T., Silverstein, S., and Axel, R., 1979, Transformation of mammalian cells with genes from procaryotes and eucaryotes, Cell, 16:777.

TARGETING OF LIPOSOMES : STUDY OF INFLUENCING FACTORS

Gregory Gregoriadis, Christopher Kirby, Pamela Large,
Anne Meehan and Judith Senior

Division of Clinical Sciences, Clinical Research Centre
Watford Road, Harrow, Middx. HA1 3UJ, U.K.

INTRODUCTION

A decade has now elapsed since liposomes were first proposed[1-3] as vehicles for drug delivery in biology and medicine.
During this time extensive studies have revealed a multitude of
uses[4] and at the same time established many of the principles
governing the system's behaviour within the biological milieu.[5-7]
Among the advantages that liposomes offer as a drug carrier system,
versatility in structural characteristics is most prominent. For
instance, appropriate choice of lipid composition, size, surface
charge and also of surface ligands that can recognise and associate
with, target cells selectively can all profoundly influence the
fate and behaviour of the carrier and thus contribute towards
optimising the action of its drug contents. One of the major
objectives in the use of liposomes in vivo is interaction with
accessible cells i.e. those in the blood circulation, lining the
capillaries and, in certain cases, cells in extravascular areas
separated from the circulation by leaky membranes. There is,
therefore, a need for drugs to be retained by the carrier for
periods of time necessary for effective access to, and association
with the target. Here we have attempted to understand factors that
influence (a) quantitative retention of drugs by liposomes in vitro
and in vivo, (b) rates of liposome clearance from the circulation
and (c) targeting of liposomes to specific cells.

RETENTION OF DRUGS BY LIPOSOMES IN VITRO

Initial work from this laboratory showed[8] that despite quantitative retention of drugs by liposomes in the presence of buffer,
there was augmented leakage of drugs through the bilayers in the

155

circulation of injected animals. Such leakage was subsequently attributed[9] to the removal of liposomal phospholipid by plasma high density lipoproteins (HDL). This action of HDL on liposomes has now been confirmed in several laboratories.[10-14] In parallel work related to the use of liposomes as models of cell membranes it was shown[15-17] that the presence of cholesterol in liposomal membranes above the liquid-crystalline phase transition temperature (Tc) of the phospholipid component, leads to the packing of phospholipid molecules and reduction of bilayer permeability to solutes. Indeed, on this basis (i.e. reduced permeability because of molecular packing), several workers[4] with interest in preventing leakage of drugs in the presence of blood have used cholesterol-rich liposomes. It was, however, reasoned[18,19] that such packing could, in addition, prevent the removal of phospholipid molecules by HDL an event which, as it will be shown later, proved to be of central importance in controlling liposomal stability in the presence of blood. In work described below, all liposomes used were small unilamellar prepared by sonication followed by molecular sieve chromatography.[19-21] The choice of size was based on the ability of small liposomes to circulate in the blood longer than larger vesicle versions and on their anticipated freedom of passage through membranes with pores of a diameter down to 25-30 nm (the size of the smallest liposomes). Furthermore, carboxyfluorescein (CF) was used as a model solute in studies of bilayer permeability because, when entrapped at high concentrations (e.g. 0.1 M), CF self-quenches. However, the dye fluoresces upon leakage and dilution in the excess volume of the surrounding medium thus providing a rapid and direct method for the estimation of solute leakage.[19] Latent (non-leaked) CF is derived from $100 \, (Dye_t - Dye_f)/Dye_t$ where t and f denote total (measured in the presence of Triton X-100) and free dye respectively.[19] In addition to CF we have used two phase-specific anti-cancer drugs, namely melphalan and vincristine.

Table 1 shows that in the presence of buffer at 37°C, CF entrapped in small unilamellar liposomes composed of egg phosphatidylcholine (PC) retains most of its latency irrespective of the liposomal cholesterol content. In the presence of serum, however, CF latency is rapidly reduced to very low values when liposomes are devoid of cholesterol, presumably because of phospholipid loss to HDL.[9-14] Addition of some cholesterol (PC:cholesterol molar ratio 7:2) enables liposomal CF to retain a considerable proportion of its latency in the presence of serum whilst in liposomes composed of equimolar amounts of phospholipid and cholesterol CF latency is maintained fully (Table 1). This effect of cholesterol in reducing CF leakage from liposomes is also apparent when two other unsaturated phospholipids, dioleoyl phosphatidylcholine (DOPC) and sphingomyelin (SM) are used (Table 1). However, there are quantitative differences. In the presence of buffer, for instance, leakage of CF from cholesterol-free SM liposomes is much more extensive (latency down to 54%) than it is

Table 1. The effect of cholesterol content of liposomes on
their stability in the presence of serum.*

| | CF latency (%) | | | |
| Liposomes | Buffer | | Serum | |
	3 min	60 min	3 min	60 min
PC	98.0	85.6	5.1	0.0
PC:CHOL(1:0.28)	95.1	93.0	32.2	0.0
PC:CHOL(1:1) **	96.5	96.0	100.0	98.7
DOPC	92.3	70.4	58.4	0
DOPC:CHOL(1:0.28)	94.3	80.4	95.1	25.4
DOPC:CHOL(1:1)	99.7	96.6	96.6	86.3
SM	61.4	54.0	57.8	35.4
SM:CHOL(1:0.28)	99.1	89.8	90.4	93.2
SM:CHOL(1:1)	93.6	89.6	100.0	95.0

*Liposomes containing 0.25 M CF and composed of PC, DOPC or SM
without or with cholesterol (CHOL) (phospholipid : cholesterol
molar ratios shown in parentheses) were incubated in the presence
of phosphate buffer or mouse serum at 37°C. CF latency values at
3 and 60 min are expressed as % of latencies (90-98%) in the
preparations before use. Similar values to those in the presence
of serum were obtained when liposomes were incubated in the
presence of mouse whole blood.[21]
**After incubation in the presence of whole blood for 2 h CF
latency value was 98.0%.

for similar PC and DOPC vesicles. Since SM forms liposomes with a
broad Tc of 25-40°C, destabilisation of membranes is expected to
occur at the temperature of incubation (37°C). On the other hand,
in the presence of serum, leakage from SM, and to some extent from
DOPC cholesterol-rich liposomes, is not as drastic as in similar PC
liposomes. Thus, CF latency of SM liposomes is reduced to only 35%
after 60 minutes (Table 1). Indeed, serum-induced latency loss may
be even lower if one considers the loss contributed by the temperature of the experiment (i.e. CF latency of 54% on incubation in
buffer at 37°C, Table 1). Furthermore, the action of the sterol
content (e.g. 1:0.28 molar ratio) in reducing leakage of CF from SM
and DOPC liposomes is more pronounced than it is for PC liposomes
(Table 1) suggesting that the anticipated[22] removal of liposomal SM
and DOPC by serum HDL is less efficient. A similar action of
cholesterol in reducing permeability of liposomes to CF is observed
in vesicles composed of a variety of other phospholipids[20,21]

Table 2.   The effect of the cholesterol content of liposomes
on their stability in the presence of whole blood.*

Lipid composition	CF latency (%)	
Dilauroyl phosphatidylcholine	Nil	(58.0)
Dimyristoyl phosphatidylcholine	Nil	(66.8)
Distearoyl phosphatidylcholine	86.5	(93.5)
Dioleoyl phosphatidylcholine	Nil	(90.1)
Egg phosphatidylcholine	Nil	(81.1)
Sphingomyelin	27.5	(96.6)
Dilauroyl phosphatidylcholine, cholesterol	49.4	(96.7)
Dimyristoyl phosphatidylcholine, cholesterol	94.7[a]	(99.2)
Distearoyl phosphatidylcholine, cholesterol	32.4[c]	(98.9)
Dioleoyl phosphatidylcholine, cholesterol	88.4	(97.5)
Egg phosphatidylcholine, cholesterol	86.3	(97.0)
Sphingomyelin, cholesterol	97.6[b]	(98.8)

[a]Incubated for 6 h; [b]incubated for 12 h; [c]1:0.25
phospholipid:cholesterol molar ratio

*Small unilamellar liposomes (2 μmol phospholipid) composed of
various phospholipids without or with cholesterol (1:1 molar ratio)
and containing 0.25 M CF, were incubated with 10 volumes mouse
heparinized fresh blood at 37°C for 1 h unless otherwise stated.
Typical CF latency values shown here are means of duplicate readings
and are expressed as % of the latencies (shown in parentheses) of the
respective liposomal preparations[20]

(Table 2). However, with phospholipids (e.g. distearoyl phosphatidylcholine (DSPC) (Table 2), dipalmitoyl phosphatidylcholine and
other phospholipids with saturated fatty acid esters of more than 16
carbon atoms[20,21]) that have a Tc above or at 37°, incorporation of
excess cholesterol renders the bilayers fluid. This, at 37°C (incubation temperature), enhances CF latency loss presumably because
fluid bilayers are conducive to the removal of phospholipid molecules
by HDL.

The proposition[9-14] that cholesterol reduces solute leakage
through prevention of liposomal phospholipid loss to HDL was tested
with CF-containing liposomes labelled with tritiated PC, incubated

in the presence of serum and the mixture passed through an Ultrogel
column.[12] It was shown that, with cholesterol-free liposomes, only
a fraction of ^{3}H-PC and CF markers applied to the column elutes as
intact vesicles the remainder being recovered in a peak (as ^{3}H-PC)
containing HDL and as a free CF respectively. The presence of increasing amounts of cholesterol in the liposomal membrane proportionally reduces the amounts of ^{3}H-PC appearing with HDL and of free CF.
Indeed, fractionation of lipoproteins in the above liposome-serum
mixture revealed[12] that with decreasing liposomal cholesterol content
increasing amounts of tritiated PC are found associated with HDL.
Although the mode by which HDL remove phospholipid from liposomes is
not well understood at present, it is thought[11] that hydrophobic
regions of HDL are inserted into the bilayer prior to binding with
the phospholipid and that packing of bilayers by the sterol is likely
to obstruct this insertion.

Destabilisation of liposomes by plasma HDL is believed to be
synonymous with their total destruction.[23] However, the quantitative
release of solutes from liposomes observed in the presence of serum
(Tables 1 and 2) could also be compatible with the formation in otherwise intact membranes of pores through which solutes up to a certain
size can pass freely.[18] Recently, we have attempted[24] to establish
which of the two events occurs, in two ways: (a) radiolabelled solutes of various molecular weights were incorporated into PC liposomes
and their release in the presence of plasma was measured. If liposomes do indeed break down, release of contents into the media would
then occur independently of solute size. On the other hand, preferential release of solutes favouring those of smaller size would be
accounted for by pore formation;   (b) buffer-loaded PC liposomes

Table 3. Release of solutes from liposomes in the presence of
          plasma*

Liposomes	Sucrose	Inulin	Polyvinyl-pyrrolidone
Cholesterol-free	80.6±10.4(3)	68.9±6.9(3)	26.9±3.7(3)
Cholesterol-poor	42.2±2.8(3)	31.1±7.2(3)	26.1±3.0(3)
Cholesterol-rich	4.1±2.1(3)	7.7±0.9(3)	6.6,7.7

*Small unilamellar liposomes containing radiolabelled sucrose,
inulin and polyvinylpyrrolidone were incubated in the presence of
mouse plasma at 37°C for 30 min. Samples were then chromatographed
on Ultrogel AcA 34 columns. Radioactivity released from liposomes
and eluted in corresponding fractions was pooled and expressed
as a percentage of the total applied. Results are means ±
S.D. for the numbers of experiments indicated in parentheses.[24]

were exposed to plasma containing 0.2M CF.   At this concentration
the dye is, as already mentioned, fully quenched and should there be
formation of pores in the vesicles, CF would diffuse into their
interior.   Upon re-isolation, liposomes should then contain self-
quenched dye.   Table 3 showing the extent of release of sucrose,
inulin and polyvinylpyrrolidone after incubation of the liposome-
entrapped markers in the presence of plasma, confirms that solute
release is dependant on size. With cholesterol-free liposomes, for
instance, 80.6, 68.9 and 26.9% of sucrose, inulin and polyvinylpyrrolidone respectively are released (Table 3).   Such preferential
loss of the smaller sucrose and inulin molecules argue against membrane fragmentation or major disruption and are consistent with the
retention of a closed, albeit leaky, vesicle structure. Because of
the similarity of loss of the two smaller solutes (Table 3), pores
formed are likely to be wide enough to allow relatively free passage
of sucrose and inulin but not of polyvinylpyrrolidone.   Enrichment
of liposomes with some cholesterol (PC: cholesterol molar ratio 7:2),
reduces the size of pores to the extent that inulin loss (31.1%) is
now similar to that of polyvinylpyrrolidone (26.1) whereas that of
sucrose (42.2) is still relatively high (Table 3). The size of pores
in such cholesterol-poor liposomes is now small enough to restrict
the passage of inulin and polyvinylpyrrolidone more than it does with
that of sucrose. With liposomes composed of equimolar PC and cholesterol, release of all solutes is low (4.1 - 7.7%) and any pores
present must be too small even for sucrose (Table 3). Results from
the reverse experiment i.e. incubation of buffer-loaded liposomes
with or without cholesterol in the presence of plasma containing
quenched CF showed[24] that after chromatography of the incubation
mixtures, fractions expected to contain liposomes also contained
latent CF indicating entry of dye into vesicles, presumably through
formed pores.

     In subsequent work, the effect of the cholesterol content
of liposomes on the release of entrapped ^{14}C-melphalan and
[3]H-vincristine in the presence of plasma was also investigated[25].
Cholesterol-free and cholesterol-rich liposomes containing the two
drugs were incubated with mouse plasma at 37°C and aliquots removed
at time intervals fractionated on Ultrogel AcA 34 columns. Fig. 1
shows drug elution profiles after incubation for 2.5 minutes. With
each type of liposome (both drugs), portions of the radiolabel are
eluted with liposomes in peak a corresponding to the void volume of
the columns and as additional peaks, peak d representing released
free drug and peaks b and c representing drug probably bound to plasma
proteins[25]. Indeed, the involvement of plasma in both release of
drug from liposomes and drug appearance in peaks b and c is supported
by the finding[25] that after incubation with PBS[25] and chromatography
more than 95% of the radioactivity applied is recovered with peak a
and none with fractions related to peaks b and c (not shown). A large
number of anti-cancer drugs bind non-specifically to plasma proteins
(an event often paralleled by high drug lipophilicity) and although

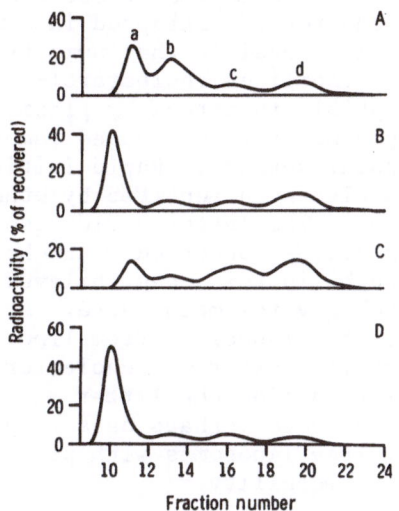

Fig. 1.   The effect of liposomal cholesterol on drug release from
           PC liposomes during incubation with plasma. Cholesterol-
           free (A,C) and cholesterol-rich (B,D) liposomes containing
           ^{3}H-vincristine (A,B) or ^{14}C-melphalan (C,D) were incubated
           with mouse plasma at 37°C. After 2.5 min. samples were
           removed and chromatographed on Ultrogel AcA 34 and fractions
           collected analysed for radioactivity. Values in each of
           the peaks obtained are expressed as % of total radioactivity
           recovered from the columns. Recoveries were 95-100% of the
           quantities applied[25].

many of these drugs have a greater affinity for plasma albumin,
vincristine is unusual in that it binds more strongly to α and β
globulins[26]. It seems, therefore, likely that peak b corresponds to

the fractions where these globulins are eluted and that peak c is
associated with the presence of some other component (e.g. albumin).
Quantitation of drug release from liposomes (Table 4) showed that as
with CF (Table 1), loss of the two drugs from cholesterol-free liposomes soon after mixing with plasma was pronounced especially in the
case of melphalan (85.5% total released as peaks b, c and d, Table 4).
On the other hand, total (peaks, b, c and d) drug loss from cholesterol-rich liposomes was less and amounted to 31.8 (melphalan) and
50.1% (vincristine) of the applied radioactivity (Table 4). Such
losses were, however, much greater than those (less than 5%) observed
under identical conditions for CF entrapped in similar PC liposomes
(Table 1). Although it is possible that some type of drug-lipid
interaction partially destabilises cholesterol-rich liposomes or
renders them more susceptible to attack by plasma HDL, we subscribe
to the possibility of plasma protein-induced removal of drugs weakly
adsorbed onto the liposomal surface. Rapid initial loss of vincristine from liposomes has also been reported by others[27] and attributed
to reversal of adsorption. The latter could also account for some of
the plasma-induced drug release observed with cholesterol-free liposomes (see below) although, in this case, bilayer destabilization
by plasma HDL[9-14] is probably the main cause. At subsequent time
intervals drugs continue to dissociate from liposomes at rates which
for up to 15 min. are still greater for cholesterol-free liposomes.
Thereafter, drug association from the latter parallels that observed
with cholesterol-rich liposomes perhaps as a result of gradual enrichment of the cholesterol-free liposomes with plasma cholesterol in
turn reducing membrane permeability.[25]

Table 4. Release of melphalan and vincristine from cholesterol-free
          and cholesterol-rich liposomes in the presence of plasma.*

Drug	Liposomes	Peaks b and c		Peak d	
		2.5 min	65 min	2.5 min	65 min
Melphalan	PC	44.0	48.0	38.5	45.0
	PC:CHOL	20.7	26.1	11.1	17.0
Vincristine	PC	50.0	55.4	19.3	32.9
	PC:CHOL	21.0	24.1	29.1	34.5

*Cholesterol-free or cholesterol-rich (molar ratio 1:1) small unila-
mellar PC liposomes contained ^{14}C-melphalan or ^{3}H-vincristine. Liposomes were incubated in the presence of mouse plasma at 37°C for 2.5
and 65 min and samples were subsequently chromatographed. Released
^{14}C and ^{3}H radioactivity in peaks b, c and d was then measured and
expressed as % of total recovered. Recoveries were 94.6-99.1% of the
radioactivity applied.[25]

RETENTION OF DRUGS BY LIPOSOMES <u>IN VIVO</u>

Reduction of solute leakage from liposomes as a result of
the presence of cholesterol in the bilayers is also observed in the
blood circulation of animals after intravenous injection.[19]
For instance, with PC liposomes containing equimolar amounts of
cholesterol, CF clearance is linear, probably reflecting the rate of
clearance of its carrier. This was, in fact, established in
experiments[19] in which CF-containing liposomes were labelled with
[14]C-cholesteryl oleate : CF/^{14}C ratios in blood samples obtained at
time intervals were almost identical to that (unity) in the injected

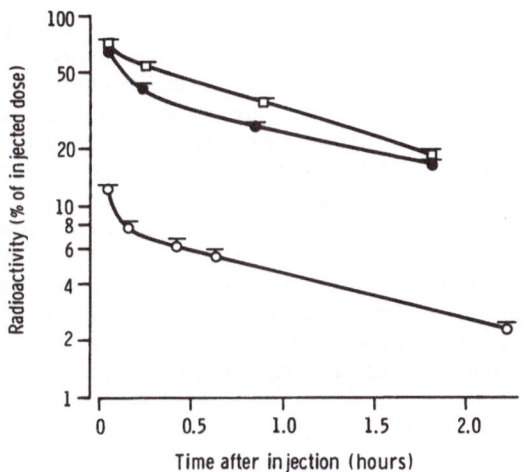

Fig. 2. The effect of the cholesterol content of liposomes contain-
         ing ^{14}C-melphalan on drug clearance from the blood of
         injected mice. Melphalan was administered intravenously in
         the free form (O) or entrapped in cholesterol-free (●)
         or cholesterol-rich (□) PC liposomes. Mice were bled
         from the tail vein at time intervals and plasma analysed
         for radioactivity. Values (means from 4 animals) are
         expressed as % ± S.E. of the injected dose per total mouse
         plasma.[25]

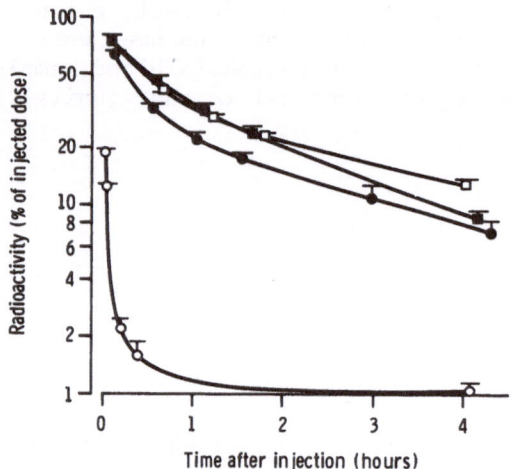

Fig. 3. The effect of the cholesterol content of liposomes containing ^{3}H-vincristine on drug clearance from the blood of
injected mice. Vincristine was administered intravenously
in the free form (O) or entrapped in cholesterol-free PC
liposomes or in PC liposomes also containing varying amounts
of cholesterol. Clearance values for drug administered in
cholesterol-free or cholesterol-containing (molar ratio
1:0.2) liposomes (●) and in cholesterol-containing liposomes with molar ratios of 1:0.4, and 1:0.6 (■) and of
1:0.8 and 1:1 (□) were pooled because of value similarity
within pairs. Values (means from 8 animals; 4 of each of
the two liposome types) are expressed as % ± S.E. of the
injected dose per total mouse plasma.[25]

preparation. As expected from the in-vitro work,[12] cholesterol was
found to act similarly _in vivo_ by preventing PC loss to HDL.[13]

We have, in addition, studied[25] the effect of cholesterol
presence in ^{14}C-melphalan and ^{3}H-vincristine-containing liposomes on

drug clearance from the blood of injected animals. Figs. 2 and 3
show that the rapid (5% of injected radioactivity retained in blood
in 1 h) clearance of the radiolabelled drugs administered as free is
reduced considerably (25% retained) by their previous entrapment in
cholesterol-free liposomes. Clearance rates are further reduced
(35% retained) when drugs are entrapped in cholesterol-rich liposomes.
However, such reduction in clearance rates promoted by the presence
of cholesterol were measurable only above a certain phospholipid :
cholesterol molar ratio (e.g. 1:0.4 in the case of vincristine, Fig. 3)
and did not appear to be as great as when CF was the entrapped solute
(5 and 65% of the injected dye retained in 1 h for cholesterol-free
and cholesterol-rich liposomes respectively).[19] Furthermore, whereas
clearance of CF administered in cholesterol-rich liposomes was
linear[19] i.e. identical to that of its carrier, clearance of melphalan
and vincristine entrapped in similar liposomes was biphasic showing a
rapid initial phase followed by a prolonged linear one (Figs. 2 and 3).
In contrast to the highly polar CF, melphalan and vincristine are
lipophilic and, therefore, likely to leak through the bilayers. This
and the anticipated drug binding to plasma proteins (Fig. 1) would be
expected to influence overall clearance rates considerably. It is
thus apparent from data shown in Figs. 2 and 3 and Table 4 that
patterns of drug clearance observed in vivo are the sum total of
clearances of entrapped, protein-bound and free drugs. To accurately
estimate the effect of the cholesterol content of injected liposomes
on the extent to which drugs circulate at any given time in association with the carrier, cholesterol-free and cholesterol-rich liposomes
containing ^{3}H-vincristine were injected intravenously into mice which
were then bled at time intervals and blood plasma fractionated on
Ultrogel. Liposome-associated drug values (peak a) plotted in Fig. 4
are now free of interference from leaked protein-bound or free drug
and reveal the considerable effect of cholesterol in reducing the
rate of clearance of vincristine from the circulation (compare with
data in Figs. 2 and 3). They also suggest that intermediate concentration of cholesterol as used in Fig. 3 may lead to distinct corresponding rates of drug clearance.

CONTROL OF THE RATE OF CLEARANCE OF LIPOSOMES FROM THE CIRCULATION

     A possible role of the phospholipid component of liposomes on
their rate of clearance from the blood circulation has been recently
investigated[20,21]. CF was again used as a model solute since with
liposomes from which dye leakage in the circulating blood is nil or
minimal, clearance rates of quenched CF should closely represent
that of the carrier. Therefore, liposomes showing (Table 2) very
little permeability to CF in the presence of whole blood at 37°C,
were used. Data in Fig. 5 and in published work[20,21] reveal that
quenched CF clearance rates from the blood of intravenously injected
mice correspond to half-lives ranging from 0.1 h (cholesterol-rich
DLPC liposomes) to a maximum of 16 h (cholesterol-rich SM liposomes). An almost identical half-life of small unilamellar liposomes made of sphingomyelin and cholesterol has also been observed

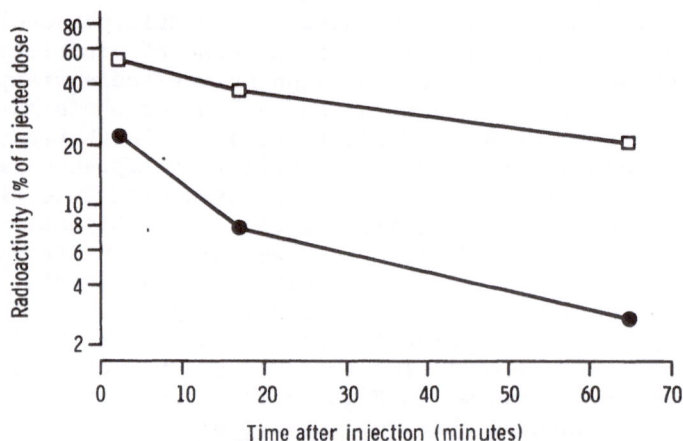

Fig. 4.   The effect of liposomal cholesterol on the clearance of
          entrapped vincristine. Cholesterol-free (●) and choles-
          terol-rich (□) PC liposomes containing ^{3}H-vincristine
          were injected intravenously into mice (3 in each group).
          Animals were bled at time intervals and plasma samples
          chromatographed on Ultrogel AcA 34 columns. Radioactivity
          eluting in the fractions corresponding to the liposomal
          peak (peak a) was then estimated and expressed as % (mean)
          of the total radioactivity injected per total mouse plasma.
          Recovery of radioactivity from the columns was 96-99% of the
          quantities applied.[25]

by others.[28] Since there is inevitably some leakage of CF into the
circulation, especially for liposomes made of DLPC (see Table 2),
half-lives shown (Fig. 5 and legend) may be underestimates of those
of the vesicles themselves. However, with cholesterol-rich PC,
DMPC and SM liposomes exhibiting nearly full CF retention in the
presence of blood (Table 2) the use of tritiated PC as a marker of
the lipid phase shows that both CF and the marker ^{3}H are cleared at
nearly identical rates (Fig. 6). These data confirm that such
cholesterol-rich liposomes retain much of their integrity while in
the circulation. Furthermore, after intraperitoneal injection,

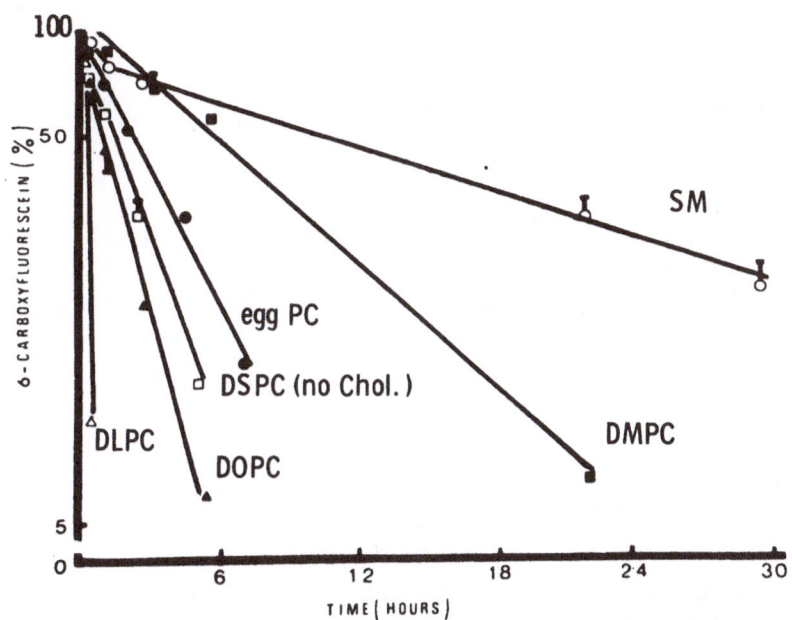

Fig. 5.   The effect of the phospholipid component of liposomes on the
          clearance of entrapped CF from the blood of injected mice.
          Mice were bled at time intervals after intravenous injection
          with CF entrapped in small unilamellar liposomes (3 mg
          phospholipid) composed of dilauroyl phosphatidyl choline
          (△), dioleoyl phosphatidylcholine (▲), distearoyl
          phosphatidylcholine (□), egg phosphatidylcholine (●),
          dimyristoyl phosphatidylcholine (■) or sphingomyelin (○).
          With the exception of liposomes made of distearoyl phospha-
          tidylcholine, all preparations contained cholesterol (1:1
          molar ratio). Latent CF values (means from 3 animals) in
          total mouse plasma are expressed as % of latent CF injected
          (SE ⟨3% are shown). Half-lives estimated from slopes were
          DLPC, 0.1; DOPC, 1; DSPC, 1.5; egg PC, 2; DMPC, 6;
          sphingomyelin, 16h.[20]

cholesterol-rich liposomes enter the circulation quantitatively and
in intact form[21] probably through the lymphatics. Fig. 6 shows that
although rates of entry are not dependant on the phospholipid
composition of liposomes, clearance rates from the circulation
corresponded to those (Fig. 5) measured after intravenous injection.
As discussed elsewhere[20,21] half-lives of liposomes bear no obvious
relationship to the physical characteristics (e.g. Tc) of the phospholipid component. However, whatever the liposomal surface

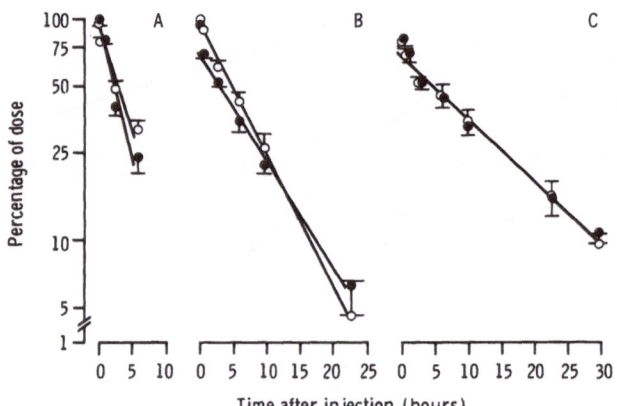

Fig. 6. Clearance of cholesterol-rich liposomes from the blood of
injected mice. Mice in groups of 3 were injected into the
tail vein with cholesterol-rich (phospholipid:cholesterol
molar ratios 1:1) small unilamellar liposomes composed of
PC (A), DMPC (B) or SM (C). All preparations contained
0.25 M CF and were labelled with tracer ^{3}H-PC. Values of
latent CF (O) and ^{3}H (●) in total blood are expressed as
% ± S.D. of the injected dose. In one experiment in which
mice were injected with cholesterol-rich SM liposomes
labelled with ^{14}C-SM, half-life was identical to that of
^{3}H in C.[21]

properties that enable some preparations to persist in the blood
longer than others, these must be considered in conjunction with the
mechanism(s) responsible for the recognition and uptake of liposomes
by the liver and spleen. It is known, for instance, that plasma
components such as α_1-macroglobulin[29] and other proteins[30] coat
liposomes upon contact and it may be that this opsonizes them for
phagocytosis by the reticuloendothelial system. It is conceivable
that the efficiency of this process is reduced by certain phospho-

lipids and augmented by others.

As expected, variation in the half-lives of liposomes is reflected in the extent of uptake of entrapped solute by the liver and spleen.[20]   Here, we have used as a model solute ^{111}In-labelled bleomycin because ^{111}In, unlike CF, persists in tissues for several days[31] thus allowing measurement of tissue radioactivity content at a time (e.g. 72 h after injection) when blood radioactivity is very low.[31] Therefore, the total amount of solute carried to tissues by a given liposomal preparation can be determined. Our data[20] show that injection of mice with liposomes of increasing half-lives is associated with decreasing transport of radioactivity to the liver and spleen. Thus, hepatic uptake of ^{111}In is reduced from 32% (PC) to 23% (DMPC) and 16% (SM liposomes) per g tissue.

More recent results[25] suggest that the effect[20,21] of the phospholipid component of liposomes on entrapped CF clearance from the circulation may not be as distinct with other solutes (e.g. melphalan and vincristine). Fig. 7 shows that, as with CF (Fig. 5), drugs administered in cholesterol-rich SM liposomes remain in the circulation of intravenously injected mice for a considerably longer period than when given in similar PC or DMPC liposomes. However, whereas CF clearance is for all three types of liposomes, linear throughout (Fig. 6), those of melphalan and vincristine are biphasic with a rapid initial phase followed by a slower linear one (Fig. 7). The rapid loss of drugs during the initial phase may, as discussed above, reflect dissociation of drugs adsorbed onto the liposomal membrane and their subsequent rapid distribution into extravascular compartments. This and an increased leakage (and ensuing clearance) of the lipophilic drugs from liposomes during the second slower phase may have contributed to the overall drug clearance rates which are considerably lower than those of CF in liposomes of corresponding phospholipid composition. Furthermore, and in contrast to the behaviour of CF (Fig. 5), drug clearance rates for PC and DMPC liposomes are nearly identical (Fig. 7). Again, it could be that any existing differences in drug clearance between the two types of liposomes have been (as in the case of liposomes with varying cholesterol content; Figs. 2 and 3) masked by the binding of released drug to plasma proteins.

As treatment of experimental tumours is often carried out through the intraperitoneal route, it was of interest to see whether liposomal drugs behave similarly to CF (i.e. entry of entrapped solute into the periphery via intact liposomes) and if so, to study their rates of clearance from the circulation. Results in Fig. 8 show that after intraperitoneal injection of mice with cholesterol-rich liposomes composed of PC, DMPC or SM and containing vincristine, patterns of drug entry into the circulation are very similar for the three preparations each showing a peak of blood radioactivity (24.1 - 29.5% of the dose) at 2 h. This compares with a peak concentration

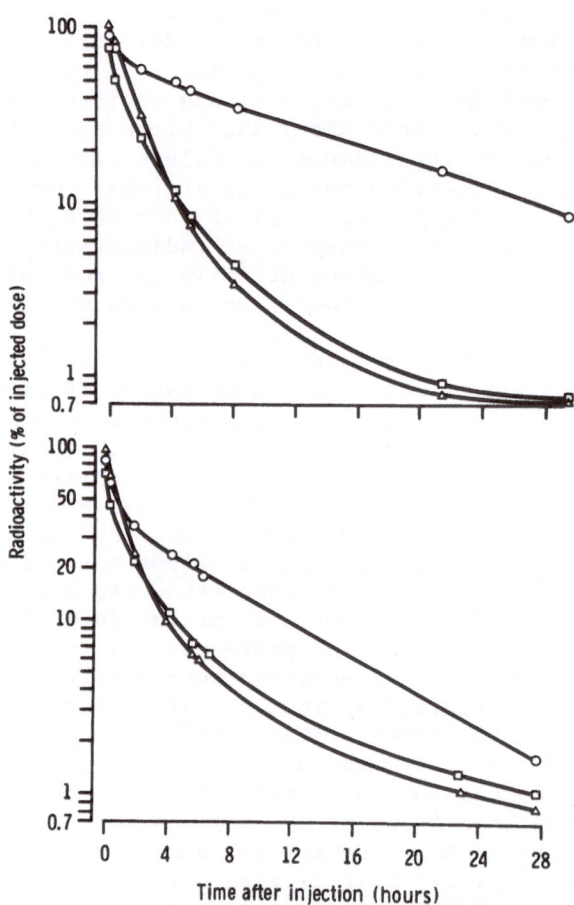

Fig. 7. The effect of phospholipid composition of liposomes containing ^{14}C-melphalan or ^{3}H-vincristine on drug clearance from the blood of injected mice. Cholesterol-rich PC ($\triangle$), DMPC ($\square$) and SM ($\bigcirc$) liposomes containing ^{14}C-melphalan (upper) or ^{3}H-vincristine (lower) were injected intravenously into mice which were bled at time intervals. Plasma was analysed for radioactivity and values (means from 4 animals) are expressed as % of the injected dose per total mouse plasma. Standard errors (not shown) were all less than 4%.[25]

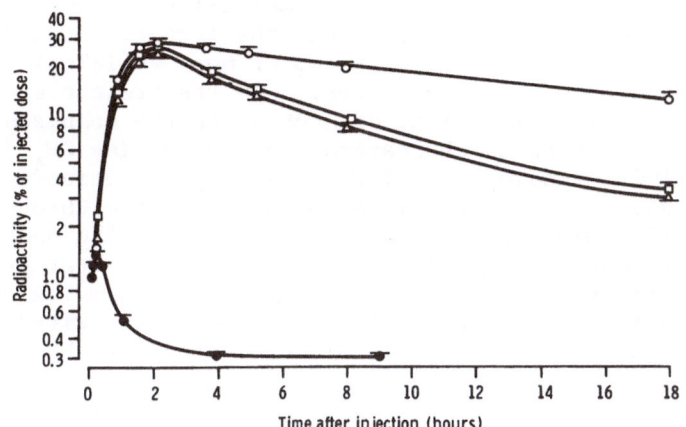

Fig. 8.   The effect of phospholipid composition of liposomes containing ^{3}H-vincristine on drug clearance from the blood
of injected mice.   Vincristine in the free form (●) or
entrapped in cholesterol-rich PC (△), DMPC (□) or SM (○)
liposomes was injected intraperitoneally into mice which
were then bled at time intervals.   Plasma was analysed for
radioactivity and values (means from 4 animals) are
expressed at % ± S.E.[25]

of 1.4% at 9 min for the free drug (Fig. 8) of which the rate of
entry into the blood is, apparently, lower than its rate of clearance.   On the other hand, rates of clearance of liposomal vincristine from the blood (Fig. 8) differed according to the phospholipid component of the carrier and patterns were similar to those
observed after intravenous injection (Fig. 3).   Overall clearance
rates were, however, reduced presumably because of a more rapid
liposomal drug entry into the periphery than exit from it.

EFFECT OF STORAGE ON SOLUTE RETENTION BY LIPOSOMES AND SOLUTE
CLEARANCE FROM THE CIRCULATION

Application of liposomes in the clinic will only be widely
accepted when some of the more practical aspects of this carrier

system are considered. These include the effect of prolonged
storage on liposomal stability. Stability is defined here as (a)
the extent to which liposomes retain entrapped drugs and (b) the
extent to which liposomal drugs upon intravenous injection retain
their clearance rates (as measured before storage). The former is
intended to show changes in bilayer permeability of stored liposomes
as such or in the presence of blood and the latter, changes in liposomal size (e.g. through fusion of two or more vesicles) in turn
leading to changes in clearance rates.[4] In the present studies[32]
liposomes were small unilamellar of neutral charge composed of PC,
DMPC or SM with or without cholesterol and containing CF, [3]H- vincristine and ^{14}C-melphalan. Following their preparation[32] drug-
containing liposomes were sterilised by passing them through Milli-
pore filters (0.22 μm pore diameter) and stored at 4°C under nitrogen
in sealed vials until required. At time intervals after preparation
aliquots (50 μl) of the liposomal suspensions (0.5 μmoles of phospholipid and 0, 0.14 or 0.5 μmoles of cholesterol) were withdrawn and
diluted to 0.5 ml with mouse whole blood or phosphate buffered 1%

Table 5. The effect of storage on drug retention by
cholesterol-rich liposomes*

Drug	Storage (days)	Retention (%)		
		PC CHOL	DMPC CHOL	SM CHOL
CF	6	98.1		
	16	92.3		
	40	85.8		
	78	86.9		
Vincristine	6	95.6		
	16	98.6	97.5	97.4
	40	94.2	95.8	95.1
	78	93.1	94.2	93.7
Melphalan	6	99.3		
	18	91.7	97.0	94.8
	38	96.3	98.1	95.3
	80	67.3	96.2	97.1

*Small unilamellar liposomes composed of PC, DMPC or SM and equi-
molar cholesterol (CHOL) and containing CF, ^{3}H-vincristine or
[14]C-melphalan were stored as described in the text. At time
intervals, solute retention was estimated and expressed as % of
drug contained in liposomes on the day of preparation.[32]

NaCl (PBS).[19,32] Drug retention by liposomes was determined before
and after 30 minutes incubation at 37°C in either PBS or whole blood.
In each case, released drug was separated from entrapped drug by
gel filtration on a Sephadex G-200 column and expressed as % of drug
contained in liposomes on the day of their preparation. The effect
of storage on the clearance rates of liposomes was investigated by
injecting 50 μl liposomes stored for various periods of time, into
the tail vein of mice which were then killed 10 minutes later. In
control experiments, mice were injected with equivalent amounts of
free drug. Drug content in blood samples was expressed as % of the
injected dose per ml blood.

Table 5 and Figs. 9 and 10 show respectively drug retention by
cholesterol-rich liposomes after storage for up to 80 days and the
effect of such storage on drug retention upon exposure to PBS or
whole blood for 30 minutes at 37°C. It is apparent that storage of
PC liposomes for the period of time studied leads to only minor
leakage of CF and vincristine (86.9 and 93.1% retained respectively;
Table 5). On the other hand, leakage of melphalan is more pronounced
(67.3% retained; Table 5). With the other two types of cholesterol-
rich liposomes (DMPC and SM) retention values of vincristine and
melphalan are high (93.7% after 78 days of storage; Table 5). Such
pronounced retention of drugs is maintained fully after incubation
of stored PC and SM liposomes in the presence of PBS at 37°C (Figs.
9 and 10). However, after exposure to whole blood, whilst retention
values for vincristine and melphalan are reduced considerably those
of CF remain virtually unchanged (Fig. 9). This blood induced loss
of vincristine and melphalan from cholesterol-rich liposomes is
constant throughout the entire storage period (Fig. 9) and can be
largely attributed to reversal of drug absorption onto the liposomal
surface (see above). It also appears that SM liposomes (Fig. 10)
are more effective in retaining vincristine and melphalan than are
PC liposomes (Fig. 9). This finding is consistent with previous data
obtained with the two types of liposome containing CF (Table 1). In
other storage experiments in which cholesterol-free or cholesterol-
poor liposomes were used, drug retention values after incubation in
PBS retained their initial high levels throughout the 80-day storage
period. However, after incubation in whole blood, values were lower
than those observed with cholesterol-rich liposomes but, again remained constant[32] i.e. independant of storage time.

The effect of storage on the rates of clearance of entrapped
drugs (e.g. vincristine) after intravenous injection is shown in
Fig. 11. As expected from work discussed earlier (Figs. 2 and 3),
liposomal drug levels in the blood are directly proportional to the
cholesterol content of (PC) liposomes. In the case of cholesterol-
rich liposomes, such levels also depend on the phospholipid component. For instance drug levels for PC, DMPC and SM liposomes
increase in that order. Fig. 11 shows in addition that storage
of all types of liposomes studied does not significantly influence
drug level values in the blood.

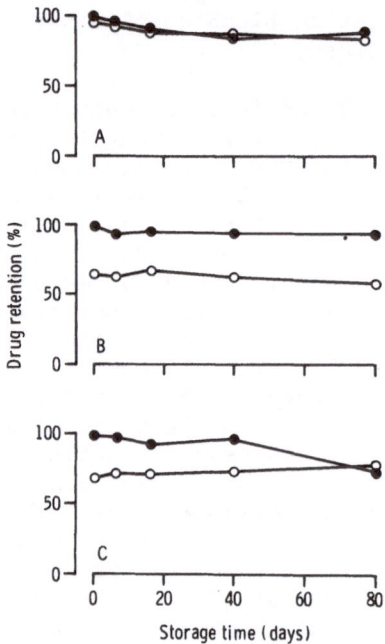

Fig. 9. The effect of storage on drug retention by liposomes
         exposed to blood. Small unilamellar liposomes composed
         of PC and cholesterol (molar ratio 1:1) and containing CF
         (A) ^{3}H-vincristine (B) or melphalan (C) were stored as
         described in the text. At time intervals samples were
         exposed to PBS (O) or mouse whole blood (●) for 30 min
         at 37°C. Drug retention by liposomes was then estimated
         and expressed as % of the drug contained on the day of
         preparation.[32]

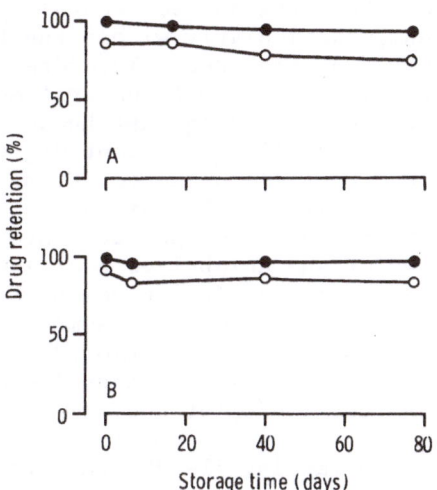

Fig. 10. The effect of storage on drug retention by liposomes
          exposed to blood. Small unilamellar liposomes composed
          of SM and cholesterol (molar ratio 1:1) and containing
          ^{3}H-vincristine (A) or ^{14}C-melphalan (B) were stored as
          described in the test.[32] For other details see legend
          to Fig. 9.

TARGETING OF LIPOSOMES

    Effective use of liposomes as drug carriers will require access
to, and interaction with, cell targets.[4] However, with the exception of cells associated with the reticuloendothelial system and
which show an increased avidity for injected liposomes, other cells
take up liposomes only poorly and non-selectively.[4] Early
attempts[31,33] to target liposomes have shown that IgG raised against
tumours and subsequently incorporated on the surface of drug-containing liposomes can mediate uptake of the carrier and its contents by

the respective target cells. Although there is now convincing evidence[34-39] that liposomes coated with antibodies in a variety of ways interact with target cells selectively, understanding of factors that influence such interaction is poor. It would be of interest, for instance, to know the relative importance in targeting of antibody purity, stability of antibody-coated liposomes, availability of the antigen-recognising regions of IgG on the liposomal surface and ability of these regions to recognise and interact with the respective antigens, particularly within the biological milieu. Some of these questions have been recently addressed[40,41] by using small unilamellar liposomes coated with unpurified or affinity chromatography purified IgG raised against human IgM and human kappa chain by two methods[40] which allow different degrees of IgG availability on the liposomal surface: (A) quenched CF and anti-human IgM or anti-human kappa chain rabbit ^{131}I-IgG as such or after purification by affinity chromatography were incorporated into cholesterol-rich liposomes; (B) quenched CF and unlabelled goat IgG raised against rabbit IgG were entrapped as in (A), in liposomes which were then mixed with anti-human IgM rabbit ^{131}I-IgG. Liposome-bound rabbit IgG was separated from unbound IgG by gel filtration.[40] Liposomes obtained by both methods were highly stable for several weeks and contained about 20-40% (method A) and 63-70% of the IgG used (method B).[40]

After digestion with papain, 71-82% (in terms of radioactivity) of the IgG (method A) could be released, implying that for most liposomal IgG, Fab fragments were extraliposomal.[40] This was confirmed by the immunoelectrophoretic detection in the papain-released products of Fab but not of Fc (Fig. 12). In addition, increased CF latency values (>97%) in these liposome preparations indicate that IgG incorporation by either method does not affect vesicle stability.[40]

Further experiments showed that anti-IgM and anti-kappa chain IgG incorporated onto liposomes by either method could interact with their respective antigens.[40] For instance, liposomes bearing anti-IgM IgG (method A) were able to bind about 30% of added IgM. This value was 6-fold greater than that (5%) observed with liposomes bearing unpurified anti-IgM IgG. Binding of IgM to liposomes coated with a similar amount of anti-IgM IgG by method B was even more pronounced (about 45% of the IgM added) and again, 6-fold greater than that (7.6%) achieved with liposomes coated with unpurified anti-IgM IgG.[40] Interaction between liposomal (purified) IgG and IgM also occurred in the presence of mouse blood with no significant loss of stability and although the extent of interaction was diminished to about 24% (method A) and 30% (method B), binding values were now 25-30-fold greater than those (nearly nil) obtained with unpurified liposomal IgG. The specificity of interaction was supported by the total absence of IgM binding in the presence of excess IgM (human serum).[40] In addition, in-vivo work revealed that liposomes coated with anti-IgM IgG could interact with the antigen within the intra-

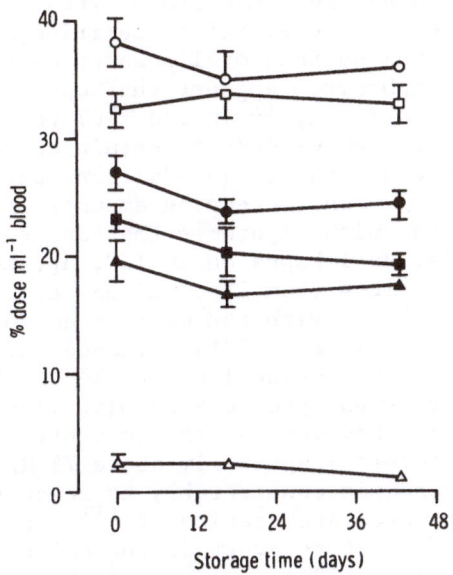

Fig. 11. The effect of storage on liposomal drug clearance. Mice
         (T.O. strain) were injected intravenously with liposomes
         containing ^{3}H-vincristine and stored for various periods
         of time as described in the text. Animals were killed
         10 min after injection and drug values in 1 ml blood are
         expressed as % of injected dose. Liposomes were composed
         of PC (▲), PC and cholesterol with molar ratios of
         1:0.28 (■) and 1:1 (●), and of DMPC (□) or SM (O) and
         cholesterol with molar ratios of 1:1.[32]

vascular space of mice previously injected with human IgM.[40] Thus,
of the human IgM injected intravenously into mice, about 36% and 43%
bound to the subsequently injected liposomes coated with anti-IgM
IgG by method A and B respectively. In-vivo association of IgM with

liposomes bearing unpurified IgG (either method) was nil.[40]

   Availability as well as frequency of receptor-recognising molecules (e.g. IgG) on the liposomal surface and of receptor molecules
(e.g. antigens) on the cellular surface are likely to influence the
extent of interaction between targeted liposomes and respective
cells. We have studied[41] such factors by using ^{111}In-bleomycin-
containing liposomes labelled with ^{14}C-PC and coated with anti-kappa
chain ^{131}I-IgG (method A) and human lymphocytes coated with kappa
chain. Data[41] related to the effect of purified anti-kappa chain
IgG concentration on the surface of liposomes on their affinity for
kappa chain-coated lymphocytes suggest that optimal binding of the
three liposomal markers (^{131}I, ^{111}In and ^{14}C) to the cells is
obtained when liposomal IgG exceeds a certain concentration (90 μg
per sample in the case studied). In addition, patterns of liposomal
binding to cells coated with increasing amounts of kappa chain
(Fig. 13) indicate that with liposomes that are either devoid of
IgG or bear unpurified anti-kappa chain IgG, uptake of the liposomal
marker (^{111}In) is low (less than 1% of added radioactivity) and
remains so for cells coated with the maximum amount of kappa chain
(i.e. 85 μg per 10^7 cells) (Fig. 13B). Indeed, even with liposomes
bearing purified anti-kappa chain IgG, uptake of the marker is only
slightly improved for lymphocytes coated with less than 10 μg kappa
chain (per 10^7 cells). However, as the concentration of kappa chain
increases to higher levels (especially above 75 μg per 10^7 cells),
[111]In uptake also increases considerably to reach values of 30%
(Fig. 13B). Such improved association of ^{111}In with the cells is
paralleled by a concomitant recovery in the cells of the liposomal
anti-kappa chain IgG (Fig. 13A), supporting the latter's role as a
mediator of liposome uptake.[41]

   The present model studies show that both purity and concentration of antibody on the liposomal surface as well as concentration of
antigen on the cell's surface are instrumental for efficient targeting. However, according to our findings[41], uptake values for the
three liposomal markers (^{111}In, ^{14}C-PC and ^{131}I-IgG) differed and,
under optimal conditions, ranged from 25.8% (^{111}In) to 60.9% (^{131}I)
of the quantity added with ^{14}C-PC, having an intermediate value of
49.5%.[41] Such varied behaviour of the markers is not surprising,
since, for instance, [111]In- labelled bleomycin would be expected[7]
to leak even from liposomes that have been slightly destabilised
through contact with cells. As bilayer destabilisation can also
lead to some phospholipid loss from liposomes,[13] it is conceivable
that values of liposomal IgG uptake (44.5 and 60.9%; see ref. 41 and
Fig. 13 respectively) reflect more faithfully true liposomal binding
to cells. On this assumption, it would appear that under the present
conditions either the liposome-binding capacity of the number of
cells used is somewhat limited or, only a (major) fraction of the
liposomes used exhibit affinity for the antigen-coated cells. However, the former possibility can be excluded since after exposure

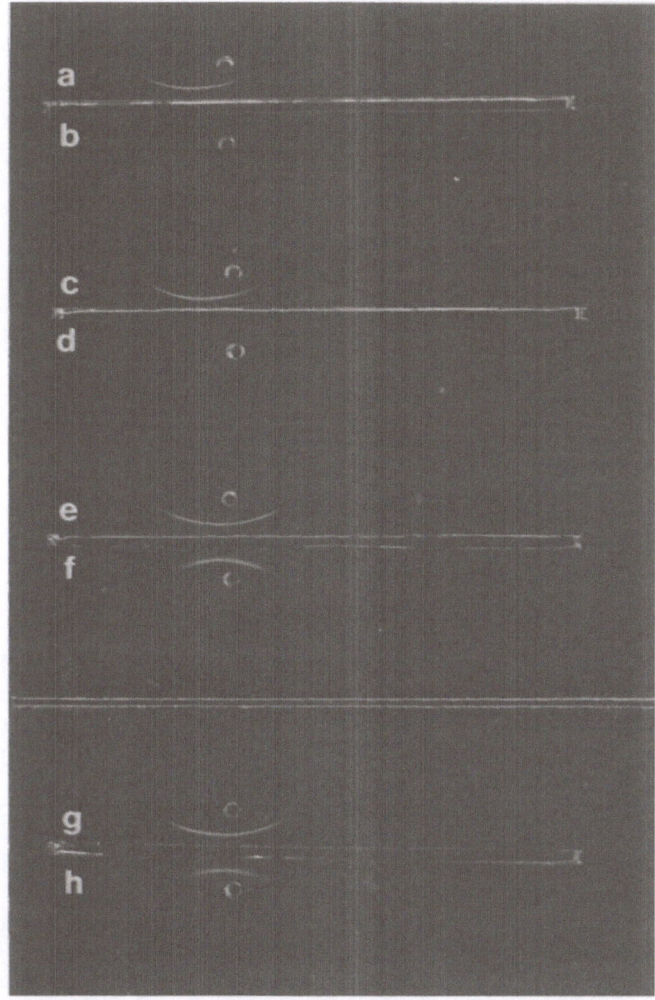

Fig. 12.   Immunoelectrophoresis of products released after treatment
            of IgG-bearing liposomes with papain. Liposomes bearing
            anti-IgM or anti-(kappa chain) IgG were incubated with pap-
            ain. Released products were then immunoelectrophoresed
            using anti-Fab and anti-Fc antiserum. (a) Fc standard
            (against anti-Fc), (b) products released from liposomes
            bearing anti-IgM IgG (against anti-Fc), (c) as in (a), (d)
            products released from liposomes bearing anti-(kappa chain)
            IgG (against anti-Fc), (e) Fab standard (against anti-Fab,
            (f) products as in (b) (against anti-Fab), (g) as in (e),
            (h) products as in (d) (against anti-Fab). Since both anti-
            Fab and anti-Fc cross-react with IgG, the absence of react-
            ion in (b) and (d) suggests the absence of IgG in the papain-
            released products[40].

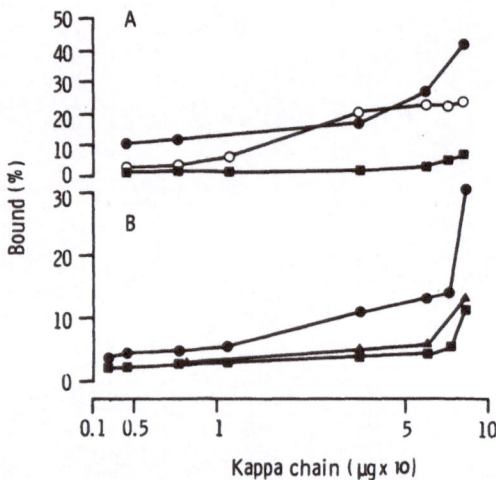

Fig. 13. Interaction of kappa chain-coated lymphocytes with liposomes.
Human blood lymphocytes (10^7) coated with increasing amounts
of kappa chain (2–85 μg/10^7 cells) were exposed to liposomes
(about 1 mg of phospholipid) composed of egg phosphatidylcholine, cholesterol and phosphatidic acid (7:7:1 molar
proportion). Liposomes devoid of IgG (■) or bearing non-
purified (▲) or affinity chromatography-purified (●) ^{131}I-
labelled anti-(kappa chain) IgG (1–2) x 10^3 c.p.m., 60–90
μg contained a tracer of ^{111}I-labelled bleomycin (1–5)
x 10^4 c.p.m. . In one experiment lymphocytes were exposed
to free anti-(kappa chain) IgG (72μg) (○). (a) ^{131}I radioactivity, (b) ^{111}In radioactivity. Results from three to
four experiments are expressed as percent ($\pm$S.D.) of added
label bound to 10^7 lymphocytes. In one experiment, after
exposure of 10^7 lymphocytes coated with 85μg kappa chain
to liposomes bearing purified anti-(kappa chain) IgG as
above but in the presence of 0.5 mg of free kappa chain,
uptake of liposomal ^{111}In and ^{131}I radioactivity by the
cells was 5.6 and 3.5% respectively.[41]

of the same number of cells to the tenth of the quantity of liposomes used in Fig. 13 uptake values (%) for all markers remained practically unaltered.[41] It seems, therefore, that IgG is distributed on the liposomal surface in a way that does not confer targeting capacity to all vesicles. It may be that a critical number of IgG molecules on the liposomal surface is required for successful association of the carrier with the cells and some of the vesicles are probably antibody "deficient". Such limited targeting capacity of a liposomal population is unlikely to relate to our method of IgG incorporation into liposomes or to the carrier's size. Indeed, other workers[36,37] using alternate techniques to link IgG with vesicles of various sizes have also reported limited uptake. Even with the use of monoconal antibodies, uptake of markers by cells carrying the respective antigens was only 10–13%.[36,37] On the other hand, in recent work[38] showing elevated (60–70%) uptake of liposomal marker, the $F(ab')_2$ conjugated onto liposomes was derived from non-purified anti-erythocyte cells IgG. Uptake values were, however, reduced to about 10% when a smaller number of erythrocytes was exposed to a proportionally smaller number of liposomes.[38] The significance of such findings in terms of methods of antibody incorporation, its state of purity and the type of target cell used remain unclear.

Work already published[31,33–41] and present results suggest that successful (quantitative) targeting may be less critically dependant on the type of specific antibody used (affinity chromatography-purified or monoclonal) or its method of incorporation onto liposomes and more on the concentration and mutual accessibility of the reacting moieties on liposomes and cells. Concentration and availability of receptor molecules on cellular surfaces are especially relevant and could become a decisive factor in selecting types of cells as candidates for targeting. Regarding targeting in vivo, an essential prerequisite for success is effective contact of liposomes with respective cells. Obviously, this can only be achieved by vesicles that are stable in the blood, circulate for controlled periods of time and can, if needed, cross membranes. Data presented here indicate that judicious manipulation of the lipid composition, size and surface charge can produce "educated" liposomes with defined characteristics in terms of solute retention and vesicle survival in the circulation. This and acquired homing properties could influence liposomal drug fate and, hopefully, efficacy.

ACKNOWLEDGEMENTS

This work was supported in part by a NIH National Cancer Institute contract (NO I–CM–87171). We thank Mrs. M. Moriarty for unrivalled secretarial work.

REFERENCES

1. G. Gregoriadis and B.E. Ryman, Liposomes as carriers of enzymes
   or drugs: A new approach to the treatment of storage diseases,
   Biochem. J. 124: 58P (1971).
2. G. Gregoriadis and B.E. Ryman, Fate of protein-containing liposomes injected into rats. An approach to the treatment of
   storage diseases, Eur. J. Biochem. 24: 485 (1972).
3. G. Gregoriadis and B.E. Ryman, Lysosomal localization of enzyme-
   containing liposomes injected into rats, Biochem. J. 128: 142
   (1972).
4. G. Gregoriadis, Targeting of Drugs : Implications in Medicine,
   Lancet, 2: 241 (1981).
5. G. Gregoriadis, The carrier potential of liposomes in Biology
   and Medicine, New Engl. J. Med. 295: 704 (1976).
6. G. Gregoriadis, The carrier potential of liposomes in Biology
   and Medicine, New Engl. J. Med. 295: 765 (1976).
7. B.E. Ryman and D.A. Tyrrell, Bags of potential, Essays Biochem.
   16: 49 (1980).
8. G. Gregoriadis, Drug entrapment in liposomes, FEBS Lett., 36: 292
   (1973).
9. L. Krupp, A.V. Chobanian and I.P. Brecher, The in-vivo transformation of phospholipid vesicles to a particle resembling
   HDL in the rat, Biochem. Biophys. Res. Comm. 72: 1251 (1976).
10. G. Scherphof, F. Roerdink, M. Waite and J. Parks, Disintegration
    of phosphatidylcholine liposomes in plasma as a result of
    interaction with high density lipoproteins, Biochim. Biophys.
    Acta. 542: 296 (1978).
11. T.M. Allen, A study of phospholipid interaction between high
    density lipoproteins and small unilamellar vesicles, Biochim.
    Biophys. Acta. 640: 385 (1981).
12. C. Kirby, J. Clarke and G. Gregoriadis, Cholesterol content of
    small unilamellar liposomes controls phospholipid loss to
    high density lipoproteins in the presence of serum, FEBS
    Lett. 111: 324 (1980).
13. C. Kirby and G. Gregoriadis, The effect of the cholesterol
    content of small unilamellar liposomes on the fate of their
    lipid components in vivo, Life Sciences, 27: 2223 (1980).
14. L.S.S. Guo, R.L. Hamilton, J. Goerke, J.N. Weinstein and
    R.J. Havel, Interaction of unilamellar liposomes with serum
    lipoproteins and apolipoprotein, J. Lipid Res. 21: 993 (1980).
15. P.D. Ladbrooke, R.M. Williams and D. Chapman, Studies on
    lecithin-cholesterol-water interactions by differential
    scanning calorimetry and X-ray diffraction, Biochim. Biophys.
    Acta, 150: 333 (1968).
16. R.A. Demel and B. Kruyff, The function of sterols in membranes,
    Biochim. Biophys. Acta. 457: 109 (1976).
17. D. Papahadjopoulos, K. Jacobson, S. Nir and T. Isac, Phase
    transitions in phospholipid vesicles. Fluorescence polariza-
    tion and permeability measurements concerning the effect of

temperature and cholesterol, Biochim. Biophys. Acta., 311: 330 (1973).

18. G. Gregoriadis and C. Davis, Stability of liposomes in vivo and in vitro is promoted by their cholesterol content and the presence of blood cells, Biochem. Biophys. Res. Comm. 89: 1287 (1979).

19. C. Kirby, J. Clarke and G. Gregoriadis, Effect of the cholesterol content of small unilamellar liposomes on their stability in vivo and in vitro, Biochem. J. 186: 591 (1980).

20. G. Gregoriadis and J. Senior, The phospholipid component of small unilamellar liposomes controls the rate of clearance of entrapped solutes from the circulation, FEBS Lett. 119: 43 (1980).

21. J. Senior and G. Gregoriadis, Stability of small unilamellar liposomes in serum and clearance from the circulation : the effect of the phospholipid and cholesterol components, (Submitted).

22. A.R. Tall, Studies on the transfer of phosphatidylcholine from unilamellar vesicles into plasma high density lipoproteins in the rat, J. Lipid Res., 21: 354 (1980).

23. G. Scherphof, J. Damen, D. Hoekstra, A.J.B.M. Van Renswoode and F.H. Roerdink, Fundamental studies on the cellular uptake of liposomes, in: "Cell Biological Aspects of Disease", Th. W. Daems, E.H. Burger and B.A. Afzelius, eds., Leiden University Press, The Hague (1980).

24. C. Kirby and G. Gregoriadis, Plasma-induced release of solutes from small unilamellar liposomes is associated with pore formation in the bilayers. Biochem. J., 199: 251 (1981).

25. C. Kirby and G. Gregoriadis, The effect of lipid composition of small unilamellar liposomes containing melphalan and vincristine on drug clearance after injection (Submitted).

26. D.S. Alberts, S.Y. Chang, H-S.G. Chen, T.E. Moon, T.L. Evans, R.L. Furner, K. Himmelstein and J.F. Gross, Kinetics of intravenous melphalan, Clin. Pharmacol. Ther., 26: 73 (1979).

27. R.L. Juliano and D. Stamp, Interactions of drugs with lipid membranes : Characteristics of liposomes containing polar or non-polar antitumour drugs, Biochim. Biophys. Acta., 586: 137 (1979).

28. K.J. Huang, K-F.S. Luke and P.L. Beaumier, Hepatic uptake and degradation of unilamellar sphingomyelin/cholesterol liposomes : a kinetic study, Proc. Nat. Acad. Sci. USA, 77: 4030 (1980).

29. C.D.V. Black and G. Gregoriadis, Interaction of liposomes with blood plasma proteins, Biochem. Soc. Trans., 4: 253 (1976).

30. D.A. Tyrrell, V.J. Richardson and B.E. Ryman, The effect of serum protein fractions on liposome-cell interactions in cultured cells and the perfused rat liver, Biochim. Biophys. Acta., 497: 469 (1977).

31. G. Gregoriadis, D.E. Neerunjun and R. Hunt, Fate of a liposome-associated agent injected into normal and tumour bearing rodents. Attempts to improve localization in tumour tissues,

Life Sciences, 21: 357 (1977).

32. P. Large and G. Gregoriadis, The effect of storage on the stability of drug-containing small unilamellar liposomes (Submitted).

33. G. Gregoriadis and E.D. Neerunjun, Homing of liposomes to target cells, Biochem. Biophys. Res. Comm., 65: 537 (1975).

34. V.P. Torchilin, V.G. Omel Yanenko, A.L. Klibanov, A.I. Michailov, V.I. Gol'Danskii and V.N. Smirhov, Incorporation of hydrophilic protein modified with hydrophobic agent into liposome membrane, Biochim. Biophys. Acta., 602: 511 (1980).

35. P. Ghosh, P.K. Das and B.K. Bachhawat, Selective uptake of liposomes by different cell types of liver through the involvement of liposomal surface glycosides, Biochem. Soc. Trans., 9: 512 (1981).

36. A. Huang, L. Huang and S.J. Kennel, Monoclonal antibody covalently coupled with fatty acid, J. Biol. Chem. 255: 8015 (1980).

37. L.D. Leserman, J. Barbet, F. Kourilsky and J.N. Weinstein, Targeting to cells of fluorescent liposomes covalently coupled with monoclonal antibody or protein A, Nature, 288: 602 (1980).

38. T.D. Heath, R.T. Fraley and D. Papahadjopoulos, Antibody targeting of liposomes : cell specificity obtained by conjugation of F(ab')$_2$ to vesicle surface, Science, 210: 539 (1980).

39. V.K. Jansons and P.L. Mallett, Targeted liposomes : a method for preparation and analysis, Anal. Biochem. 111: 54 (1981).

40. G. Gregoriadis, A. Meehan and M.M. Mah, Interaction of antibody-bearing small unilamellar liposomes with target free antigen in vitro and in vivo: Some influencing factors, Biochem. J. 200: 203 (1981).

41. G. Gregoriadis and A. Meehan, Interaction of antibody-bearing small unilamellar liposomes with antigen-coated cells : the effect of antibody and antigen concentration on the liposomal and cell surface respectively, Biochem. J. 200: 211 (1981).

ANTIBODY-MEDIATED TARGETING OF LIPOSOMES

John N. Weinstein (1), Lee D. Leserman (2), Pierre A.
Henkart (3), and Robert Blumenthal (1)

1. Section on Membrane Structure and Function,
Laboratory of Theoretical Biology, NCI, NIH, Bldg 10,
Rm 4B-54, Bethesda, Md 20205, USA; 2. Centre
d'Immunologie INSERM-CNRS de Marseille-Luminy, Case
906, 13288 Marseille Cedex g, France; 3. Immunology
Branch, NCI, NIH

ABSTRACT

We have studied a number of permutations on the use of antibody and antigen for targeting liposomes in vitro. Our first
strategy was to make liposomes with lipid bearing the dinitrophenyl
(DNP) hapten. These liposomes bound specifically to cells in three
experimental configurations: (i) with TNP-modified human peripheral
blood lymphocytes as targets and sheep IgG anti-TNP as cross-linking
agent; (ii) with murine myeloma MOPC 315 cells (which bear an IgA
with high affinity for nitrophenyl haptens) as target, using
endogeneous surface immunoglobulin on the cells as a point of
attachment; (iii) with Fc-receptor bearing cells as targets and
rabbit anti-TNP as an opsonizing agent. We monitored the interactions by encapsulating carboxyfluorescein and/or methotrexate in
the liposomes, and in some experiments by incorporating ^{14}C-dipal-
mitoyl phosphatidylcholine or a fluorescent marker in the lipid.
In each study large numbers of liposomes could be bound specifically
to the target cells, but they were internalized in significant
numbers only in (iii) when cells capable of Fc-mediated endocytosis
were used. The most striking internalization was found with the
mouse macrophage line P388D1. Encapsulated methotrexate had a
several-fold greater effect on the metabolism of P388D1 (as assayed
by ^3H-deoxyuridine uptake) than did an equivalent amount of methotrexate free in solution. This finding indicated that an appropriately chosen drug can escape the phagosomal system to exert its
effect in the cytoplasm.

185

Our second principal effort has been to couple immunoglobulin to liposomal phosphatidylethanolamine covalently, or else through covalently coupled Staphylococcus aureus protein A. Coupling is achieved with the heterobifunctional agent N-succinimidyl 3-(2-pyridyldithio) propionate (SPDP). This method of coupling results in minimal aggregation and little leakage of vesicle contents. Liposomes bearing covalently coupled monoclonal antibody bind with high specificity to cells with the corresponding determinants.

INTRODUCTION

Our studies on antibody-mediated targeting of liposomes have addressed three principal questions: The first is "Can liposomes be bound preferentially to cells bearing the target hapten or anti-body? The answer, at least in vitro, is clearly "yes". The more interesting and difficult questions that follow are "Does the binding increase incorporation of liposome contents into the cell?" and "If so, can those contents -- for example, a drug or a toxin -- reach sites of action in the cytoplasm or nucleus?" To address these issues we first studied the interaction of hapten-bearing liposomes with hapten-modified lymphocytes using IgG as a cross-linking agent. We then examined the interaction of hapten-bearing liposomes with the Ig-bearing murine myeloma cells MOPC 315 and TEPC 15, and with murine tumor cells P388, P388D1, and EL4. More recently, we have developed a technique for covalent coupling of immunoglobulin and other macromolecules to liposomes and are using the resulting lipo-somes to study other variations on the theme.

MATERIALS AND METHODS

Details of our liposome preparations can be found in several references (Weinstein et al., 1977: 1978; Leserman et al., 1979; 1980a; 1980b). For the most part we have used highly sonicated liposomes of 50: 47.5: 2.5 (molar) dioleoyl phosphatidylcholine (DOPC): cholesterol: haptenated phosphatidylethanolamine or 30: 30: 37.5: 2.5 dipalmitoyl phosphatidylcholine (DPPC): distearoyl phospha-tidylcholine (DSPC): cholesterol: haptenated phosphatidylethanolamine. The covalent coupling procedure will be described separately.

The haptenated lipid N-dinitrophenylaminocaproyl phosphati-dylethanolamine (DNP-cap-PE) was first synthesized by Six et al. (1973). Phosphatidylethanolamine bearing the phosphorylcholine hapten on a six carbon spacer (PC-cap-PE) was synthesized by esterification of phosphatidylethanolamine with p-nitrophenyl-6-o (phosphorylcholine)hexanoate (described in Leserman et al., 1980a).

We generally used carboxyfluorescein (CF) as a marker of the aqueous space of liposomes. In most studies the CF was encapsulated

at 10 mM, a concentration at which its fluorescence in small unilamellar vesicles is about 60% of the value obtained after release into
the medium. The CF fluorescence could therefore be taken as an index
of total cell-associated vesicle contents (whether still in vesicles
or not). In other studies we used 100 mM CF to make use of self-
quenching to distinguish material released from the liposomes into
the cell from that still in vesicles bound to the cell surface (see
Weinstein et al., 1977, and Hagins and Yoshikami, 1978, for further
explanation of the method). CF fluorescence of cells was assessed
by fluorometry, by fluorescence activated cell sorter, and by microscopy. Note: At least some batches of CF from Eastman Kodak contain
hydrophobic impurities, which we remove by adding to our older
purification method an elution with water on Sephadex LH20 (Ralston
et al., submitted). These impurities appear not to be important for
the studies described here, which involve high levels of binding and
are, for the most part, conducted in the presence of serum.

As an aqueous drug for encapsulation we chose the folic acid
analogue methotrexate (MTX). Leakage of MTX from liposomes is
commensurate with that of CF. MTX affords a sensitive assay for
delivery of encapsulated material to the cytoplasm since its action
is principally due to an only slowly reversible binding to the
cytoplasmic enzyme dihydrofolate reductase (DHFR). We assay MTX
effect by measuring reduction of the incorporation of tritiated
deoxyuridine (^{3}H-Urd).

Human peripheral blood lymphocytes were isolated and TNBS-
modified as previously described (Weinstein et al., 1977). MOPC 315
and TEPC 15 were maintained by intraperitoneal transfer in Balb/c
mice. EL4 and P388 were similarly maintained in C57BL/6 and DBA/2
mice, respectively. The macrophage-like line P388D1 was maintained
in spinner culture. Phagocytosis was assessed using latex beads, and
the presence of IgG Fc receptors was determined by a rosetting assay.
The IgG used in the initial studies with lymphocytes was obtained
from sheep hyperimmunized with TNP. It was affinity purified with
DNP. IgG for studies of Fc-mediated uptake was similarly obtained
from rabbit and affinity purified. (These preparations are termed
"anti-TNP" and "anti-DNP" interchangeably in this paper). The
method for covalent coupling of macromolecules to liposomes is
described in Leserman et al. (1980c). A similar approach has been
taken by Godfrey et al. (1981). Briefly, dithiopyridyl (DTP) groups
are placed on free amino groups of phosphatidylethanolamine by use of
the heterobifunctional cross-linking reagent N-succinimidyl 3-(2-
pyridyldithio) propionate (SPDP). The DTP-phosphatidylethanolamine
is stable and can be incorporated into sonicated or other liposomes.
The protein to be coupled is similarly modified with SPDP and its
DTP activated to the thiol derivative by reduction with dithiothreitol. The activated protein is then coupled to the DTP-liposomes
in aqueous solution. The conditions of reaction can be arranged to
minimize protein-protein and liposome-liposome coupling.

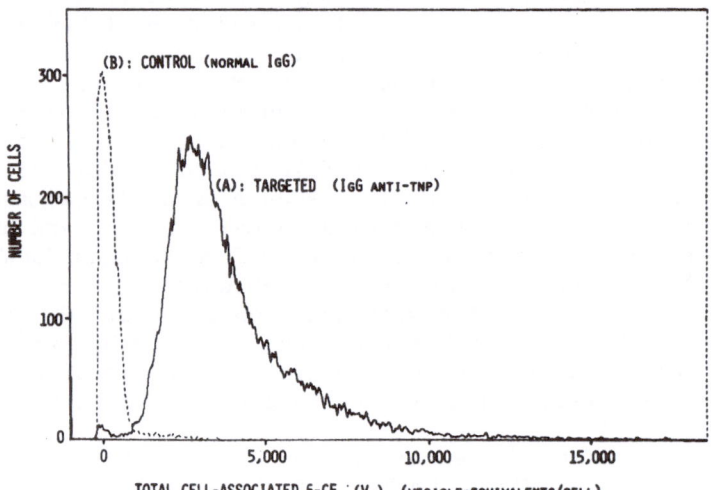

Fig. 1.   Specific binding of CF-containing, DNP-bearing liposomes
          to TNP-modified human lymphocytes. This is a frequency
          distribution of cell fluorescence obtained by flow micro-
          fluorometry. The control with irrelevant IgG shows only
          background fluorescence. The vesicles were highly sonicated
          and made of dioleoyl phosphatidylcholine: DNP-PE 95: 5.
          They contained 10 mM CF. The cells were incubated with
          vesicles in the absence of serum for 20 minutes. In each
          case, almost all cell signals fell into a single peak, with
          fewer than 1% of cells off-scale. A "vesicle-equivalent"
          is the amount of CF estimated to be in an average vesicle
          (i.e. 13 molecules at 10 mM).

RESULTS

Interaction of hapten-bearing liposomes with lymphocytes.

     The flow microfluorometric profile in Fig. 1 illustrates the
binding of CF-containing DNP-vesicles to TNP-lymphocytes (antibodies
to DNP and TNP cross-react). The immunologic specificity of the
binding was shown in a series of such experiments, whose results are
given in Figure 2a. The IgG anti-TNP, or its $F(ab')_2$ fragment, acted
as a cross-bridge binding vesicles to cells. However, as shown in
Fig. 2b, from experiments with vesicles containing self-quenched CF,
the binding led to no increase over low background values in the
amount of vesicle contents released into the cell cytoplasm. These
findings were corroborated by bulk fluorometry and microscopy
(Weinstein et al., 1978).

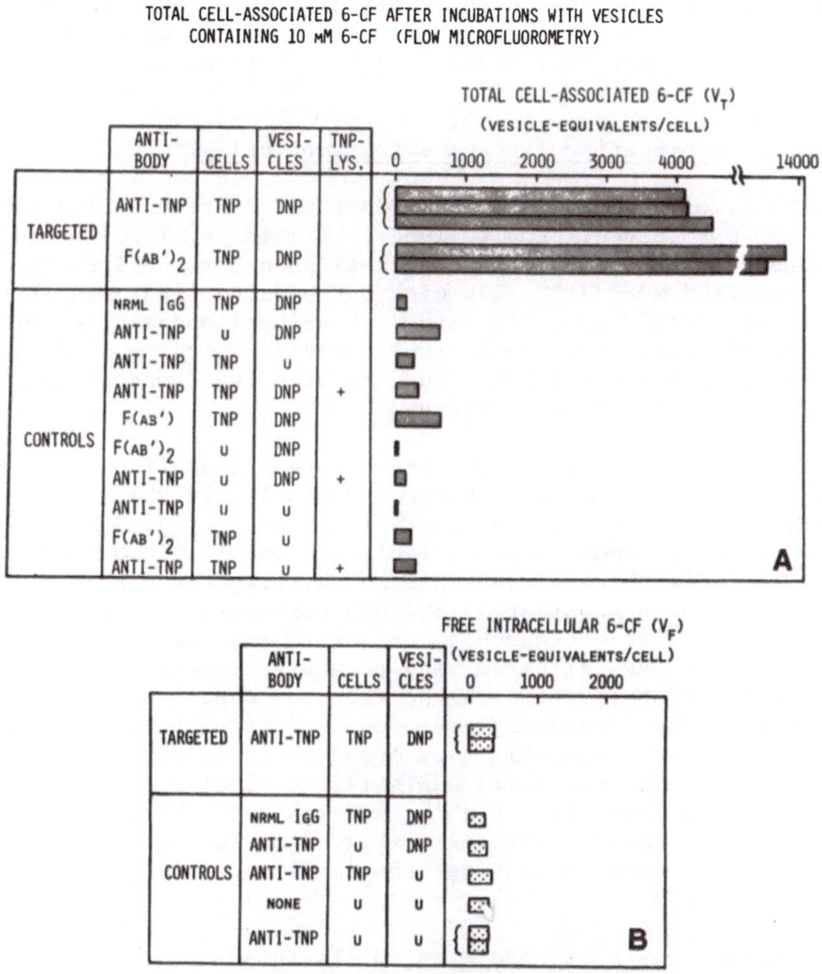

Fig. 2. Summary of flow microfluorometric data on association of
CF-containing vesicles with lymphocytes. Calculated means
from histograms such as that in Fig. 1 are shown.
u - unmodified cell; lys - lysine. (a) vesicles containing
10 mM dye, to indicate total cell-associated CF.
(b) vesicles contained 100 mM dye, to indicate entry of CF
into cells (that is, the fluorescence of CF remaining in
vesicles on the cell surface is largely self-quenched).
The targeting clearly led to little or no entry. The
already very low values for the controls in (a) and for
all cells in (b) might have been even lower if the effects
of low-level impurities in the CF had been subtracted.

At that point in our studies, we worried that the lack of
incorporation might be due to the artificiality of our system, in
which the cell surface had been chemically modified with TNP. Hence,
we turned to the tumor cell systems to be described next.

Binding of hapten-bearing liposomes to tumor cells.

MOPC 315 cells secrete and bear on their surface an IgA with
affinity for DNP (Eisen, et al., 1968). Similarly, TEPC 15 cells
secrete and bear on their surface an anti-phosphorylcholine (anti-PC).
When we incubated MOPC 315 cells with DNP-bearing liposomes (Leserman,
et al., 1979) or TEPC 15 cells with PC-bearing liposomes (Leserman,
et al., 1980a), there was considerable specific binding, mediated by
the endogenous surface antigen. But, as with the lymphocytes, uptake
of CF into the cells was not enhanced.

We next examined the possibility of opsonizing liposomes for
interaction with Fc receptors (Leserman, et al., 1980b). One set
of results from flow microfluorometry is shown in Fig. 3, and a more
extensive series is summarized in Table 1. The 10,200,000 CF molecules associated with each P388 cell in the targeted case corresponds
to the contents of approximately 800,000 vesicles. As indicated in
Table 1, non-specific backgrounds were extremely low. As expected,
DNP-bearing liposomes failed to bind to the Fc-receptor bearing
tumors P388 and P388D1, or to the Fc-receptor negative line EL4.
However, when those liposomes were opsonized with rabbit IgG anti-
TNP (or its $F(ab')_2$ fragment), they bound in large numbers to P388
and P388D1. As expected, there was still no binding to the Fc-
receptor negative line EL4. $F(ab')_2$ and IgA anti-TNP failed to
mediate binding to any of the cells (Fig. 3). The question of uptake
will be addressed when we consider the results of microscopy.

Effect of methotrexate encapsulated in liposomes.

Uptake of ^{3}H-Urd by myeloma tumor cells was inhibited by free
MTX in solution (not shown). However, when the same amount of MTX
was encapsulated in liposomes (whether hapten-bearing or not), the
drug effect was markedly reduced. Thus, mirroring the results for
CF, binding to surface immunoglobulin was insufficient for drug
delivery. Similarly, when liposomes containing MTX and bearing DNP
were incubated with P388, P388D1, or EL4, the cells were little
affected by the drug, though they were sensitive to free MTX (Fig. 4).
In contrast, when liposomes were opsonized by IgG anti-TNP, ^{3}H-Urd
uptake by P388D1 cells was inhibited to a much greater extent than
by the free drug (Fig. 4a). EL4 was insensitive to IgG-opsonized
liposomes containing MTX, though sensitive to free MTX (Fig. 4b).
P388 was somewhat sensitive to drug in opsonized liposomes, but not
to the same extent as with free drug (Fig. 4c). None of the cells

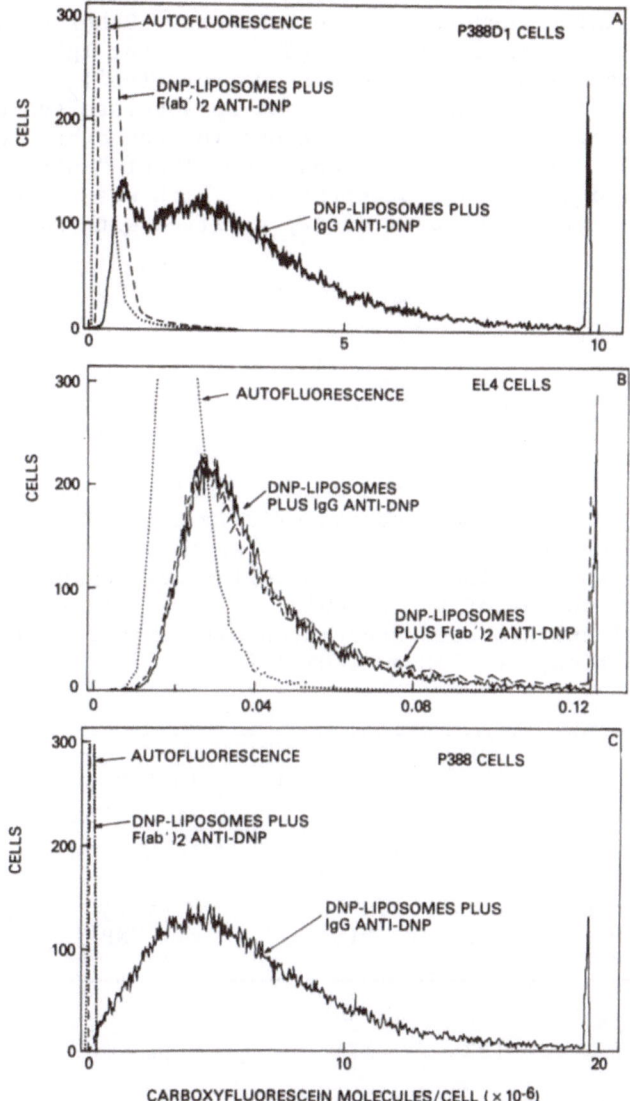

Fig. 3. Flow microfluorometric profiles of (a) P388D1, (b) EL4, and (c) P388 cells. Cells were incubated in 10% fetal calf serum with DNP-liposomes alone or in the presence of IgG, IgA, or F(ab')$_2$ anti-TNP. Liposomes contained 10 mM CF; the concentration of CF in the incubations was 1.3 M. The liposome composition was DSPC: DPPC: cholesterol: DNP-cap-PE 30: 30: 37.5: 2.5 (molar). With EL4 the CF vesicles slightly increased fluorescence over background, but targeting for Fc receptors with whole IgG did not lead

to additional binding. With P388 and P388D1, targeting led
to a large increase in fluorescence. Other controls (naked
vesicles, IgA instead of IgG, irrelevant IgG, etc.) gave
the same results as those shown for $F(ab')_2$ in the figures.
Note the very large difference in abscissa scale between
the histogram for EL4 and those for the other two cell
types. (In Figs. 3, 4, and 5 the label "anti-DNP" is
applied to this Ig preparation, which was raised by immunization with TNP but affinity purified with DNP).

Table 1. Flow microfluorometric measurements on cells incubated
          with DNP-liposomes and anti-TNP immunoglobulin. DPPC:
          DSPC: Cholesterol: DNP-cap-PE vesicles were incubated with
          cells for 20 minutes. Mean cell fluorescence is expressed
          as the number of CF molecules x 10^{-3} /cell (e.g. 3,130,000
          CF molecules became associated with each P388D1 cell during
          incubation with IgG anti-DNP).

Cell line	Temp. ^{o}C	Mean cell CF fluorescence			
		No Ig*	IgA anti-DNP (MOPC 315)	$F(ab')_2$ anti-TNP	IgG anti-TNP
P388D1	4	55	37	27	3,130
	37	183	171	86	4,530
P388	4	19	12	8	4,520
	37	17	17	17	10,200
EL4	4	3	3	3	6
	37	25	22	29	27

*Background "autofluorescence" was as follows: P388D1, P388,
60; EL4, 38. These value have been subtracted from the data
to obtain the numbers above.

were affected by liposomes carrying IgA or F(ab')$_2$ (as illustrated, for P388D1, in Fig. 5).

Fluorescence microscopy.

    In fluorescence microscopy, the targeted systems with TNP-modified lymphocytes and with myeloma cells showed patchy binding but no internalization (not shown). The findings with EL4, P388, and P388D1 cells (Fig. 6) were more complicated, but consistent with an Fc-receptor mediated binding and endoyctosis. Little or no fluorescence (above background) was seen when any of the three cell types was incubated with DNP-liposomes and IgA anti-DNP, F(ab')$_2$ anti-TNP, or no antibody. EL4 cells did not bind liposomes even when intact IgG anti-TNP was added. However, there was considerable binding when P388D1 and P388 cells were incubated at 37°C with IgG opsonized liposomes. In the case of P388, most of the liposomes remained in patches at the cell surface, but a well-localized aggregation of small fluorescent spots was seen internally, near the nucleus of many cells (Fig. 7a). Most of the bound liposomes were rapidly internalized by P388D1. Incubation at 2°C or inclusion of azide plus 2-deoxyglucose essentially prevented internalization of fluorescence but, as expected, did not block binding (Fig. 7c).

Covalent coupling of monoclonal antibody and protein A to liposomes.

    As indicated in Table 2, liposomes bearing covalently coupled mouse monoclonal antibody against human β_2-microglobulin (antibody B1.1G6 (IgG$_{2a}$,k)) showed the appropriate specificity in that they bound specifically to human cells but not to mouse cells. Conversely, liposomes bearing an antibody against mouse histocompatibility antigens (11.4.1 IgG$_{2a}$, k anti H-2 K^k) bound to mouse cells, but not to human cells (Barbet, et al., 1981). Liposomes bearing protein A bound to human cells previously incubated with the B1.1G6 antibody but not to cells incubated without antibody (not shown).

DISCUSSION

    Many of the therapeutic and cell biological applications envisioned for liposomes will require direction of the liposomes to specific target cells or tissues (Gregoriadis and Neerunjun, 1975; Weissmann et al., 1975: Magee et al., 1978; Weinstein et al., 1978; Leserman et al., 1979). The studies described here have delineated three essential steps which must be well understood if such enter-prises are to succeed:

    (1) The first is to obtain specific binding to the cell surface. In vitro, that appears not to be a problem for antibody-mediated

Table 2. Specific binding of B1.1G6-bearing liposomes to human RAJI cells and of 11.4.1-bearing liposomes to mouse RDM4 tumor cells. The total lipid concentration was 0.6 mM. The concentration of CF in liposomes was 40 mM. The specific activity of the protein was 3.3 mCi/mol for B1.1G6 and 4.8 mCi/mol for 11.4.1. The total amounts of I-protein and CF were 7,000 cpm and 510 pmol/well, respectively, for both liposome preparations. Each well contained 2.5 x 10 cells.

Antibody on liposomes	Inhibitor added (25 g/ml)	Binding to RAJI cells		Binding to RDM4 cells	
		^{125}I protein counts bound	pmol of CF bound	^{125}I protein counts bound	pmole of CF bound
B1.1G6*	–	1,030	52.8	40	0.8
B1.1G6	B1.1G6	20	1.2	N.D.**	N.D.
B1.1G6	11.4.1	1,135	58.4	N.D.	N.D.
11.4.1	–	49	0.8	262	11.2
11.4.1	B1.1G6	N.D.	N.D.	220	9.6
11.4.1	11.4.1	N.D.	N.D.	60	1.2

* The fluorescence of cells incubated with liposomes not coupled to antibody (total CF: 510 pmole) was below the limit of resolution of the measurement (0.4 pmol).

** N.D: not done.

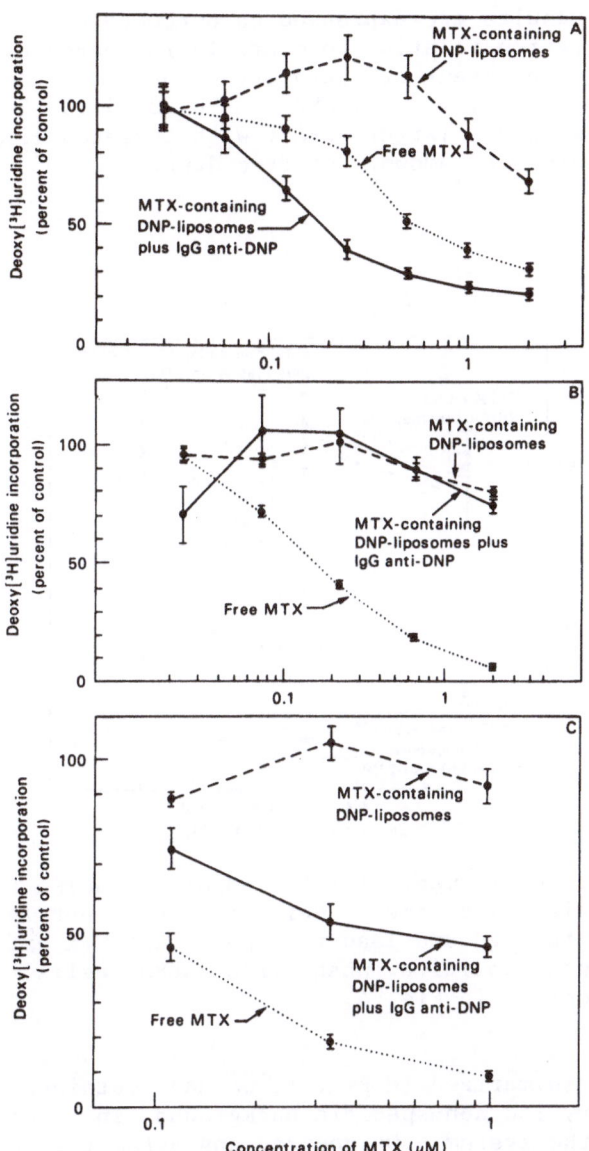

Fig. 4. Drug effect in the cytoplasmic compartment. Inhibition of
[3]H-Urd incorporation into murine tumor cells by MTX in free
solution or in TNP-bearing liposomes in the presence of
IgG anti-TNP, F(ab')$_2$ anti-TNP, or IgA anti-DNP. P388D1
(Fig. 4a), EL4 (Fig. 4b), or P388 (Fig. 4c) cells were
incubated in the presence of MTX, free or in liposomes, at
the concentration indicated. ^{3}H-Urd was added after three

hours, and cultures were harvested after overnight incubation. Results are expressed as percentage of ^{3}H–Urd
incorporation relative to controls incubated without MTX.
The bars represent standard errors of the mean. Liposomes
were DOPC: cholesterol: DNP–cap–PE 50: 47.5: 2.5 (molar).
P388D1 showed a larger effect with targeted liposomes than
with equivalent amounts of free drug.

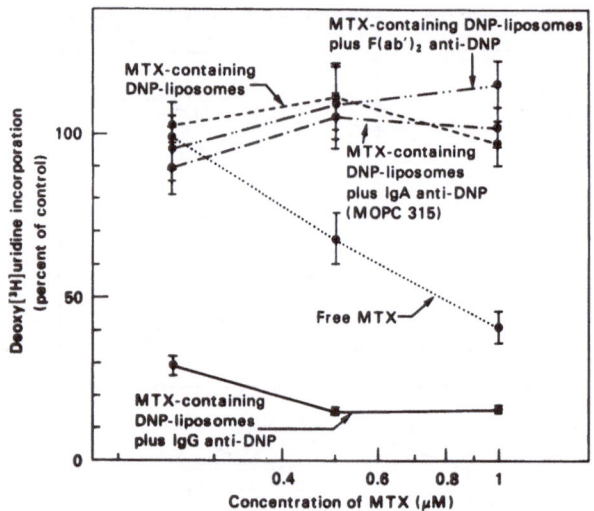

Fig. 5. Specific requirements for Fc–mediated binding and uptake
of opsonized liposomes. Neither F(ab')$_2$ nor IgA could
replace the IgG and lead to significant MTX effect in the
Fc–receptor positive, phagocytic P388D1 cells. Same
conditions as in Fig. 4.

interaction. As summarized in Fig. 8, we have obtained the expected
binding, with very low non-specific background, in a number of
permutations of the system. Of course, any attempt to bind targeted
liposomes in vivo would encounter additional problems: the sequestra-
tion of most interesting determinants behind endothelial or other
physiological barriers; the plasticity cells show in modulating their
surfaces; the immunogenicity of the proteins used; the tendency of
opsonized liposomes to be removed rapidly from the circulation; and
the limitation in numbers which could be bound before saturation of
cell surface sites.

P388D, AND EL4 CELLS INCUBATED WITH
CARBOXYFLUORESCEIN−CONTAINING LIPOSOMES

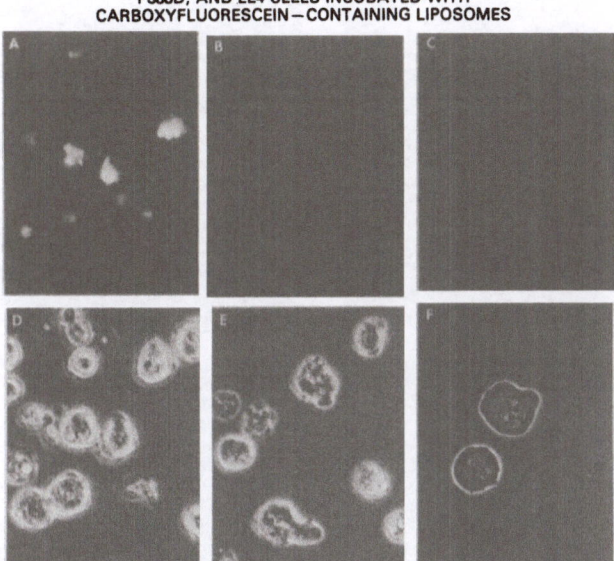

Fig. 6.   Micrographs of cells incubated at 37°C for 20 minutes with
          DNP-liposomes containing 10 mM CF. Liposomes were of DSPC:
          DPPC: cholesterol: DNP-cap-PE 30: 30: 37.5: 2.5 (molar).
          A-C are fluorescence micrographs. D-F are phase micro-
          graphs.

               A,D - P388D1 in the presence of IgG anti-TNP
               B,E - P388D1 in the presence of F(ab')$_2$ anti-TNP
               C,F - EL4 in the presence of IgG anti-TNP

     (2) The second major issue is entry into the cells. In
limited contexts such as that of encapsulated radio-diagnostics or
alpha-emitters, delivery of liposomal material into the cells might
not be important, but more often it would be. In the absence of
endocytosis, we saw no incorporation of vesicle contents into the
cells secondary to specific binding -- as assessed either by the
morphology of CF distribution or by the functional effect of encapsulated MTX. Thus, the proximity of bound vesicles to the cell
surface did not lead to significant fusion or similar spontaneous
transfer of contents into the cells. Addition of agents such as
polyethylene glycol (Szoka et al., 1981), glycerol (Fraley et al.,
1981), or viral coat proteins (Cabantchik et al., 1980) may usefully
stimulate incorporation of targeted liposome contents in vitro.
We know of no good ideas for obtaining such incorporation in vivo.

P388 CELLS INCUBATED WITH CARBOXYFLOURESCEIN-
CONTAINING LIPOSOMES

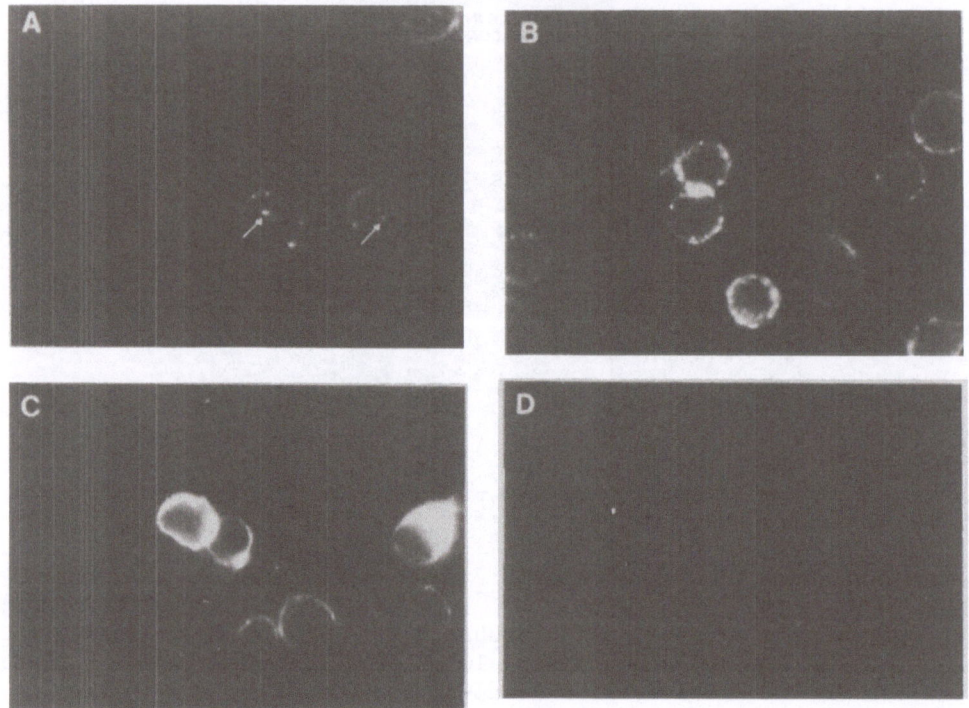

Fig. 7. Fluorescence micrographs of P388 cells incubated as
described in the legend of Fig. 5. A. Incubated at 37°C
with IgG anti-TNP. Arrows indicate fluorescent specks near
nucleus; B. Incubated at 37°C with IgG anti-TNP, plus
0.2% sodium azide and 50 mM 2-deoxyglucose. Contrary to
the impression created by this particular photograph, the
inhibitors did not appear to increase the fluorescence of
the population; C. Incubated at 2°C with IgG anti-TNP;
D. Incubated at 37°C with F(ab')$_2$ anti-TNP.

With the Fc-receptor positive, phagocytic cell line P388D1, on
the other hand, hundreds of thousands of opsonized vesicles could be
bound and their contents of CF internalized. The morphological
pattern strongly suggested phagocytosis. Similar, but much less
striking, internalization was seen with the Fc-receptor positive,
minimally phagocytic line P388.

CONFIGURATIONS OF ANTIBODY-MEDIATED
TARGETING

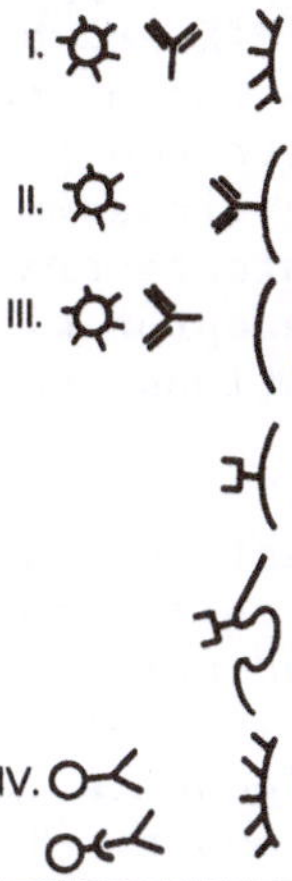

		Binding	Incor-poration	MTX Effect
I.	Hapten-Modified Lymphocyte	+	–	N.D.
II.	Myeloma Cell	+	–	–
III.	Fc-Receptor Negative	–	–	–
	Fc-Receptor Positive "Non-Phagocytic"	+	+/–	+/–
	Fc-Receptor Positive Phagocytic	+	+	+
IV.	Lymphocyte	+		

N.D. — Not Done.

Fig. 8. Summary of experimental systems used and the results.

I: Cross-linking of DNP-liposomes to TNP-modified human peripheral blood lymphocytes with sheep IgG anti-TNP.

II: DNP- or PC-liposome bound to MOPC 315 or TEPC 15 myeloma cell via endogenous surface IgA with high affinity for the nitrophenyl haptens.

IIIa: DNP-liposome; rabbit IgG anti-TNP; Fc-receptor negative cell (EL4).

IIIb: DNP-liposome; rabbit IgG anti-TNP; Fc-receptor positive, "non-phagocytic" cell (P388 -- actually minimally phagocytic, as indicated by these studies).

IIIc: DNP-liposome; rabbit IgG anti-TNP; Fc-receptor positive, phagocytic cell (P388D1).

IV: IgG covalently coupled to liposome or bound to covalently coupled protein A; lymphocyte or other cell bearing appropriate determinant. Incorporation and MTX effect appear to depend on whether the particular cell surface target antigen mediates endocytosis.

(3) Receptor-mediated endocytosis of liposomes then raises our
third major question: Can drug escape the phagolysosomal apparatus
to affect cellular function in cytoplasm or nucleus? Our experiments
with P388D1 and liposomal MTX indicate that they can. Further
studies will be required to assess the efficiency of this process,
the degree to which it depends on cell and liposome type, and the
range of drugs for which it is useful. CF and MTX are both weak
organic anions, which would be expected to pass out of the relatively
acidic lysosomal environment. Would we have obtained the same
functional effect for a cationic agent? Do the liposomes reach
lysosomes in the first place? Before their contents are released?
And what surface determinants besides the Fc-receptor will mediate
endocytosis of liposomes. These important questions indicate the
degree of our present ignorance.

One clear requirement before the above questions can be
answered is the ability to couple a variety of molecules covalently
to liposome surfaces. The SPDP method described here results in
efficient binding of ligand to liposomes, with minimal aggregation
and without denaturation of the ligand. The liposomes remain intact
and do not leak encapsulated CF during the procedure. Thus far, it
has been applied with mouse and rat monoclonal IgG, affinity purified
rabbit IgG, protein A, and albumin. In principle, it should be
applicable to most peptides, proteins, and other molecules having
free amino groups. Several other procedures for attachment of antibody have recently been described (Gregoriadis and Neerunjun, 1975;
Huang and Kennel, 1979; Huang et al., 1980; Godfrey et al., 1981;
Heath et al., 1981; Martin et al., 1981). The method described here
is versatile and does not appreciably degrade liposome or antibody.
However, only further experience will determine the range of functions
most appropriate for each approach. The combination of covalent
ligand coupling and drug encapsulation, as described here, makes it
immediately possible to design a large number of interesting immunological and cell biological studies in which selected cells are
killed or otherwise altered. Several such projects are underway.

REFERENCES

Barbet, J., Machy, P., and Leserman, L.D., 1981, Monoclonal antibody
     covalently coupled to liposomes: Specific targeting to cells,
     J. Supramolec. Struct. Cell Biochem., in press.
Cabantchik, Z.I., Volsky, D.J., Ginsberg, H., and Loyter, A.,
     Reconstitution of the erythrocyte anion transport system: in
     vitro and in vivo approaches, Ann. N.Y. Acad. Sci., U.S.A.
     341:444.
Eisen, H.N., Simms, E.S., and Potter, M., 1968, Mouse myeloma pro-
     teins with anti-hapten antibody activity. The protein produced
     by plasma cell tumor MOPC-315, Biochemistry 7:4126.
Fraley, R., and D. Papahadjopoulos, D., 1981, New generation lipo-

    somes: the engineering of an efficient vehicle for intra-
    cellular delivery of nucleic acids, T.I.B.S. 9: 467.
Godfrey, W., Doe, B., Wallace, E.F., Bredt, B., and Wofsy, L.,
    1981, Affinity targeting of membrane vesicles to cell surfaces,
    Exptl. Cell Research, in press.
Gregoriadis, G., and Neerunjun, D.E., 1975, Homing of liposomes to
    target cells, Biochem. Biophys. Res. Commun. 65: 537.
Hagins, W.A., and Yoshikami, S., 1978, In: "Vertebrate Photo-
    receptors," Fatt, P., and Barlow, H.B., eds., Academic Press,
    N.Y.
Heath, T.D., Macher, B.A., and Papahadjopoulos, D., 1981, Covalent
    attachment of immunoglobulins to liposomes via glycosphingo-
    lipids, Biochem. Biophys. Acta, 640: 66.
Huang, L., and Kennel, S.J., 1979, Binding of immunoglobulin G to
    phospholipid vesicles by sonication, Biochemistry, 18: 1702.
Huang, A., Huang., L., and Kennel, S.J., 1980, Monoclonal antibody
    covalently coupled with fatty acid, J. Biol. Chem., 255: 8015.
Leserman, L.D., Weinstein, J.N., Blumenthal, R., Sharrow, S.O.,
    and Terry, W.D., 1979, Binding of antigen-bearing fluorescent
    liposomes to the murine myeloma tumor MOPC 315, J. Immunol.
    122: 585.
Leserman, L.D., Weinstein, J.N., Moore, J.J., and Terry, W.D.,
    1980a, Specific interaction of myeloma tumor cells with hapten-
    bearing liposomes containing methotrexate and carboxyfluorescein,
    Cancer Res., 40: 4768.
Leserman, L.D., Weinstein, J.N., Blumenthal, R., and Terry, W.D.,
    1980b, Receptor-mediated endocytosis of antibody opsonized
    liposomes by tumor cells, Proc. Natl. Acad. Sci. U.S.A.,
    77: 4089.
Leserman, L.D., Barbet, J., Kourilsky, F.M., and Weinstein J.N.,
    1980c, Targeting to cells of fluorescent liposomes covalently
    coupled with monoclonal antibody or protein A, Nature, 288: 602.
Leserman, L.D., and Weinstein, J.N., Receptor mediated binding and
    endocytosis of drug-containing liposomes by tumor cells, in:
    "Liposomes and Immunobiology," Tom, B.H., and Six, H.R., eds.,
    Elsevier, Amsterdam (1980).
Magee, W.E., Cronenberger, J.H., and Thor, D.E., 1978, Marked
    stimulation of lymphocyte-mediated attack on tumor cells by
    target-directed liposomes containing immune RNA, Cancer Res.,
    38: 1173.
Martin, F.D., Hubbell, W.L. and Papahadjopoulos, D., 1981, Immuno-
    specific targeting of liposomes to cells: a novel and efficient
    method for covalent attachment of Fab' fragments via disulfide
    bonds, Biochemistry, 20: 4229.
Six, H.R., Uemura, K., and Kinsky, S.C., 1973, Effect of immuno-
    globulin class and affinity on the initiation of complement-
    dependent damage to liposomal model membranes sensitized with
    dinitrophenylated phospholipids, Biochemistry, 12: 4003.
Szoka, F., Magnusson, K.E., Wojcieszyn, J., Hou, Y., Derzko, Z. and
    Jacobson, K., 1981, Use of lectins and polyethylene glycol for

fusion of glycolipid-containing liposomes with eukaryotic cells, Proc. Natl. Acad. Sci. U.S.A., 78: 1685.

Weinstein, J.N., Yoshikami, S., Henkart, P.A., Blumenthal, R., and Hagins, W.A., 1977, Liposome-cell interaction: transfer and intracellular release of a trapped fluorescent marker, Science, 195: 489.

Weinstein, J.N., Blumenthal, R., Sharrow, S.O., and Henkart, P.A., 1978, Antibody-mediated targeting of liposomes; binding to lymphocytes does not ensure incorporation of vesicle contents into the cells. Biochem. Biophys. Acta, 509: 272.

Weissmann, G., Bloomgarden, D., Kaplan, R., Cohen, C., Hoffstein, S., Collins, T., Gotleib, A., and Nagle, D., 1975, A general method for the introduction of enzymes, by means of immuno-globulin-coated liposomes, into lysosomes of deficient cells, Proc. Natl. Acad. Sci. U.S.A., 72: 88.

DELIVERY OF DRUGS IN TEMPERATURE-SENSITIVE LIPOSOMES

R.L. Magin and J.N. Weinstein*

Department of Electrical Engineering
University of Illinois at Urbana-Champaign
Urbana, Illinois 61801, USA

*Section of Membrane Structure and Function
Laboratory of Mathematical Biology
National Cancer Institute, NIH
Bethesda, Maryland 20205, USA

ABSTRACT

In the presence of certain serum components, principally the lipoproteins, small unilamellar vesicles (SUV) can be made to release their contents rapidly and completely at the liquid crystalline phase transition temperature. By using a mixture of lipids with phase transition at about 42°C the SUV can be designed to release a drug preferentially in a capillary bed (for example, in a tumor) subjected to moderate local hyperthermia. We have made such "temperature-sensitive" liposomes from 7:1 to 7:3 (molar) mixtures of dipalmitoyl and distearoyl phosphatidylcholines and have characterized their interactions with serum components. All of the standard lipoprotein fractions promote release of contents at the transition, as does at least one non-lipoprotein component.

The SUV released essentially all of their contents of carboxy-fluorescein dye during a single pass through a heated capillary bed in rat intestine. When injected i.v. in mice with subcutaneous L1210 tumors, they delivered 14 times as much ^{3}H-methotrexate (MTX) to tumors heated to 42°C by water bath as compared to unheated tumors in the same animals. Inhibition studies with unlabelled MTX and with folinic acid indicated that the ^{3}H-MTX had reached its site of action in the cell cytoplasm and that it had entered the cells by its normal transport mechanisms. Local heating did not increase accumulation of MTX in other parts of the body, suggesting that an increase in therapeutic index can be achieved with temper-

ature-sensitive liposomes. Qualitatively similar results were obtained when subcutaneous Lewis lung tumors in the flanks of mice were
heated with microwaves. Using therapeutic levels of liposomal MTX
we obtained a 4- to 16-fold greater cell kill for the L1210 tumor
than could be explained by the separate effects of heat and liposome-
entrapped MTX.

Large multilamellar vesicles do not have characteristics appropriate for use as temperature-sensitive liposomes, but large unilamellar liposomes appear more favourable in that they can be made
to release their contents (carboxyfluorescein, MTX, cytosine arabinoside) rapidly in the presence of serum. Because of their much
larger ratio of internal volume to lipid, large unilamellar temperature-sensitive liposomes may prove especially useful in vivo.

INTRODUCTION

The usual strategy for targeting liposomes is to attach a
ligand specific for a determinant on the appropriate cell. Antigens,
immunoglobulins, glycoproteins, and lectins have all been used in
this way (Gregoriadis and Neerunjun, 1975; Weissmann, et al., 1975;
Cohen, et al., 1976; Juliano and Stamp, 1976; Gregoriadis, et al.,
1977; Magee, et al., 1978, Weinstein, et al., 1978 and this volume;
Leserman, et al., 1979, 1980a,b). There are a number of obvious
problems to be overcome in this type of targeting, among them the
paucity of useful binding interactions, the antigenicity of most
ligands, the difficulty of obtaining stable association of ligand
with vesicle, the possibility that drug will not reach the appropriate cellular compartment in active form, and the presence of
endothelia or other histological barriers between the liposome and
its cellular binding site.

Temperature-sensitive liposomes permit a different approach to
targeting (Fig. 1) in which the particular difficulties just enumer-
ated do not arise. Multilamellar liposomes have been found to
release encapsulated water-soluble contents much more quickly near
their liquid crystalline phase transition temperature (T_m) than at
other temperatures (Haest, et al., 1975). It seemed possible, then,
that selective release of a drug could be induced in a locally heated
region by injecting liposomes designed to have T_m a few degrees
above physiological temperatures (Yatvin, et al., 1978; Weinstein,
et al., 1979). However, when we tested for leakage at the transition,
multilamellar vesicles leaked over too broad a temperature range to
be useful, and most of the fast release observed was a function of
osmotic imbalance. Small unilamellar vesicles scarcely leaked at
all at T_m. The prospects for temperature-sensitive liposomes did
not look promising at that point because there was still another
problem to be confronted: we worried that the presence of serum
would vitiate the effort in vivo, through broadening of the tran-

sition by cholesterol and possibly other serum components. On the contrary, we found that serum makes the whole enterprise possible. Small unilamellar vesicles are relatively stable to its effects below T_m but release their contents rapidly in the presence of serum at T_m (see Fig. 1).

Local hyperthermia itself is currently under development as a tool in cancer therapy, for use alone or in conjunction with radiation (Har-Kedar and Bleehen, 1976) or chemotherapy (Hahn, 1978). Most attention has been focused on temperatures (about 43°C) at which there may be an intrinsic selective effect on tumor cell viability (discussed in Magin and Johnson, 1979). The means for producing local hyperthermia (microwave, waterbath, radiowave, ultrasound) and its possible toxicity (e.g. burns, increased metastasis) and under intensive study (see Streffer, 1978).

We will first discuss the characterization of temperature-sensitive liposomes in vitro and then consider two sets of studies in vivo which demonstrates their use in selective delivery of MTX to tumors.

MATERIALS AND METHODS

The animals, tumor systems, radiotracers, methods of heating, and chemotherapy techniques have been described in detail elsewhere (Weinstein, et al. 1979, 1980).

Liposomes

By choosing an appropriate pair of lipids (i.e. miscible in all proportions in both fluid and gel phases), one can obtain a single T_m; by varying the ratio of the two lipids, one can manipulate the T_m within a broad range of values (Yatin, et al., 1978). For the in vivo studies described here we used a 7:3 molar mixture of dipalmitoyl phosphatidylcholine (DPPC) (T_m = 41°C) and distearoyl phosphatidylcholine (DSPC) (T_m = 54°C). We have also studied mixtures containing diheptadecanoyl phosphatidylcholine, with analogous results. The solution of drug and/or fluorophore to be encapsulated was vortex-mixed with the exhaustively dried lipid mixture at 55°C, and the suspension was then sonicated for one hour at 50°C under argon. The sonicate was quickly cooled to 2°C and subjected to column chromatography, as described previously (Yatvin, et al., 1978; Weinstein, et al., 1979, 1980). The resulting suspensions were nearly clear initially but became more turbid over a period of hours, indicating a slow increase in particle size and a change in physical state (Suurkuusk et al., 1976). When we use the term "small unilamellar vesicle" (or "SUV") we are, more accurately, referring to highly sonicated vesicles, which may not be unilamellar structures of limitingly small diameter at the time of use. Except as otherwise stated, all liposomes were of the

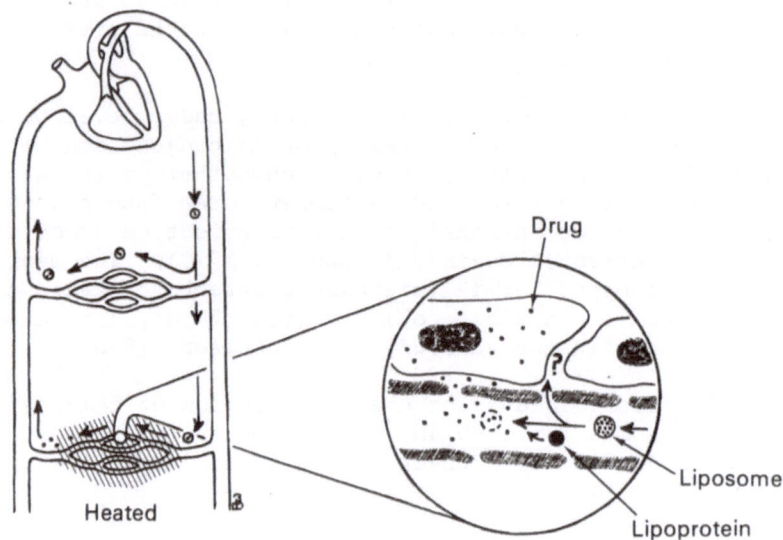

Fig. 1   Schematic view of local release from "temperature-sensitive"
          liposomes in a heated area. As liposomes enter the small
          vessels of the heated area, they release their contents at
          a rate dependent on the temperature and the action of serum
          components, principally the lipoproteins. Released drug
          equilibrates throughout the extracellular space and is trans-
          ported into cells as if injected in free form. As indicated
          by the question mark, intact liposomes might also pass into
          the extracellular space through endothelia made leaky by
          heating, and lipid molecules might be exchanged with cells
          directly or through the mediation of serum components such
          as the lipoproteins.

highly sonicated variety. Large unilamellar vesicles (LUV) were
formed in isopropyl ether and chloroform at 45°C by the method of
Szoka and Papahadjopoulos (1978). Similar preparations were found
to be largely unilamellar by derivatization studies with trinitro-
benzene sulfonate and by ^{31}P nuclear magnetic resonance with line
broadening reagents (Weinstein, et al., 1981).

     The integrity and transition release of each liposome prepara-
tion was tested using a method based on fluorescence self-quenching
of encapsulated carboxyfluorescein (CF) (Weinstein, et al., 1977;
Hagins and Yoshikami, 1977). This water-soluble fluorophore was
encapsulated at a sufficiently high concentration so that its

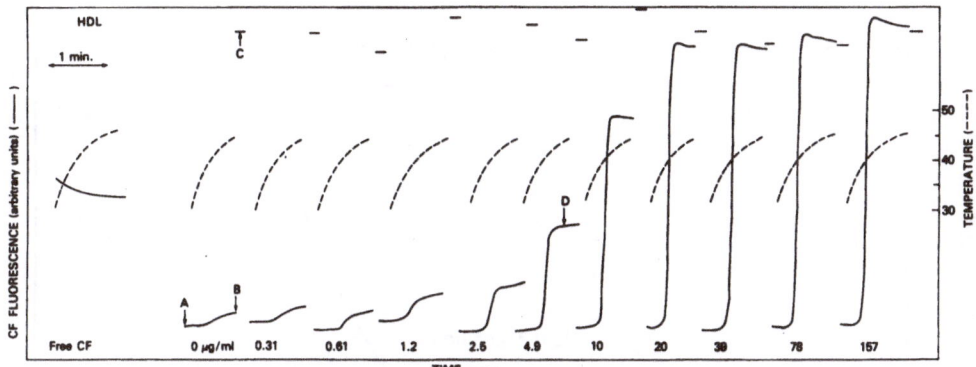

Fig. 2. "Phase transition release" profiles for small unilamellar
DPPC:DSPC (7:3 molar) vesicles as a function of HDL concentration. The letter "c" indicates 100% release (after
addition of Triton X-100, with a 4% correction for the
volumes of detergent added). The first profile is that of
free CF, indicating the temperature dependence of fluorescence. Subsequent profiles are for vesicles. The vesicle
lipid concentration was 60 μM for each scan, and the HDL
protein concentrations were varied as indicated at the
bottom of the figure.

fluorescence was largely self-quenched. Its release from the
vesicles could then be related directly to a progressive increase
in fluorescence of the suspension as the temperature was increased
through T_m. This experimental method, which we call "phase transition release" (PTR), has proved useful for study of the interaction
of a number of proteins with lipid bilayers. (Weinstein, et al.,
1981; Klausner, et al., 1981).

Serum lipoprotein fractions were prepared and characterized
by T.L. and C. Innerarity, using standard methods described by
Weinstein, et al. (1981).

RESULTS

Role of serum components

Liposomes proved to be quite stable to the effects of serum
below T_m, but could release their contents completely within a few
seconds near the transition. This effect of serum is in large part,
but not entirely, due to lipoproteins (Yatvin et al., 1978;
Scherphof et al., 1979; Weinstein et al., 1979). Fig. 2 shows
the PTR profiles obtained for release of CF from temperature-sen-

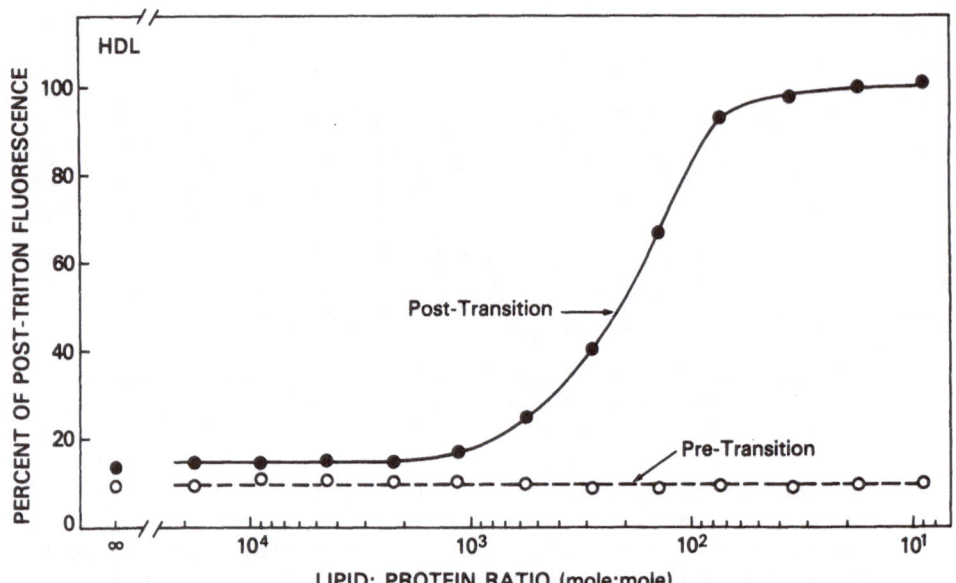

Fig. 3. Dependence of PTR on HDL concentration for small unila-
        mellar vesicles. The curves were calculated from the scans
        in Fig. 2. At high protein concentrations, release appro-
        ached 100% of the Triton-releasable CF. The point of 50%
        release was reached at a lipid:protein ratio of 200:1.

sitive liposomes in the presence of different concentrations of
human high density lipoprotein (HDL). Each scan took about 90
seconds, and almost all of the release took place within the first
5 seconds. Release was low without HDL and essentially total at
sufficiently high HDL concentrations. The data can be replotted
as in Fig. 3 to indicate that HDL releases 50% of the CF at a
lipid protein molar ratio of about 200:1. Other experiments indicated that the process, at least with apolipoproteins, involves
binding to the vesicle surface below transition and a stoichiometric
disruption of the permeability barrier at T_m. The repeated temperature cycles in Fig. 4 show the essentially stoichiometric nature
of the interaction. Effects similar to that in Fig. 3 were obtained
with whole serum, with all of the standard lipoprotein fractions,
and with some component(s) of the non-lipoprotein serum fraction.
As indicated in Table 1, we found that high density, low density,
intermediate density, and very low density lipoproteins had approximately equivalent effect per mg of protein. These studies and
their extension to apolipoproteins of HDL are described in detail
elsewhere (Weinstein et al., 1981).

TABLE I

Relative Efficacy of Human Plasma Fractions in PTR

Plasma fraction	Protein required for 50% CF release*	Protein concentration in plasma**
VLDL	10 μg/ml	170 μg/ml
LDL	9	80
LDL	15	520
HDL	8	1,100
d 1.21 infranate	210	~ 30,000
Albumin***	> 4,000	40,000
Whole plasma	0.4% ****	

* Vesicle lipid concentration 48 μg/ml.

** As measured by Lowry method on serum fractions used in this experiment.

*** Crystalline bovine serum albumin (Miles Laboratories). Crude fraction V albumin preparations often contain significant PTR-inducing contaminants.

**** That is, a 250-fold dilution of plasma will release 50% of CF from this concentration of vesicles.

Temperature-sensitive release from vesicles

LUV formed by reverse phase evaporation were osmotically sensitive at T_m but less so at lower temperatures. Osmotically balanced vesicles (Fig. 5a) showed a small amount of spontaneous release in an initial scan without lipoprotein, no further release in a second scan, and then large fractional release after addition of an appropriate serum fraction (in the case shown, apo HDL). Release continued, though at a lower rate, above T_m. With MLV, on the other hand, there was a small amount of spontaneous release (which could be very large if the vesicles were not protected against osmotic imbalance) but only a slight, rather slow additional effect with serum (Fig. 5b). MLV can be broken down by serum components but only over longer periods than those studied here.

CF FLUORESCENCE (arbitrary units)

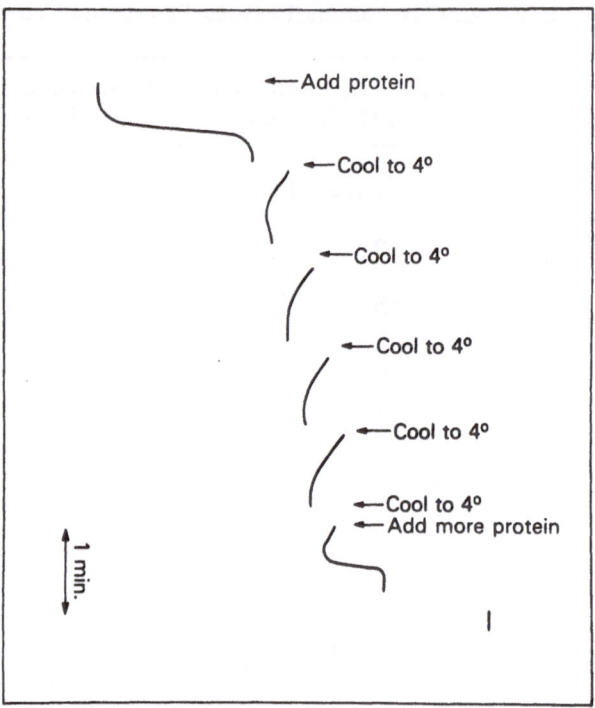

Fig. 4. Repeated temperature scans with small unilamellar DPPC
vesicles and 0.029 μM apo HDL. After the first scan, there
was subsequently little additional release of CF until
more apo HDL was added to bring the final concentration
to 0.058 μM. The downward slants in scans 2 to 5 reflect
the temperature dependence of CF fluorescence. The vesicle
lipid concentration was 36 μM.

    SUV released methotrexate (MTX) and cytosine arabinoside
(ara-C) at about the same rate as they did CF. This result is not
surprising since other studies indicate that the release process
with apolipoproteins is an all-or-nothing disruption, not a uniform
partial leakage from each vesicle (Weinstein et al., 1981). Figure
6a shows the release of ara-C as a function of temperature in a
series of one-minute incubations in 50% mouse serum. There was a
dramatic and potentially quite useful increase in rate at about 40°C
for this liposome preparation (DPPC:DSPC 5.5:1). Figure 6b corro-
borates the finding with CF (Figure 5a) that large percentage release can take place within a few seconds.

Release of liposome contents in vivo

    From the pharmacokinetic point of view, it is important to

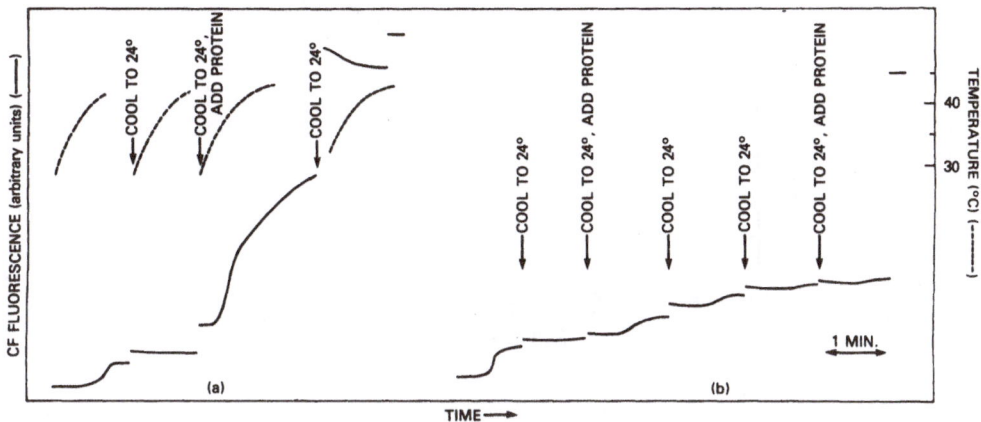

Fig. 5. PTR characteristics of reverse phase evaporation vesicles
   (a) and vortex-mixed multilamellar vesicles (b). The reverse phase vesicles showed in small spontaneous release,
   with no further release after recylcing through T_m. After
   addition of apo HDL to a final concentration of 52 μg/ml
   (lipid: protein ratio of 23:1), there was a large release.
   Recycling indicated considerable additional release even
   before the next upward temperature scan. The MLV showed
   a small spontaneous release on the first scan and only a
   slight additional release on addition of apo HDL to a
   final concentration of 52 μg/ml. This release clearly
   continued for at least two scans, and addition of more
   protein yielded no further effect. On this time scale the
   interaction was slow and incomplete.

know whether large fractional release of the liposome contents can
be obtained in a single pass through a capillary bed. To address
this question, we anesthetized rats, pulled a loop of small intestine through an abdominal incision, and bathed it in a temperature-
controlled water bath. By sampling from the arcades of mesenteric
arteries and veins serving the loop, we were able to determine from
self-quenching how much CF had been released in a single passage.
The arterial-venous difference in concentration of total CF was
small, but self-quenching indicated over 80% release in a single
pass at 42°C, whereas there was only a few percent release at 27
or 37°C (data not shown). These results were encouraging but did
not, of course, indicate what fraction of the release was taking
place in the arteries and capillaries; drug released in the veins
would be washed out of the area and redistributed without creating
a higher concentration in the medium bathing the local cells.

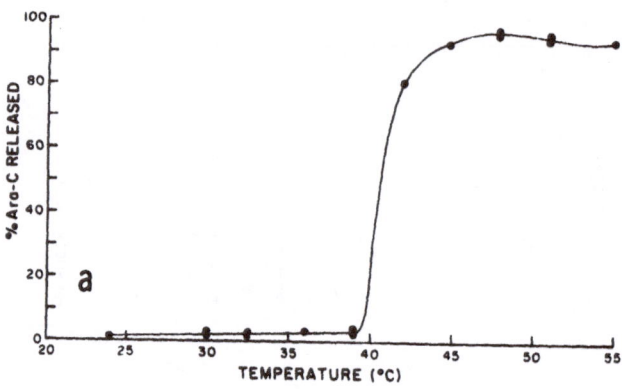

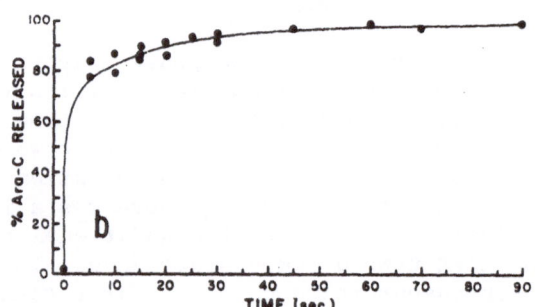

Fig. 6. Temperature-sensitive release of ^{3}H-cytosine arabinoside
        (ara-C) from DPPC:DSPC (5.5:1) large unilamellar vesicles.
   (a) Vesicles were incubated in 100 μl capillaries in 50% mouse
       serum for 1 minute. Free and encapsulated ara-C were then
       separated in a Beckman air-driven centrifuge and counted.
       A dramatic increase in release was obtained at 40°C. The
       lipid concentration was 3 mg/ml.
   (b) Time-course of ara-C release from the same vesicles.
       The bath was set at 45°C, and the time constant for
       equilibration of temperature was 1.2 seconds. Six seconds
       sufficed for near total release, and subsequent experiments
       with smaller capillary tubes have shown 2 seconds to be
       adequate.

Delivery of ^{3}H-MTX to heated Lewis lung tumors in vivo

     The liposomes were injected by tail vein during heating of a
subcutaneous Lewis lung tumor to 42°C. Heating was done with a
2450 MHz microwave apparatus, which we designed and built specifically for this purpose (Magin, 1979). Whole blood, tumor, and other
tissues were obtained for analysis at various times after a 60

minute heating period. Local tumor hyperthermia nearly doubled the
rate at which liposome encapsulated ^{3}H-MTX was cleared from the
blood (Fig. 7) and increased accumulation in the heated tumors to
an average of 4.3 times that in the unheated contralateral control
tumors on the same animals (Fig. 8). With free ^{3}H-MTX, local heating
did not increase the clearance rate or enhance accumulation in
heated tumors. High pressure liquid chromatography (by D.S. Zaharko)
showed essentially all of the ^{3}H counts in the tumors to represent
intact MTX. A large proportion of the accumulated MTX remained in
the tumors 20 hours after injection, and its accumulation was effectively blocked by competition with unlabelled free MTX (Fig. 8d).
These findings suggest that the accumulated MTX was intracellular
and bound to its target enzyme, dihydrofolate reductase. The experiment in Fig. 8e rules out the possibility that liposomes were simply
being sequestered behind endothelia made irreversibly leaky by
heating. When experiments similar to that in Fig. 8a were done
with DSPC vesicles, the ratios obtained for the two tumors were
generally less than 1.5:1.

Delivery of ^{3}H-MTX to heated L1210 tumors in vivo

     Lewis lung tumors provided a good model system in which to est-
ablish the pharmacological principles of selective release from
temperature-sensitive liposomes. However, they are not very sensitive to treatment with MTX (Zaharko et al., 1974), and our early
pilot experiments indicated that we could not substantially affect
their growth with temperature-sensitive liposomes containing MTX.
Accordingly, we switched to the L1210 murine tumor, which is more
sensitive to MTX (Chabner and Young, 1973) and which has a regular
pattern of growth previously characterized in considerable detail
(Schabel, 1977). The experiments were implemented by water bath
heating of solid L1210 tumors implanted s.c. in the hind feet of
mice. As with microwave heating of the Lewis lung tumors, ^{3}H-MTX
was cleared from the plasma more rapidly when a foot was heated to
42°C. Four hours after injection of liposomes, the heated tumors
contained an average of 14 times as much ^{3}H-MTX as did the unheated
ones (Fig. 9). A large dose of free, unlabelled MTX effectively
blocked tumor incorporation of ^{3}H-MTX (but not of ^{14}C-DPPC), indicating that the differences seen with heating did not simply represent
liposomes sequestered in the tumors. Similar inhibition was found
with dl-L-Ca leucovorin, a compound which competes with MTX for
membrane transport. This finding suggests that ^{3}H-MTX enters the
tumor cells principally by its usual molecular transport mechanisms,
not by direct interaction (e.g., fusion) of the liposomes with the
cells. A larger fraction of injected lipid than of ^{3}H-MTX remained
in the circulation after 4 or 20 hours, and there was less than a
factor of two difference in ^{14}C-DPPC uptake between heated and unheated tumors (See Fig. 10).

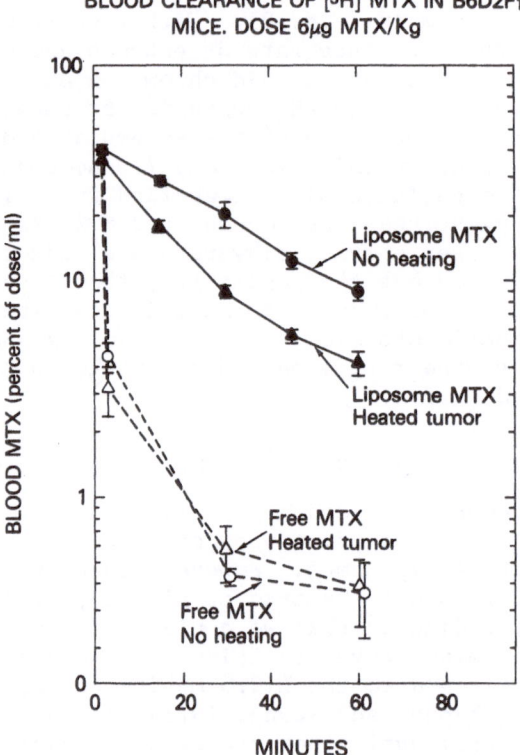

BLOOD CLEARANCE OF [3H] MTX IN B6D2F₁
MICE. DOSE 6µg MTX/Kg

Fig. 7. Clearance of ^{3}H-MTX injected by tail vein as free drug or
encapsulated in temperature-sensitive liposomes. Heating
a subcutaneous tumor to 42°C made no discernible difference
in clearance of free drug, which was largely eliminated from
the blood by redistribution within the first three minutes.
Encapsulated MTX cleared with $t_{1/2}$ = 38 minutes in the absence
of heating and $t_{1/2}$ = 23 minutes (for the first 45 minutes)
if a tumor was heated. Heating probably acts by releasing
drug from the small fraction of liposomes passing through
the area in each circulation. MTX doses were 0.006 mg/Kg.
Liposomes contained 100 mg lipid/Kg mouse. Rectal temperatures average 36.0°C and tumors were heated to 42±0.1°C.
Each point represents the mean from retroorbital collections
on four animals, and error bars represent standard errors.
Liposomal MTX was largely in serum, rather than blood cells,
after one hour.

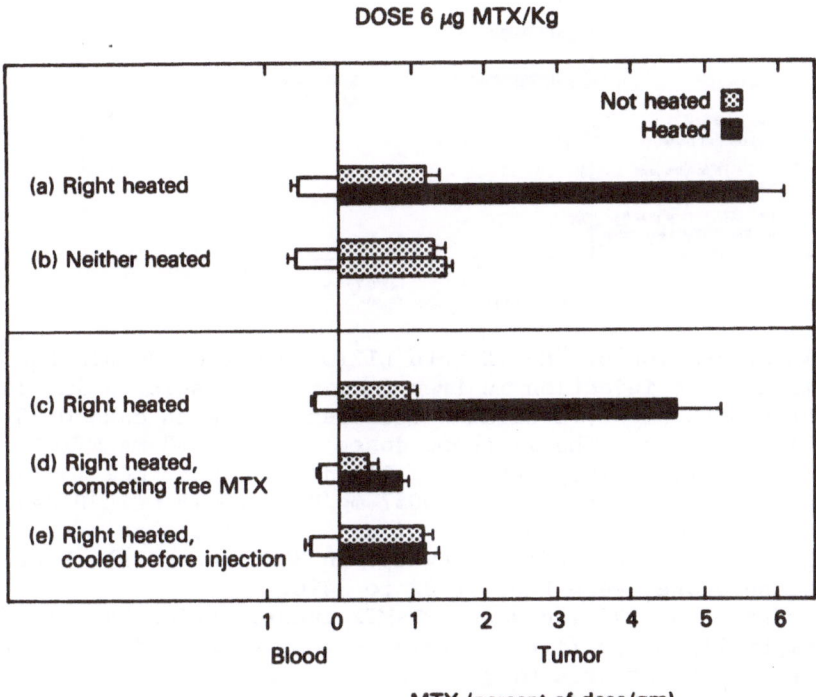

DOSE 6 μg MTX/Kg

Fig. 8. Incorporation of ^{3}H–MTX into Lewis lung tumors of "double-
tumor" mice four hours after tail-vein injection of liposome-
encapsulated MTX. Conditions were as in Fig. 7. Rectal
temperatures averaged 35.4°C.
(a) Right tumor heated: ratio = 4.8;
(b) Neither tumor heated: ratio = 1.15;
(c) Right tumor heated: ratio = 4.7;
(d) Right tumor heated, 300 mg/Kg competing dose of free
    unlabelled MTX included in injection: uptake in heated
    tumor decreased more than five-fold, indicating inhibition
    by the unlabelled MTX;
(e) Right tumor heated for one hour, liposomes then injected
    five minutes later (after tumors returned to body temper-
    ature): ratio = 1.02;
    Experiments (a)-(b) are separated from (c)-(e) to indicate
    use of different batches of liposomes and tumors. Note the
    lower, but equivalent amounts of MTX in blood under each
    condition. Abscissa numbers refer to ^{3}H–MTX (percent of
    dose/gm). Data are means±standard error from four animals.

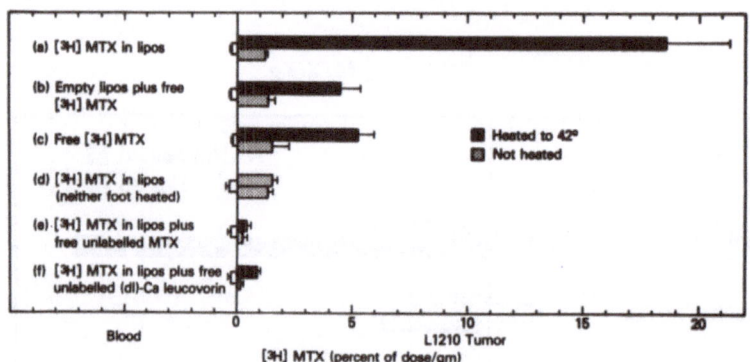

Fig. 9. Incorporation of ^{3}H–MTX into L1210 tumors of double–tumored
        mice after injection in free form or encapsulated in 7:3
        DPPC:DSPC highly sonicated vesicles. In each case 0.25 ml
        was injected. The liposome doses were 0.0058 mg MTX/Kg
        (0.0019 mCi ^{3}H/Kg) and 97 mg lipid/Kg (0.0086 mCi ^{14}C/Kg);
        the free MTX doses were 0.0057 mg/Kg (0.0018 mCi ^{3}H/Kg).
        Bars indicate mean plus or minus S.E. for groups of four mice.
        Left tumors were heated (except in 33°C controls). Rectal
        temperatures were kept at 32 to 34°C.
  (a) Heating to 42°C increased ^{3}H–MTX incorporation 14–fold;
  (b) empty liposomes (i.e. containing only buffer) did not affect
      the uptake of free MTX;
  (c) heating to 42°C increased incorporation three–fold;
  (d) immersion of the left foot in water at 33°C had no effect on
      incorporation;
  (e) free unlabelled MTX (300 mg/Kg) effectively inhibited incor-
      poration;
  (f) free dl–L–Ca leucovorin (300 mg/Kg) also inhibited incorpor-
      ation;

Treatment of L1210 Tumors

     When drug dosages were increased to the pharmacological level
of 3 mg/Kg MTX, the major results were as follows: (i) liposome-
encapsulated MTX delayed tumor growth more than did an equivalent
concentration of free MTX, with or without heating; (ii) heating
alone to 42°C for one hour delayed tumor growth for about 0.7 days,
whereas heating increased by 2.8 days the growth delay obtained with
temperature–sensitive liposomes containing MTX (Fig. 11). The "non-
additive" effect (about 2.1 days) corresponds to an extra cell kill
of 4–to 16–fold beyond that attributable to the separate effects of
heating and of the encapsulated MTX (Weinstein et al., 1980). The
effect appears to have been limited by saturation of the major cellular transport mechanism for MTX and perhaps also by saturation of
the capacity of mouse serum to disrupt liposomes. Much larger delays

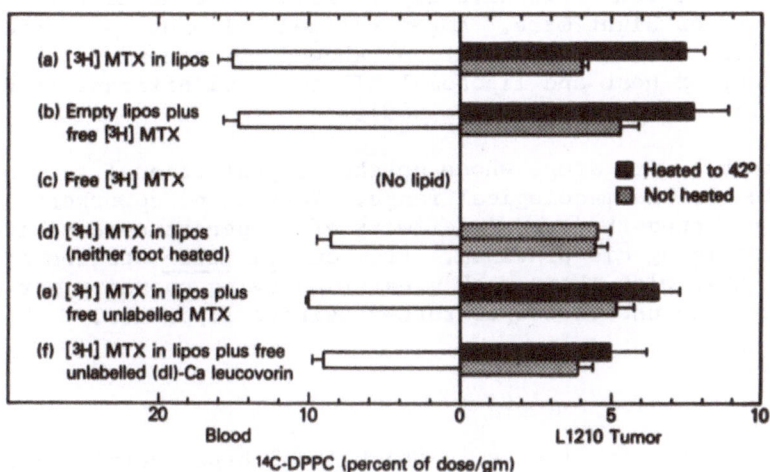

Fig. 10. Incorporation of ^{14}C–DPPC into L1210 tumors after injection in 7:3 DPPC:DSPC liposomes. Same experiment as in Fig. 9. Neither blood levels nor tumor uptakes varied by as much as a factor of 2, in contrast to the findings for ^{3}H–MTX.

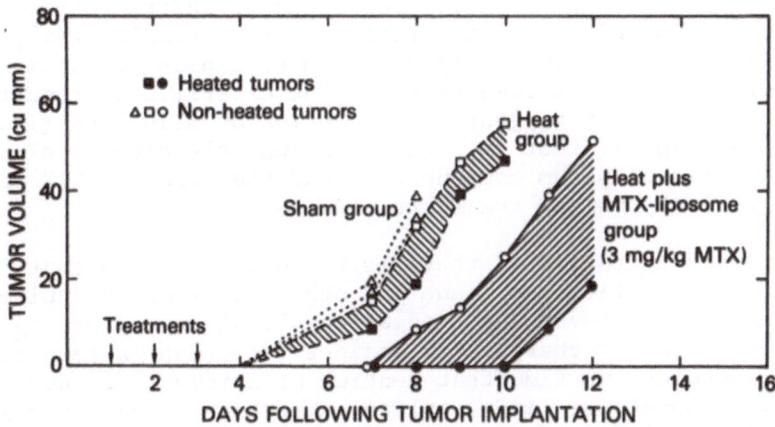

Fig. 11. L1210 tumor growth in mouse feet after treatment with hyperthermia (42°C) and/or heat–sensitive liposomes containing MTX at 3.0 mg MTX/Kg/dose (320 mg lipid/Kg/dose). There were three groups: a "sham" group, in which both tumors were at about 33°C; a "heat" group, in which the left tumor was at 42°C, the right at 33°C; a "heat plus MTX–liposome" group in which the left tumor was at 42°C, the right at 33°C, and

liposomes containing MTX were injected. Doses were given
i.v. on three successive days. Points are medians for
groups of eight mice. A generalised Wilcoxon test (two-
tailed, normal approximation) showed the non-additive
effect of heat and liposomal MTX to be significant at p =
0.015 (Weinstein et al., 1980).

may be obtainable with drugs whose uptake is proportional to concentration in the pharmacological range. Yatvin and coworkers
(1981) have reported therapeutic effects of temperature-sensitive
liposomes containing cis-platinum. From our in vitro studies it
appears that LUV, with their much greater carrying capacity per unit
of lipid, may make useful temperature-sensitive liposomes.

DISCUSSION

     There are a number of ways in which local hyperthermia might
increase the effectiveness of drug-containing liposomes (Weinstein
et al., 1979): (i) by promoting selective drug release at T_m; (ii)
by increasing local blood flow; (iii) by increasing endothelial permeability to particles, thereby enhancing accumulation of liposomes in
the target tissues; (iv) by increasing the permeability or suscept-
ibility of target cells to drug released from the liposomes; (v) by
increasing direct transfer of drug from liposomes to cells - for
example, by fusion or endocytosis; and (vi) by enhancing release from
liposomes of anions such as MTX. (This last possibility could, of
course, be realised with naturally occurring pH shifts such as those
possible in tumors and sites of infection. In a similar vein, Yatvin
et al., (1980) have developed liposomes whose lipids are designed for
selective permeability at lowered pH.) The experimental results
described in this paper suggest the operation of mechanism (i), as
schematized in Fig. 1: that is, local heating selectively releases
MTX (with the aid of serum components), and the released MTX then
enters the cells by normal transport processes.

     With regard to toxicity, there is the usual problem that lipo-
somes accumulate in liver, spleen, and other areas of reticuloendothelial function. However, heating of the local tumor, per se, is
likely to increase the therapeutic indices for drugs in temperature-
sensitive liposomes; we find that heating of a tumor does not significantly affect uptake by liver, spleen, intestine, and other sites
of potential toxicity for a drug. In the use of temperature-sensitive
liposomes, it would usually not matter if the heated field included
normal tissues, unless those tissues were highly sensitive to the
drug used. For many agents that would mean, for example, avoiding
the intestinal epithelium and other rapidly dividing cell types.
Local treatment would not deplete bone marrow cells.

     The major limitation of temperature-sensitive liposomes for

cancer chemotherapy is that they do not address the problem of metastatic disease. In this regard, they are similar to X-irradiation
and to surgery. Temperature-sensitive liposomes containing chemotherapeutic agents might be useful against local accumulations of
such tumors as melanoma, osteosarcoma, and transitional cell carcinoma
of the bladder. They might also be of use in such problems as local
infection and psoriasis. The approach is not limited to superficial
areas; selective hyperthermia of deep structures by microwaves, radio-
waves, ultrasound, and lavage is under active study.

ACKNOWLEDGEMENTS

We are grateful to others who contributed to the investigations
described here: Milton B. Yatvin, Robert Blumenthal, Daniel S.
Zaharko, Richard L. Cysyk, and Warren H. Dennis.

REFERENCES

Chabner, B.A. and Young, R.C., 1973, Threshold methotrexate concentra-
    tion for in vivo inhibition of DNA synthesis in normal and
    tumorous target tissues, J. Clin. Invest. 52:1804.
Cohen, C.M., Weissmann, G., Hoffstein, S., Awasthi, Y.C., Srivastava,
    S.K., 1976, Introduction to purified hexosaminidase A into Tay-
    Sachs leucocytes by means of immunoglobulin-coated liposomes,
    Biochemistry 15: 452.
Gregoriadis, G. and Hunt, R., 1977, Fate of a liposome-associated
    agent injected into normal and tumour-bearing rodents, Attempts
    to improve localization in tumor tissues, Life Sci. 21: 357.
Gregoriadis, G. and Neerunjun, D.E., 1975, Homing of liposomes to
    target cells, Biochem. Biophys. Res. Commun. 65:537.
Haest, C.M.W., de Gier, J.A., van Es, G.A., Verkleij, A.J. and van
    Deenan, L.L.M., 1972, Fragility of the permeability barrier
    of Escherichia coli, Biochim. Biophys. Acta 288: 43
Hagins, W.A. and Yoshikami, S., 1977, Intracellular transmission of
    visual excitation in photoreceptors: Electrical effects of
    chelating agents introduced into rods by vesicle fusion, in:
    Vertebrate Photoreception, P. Fatt, H.B. Barlow, eds. Academic
    Press, New York.
Hahn, G.M., 1978, Interactions of drugs and hyperthermia in vitro
    and in vivo., in: Cancer Treatment by Hypertheria and Radiation,
    C. Streffer, ed., Urban and Schwarzenberg, Baltimore.
Har-Kedar, I. and Bleehen, N.M., 1976, Expereimental and clinical
    aspects of hyperthermia applied to the treatment of cancer with
    special reference to the role of ultrasonic and microwave heat-
    ing, Adv. Radiat. Biol. 6:229
Juliano, R.L. and Stamp, D., 1976, Lectin-mediated attachment of
    glycoprotein-bearing liposomes to cells, Nature 261:235

Klausner, R.D., Kumar, N., Weinstein, J.N., Blumenthal, R., and
    Flavin, M., 1981, Interaction of tubulin with phospholipid
    vesicles I: Association with vesicles at the phase transition,
    J. Biol. Chem., 256: 5879.
Leserman, L.D., Weinstein, J.N., Blumenthal, R., Sharrow, S.O.,
    and Terry, W.D., 1979, Binding of antigen-bearing fluorescent
    liposomes to the murine myeloma tumor MOPC 315, J. Immunol.
    122: 585.
Leserman, L.D., Barbet, J., Kourilsky, F.M., and Weinstein, J.N.,
    1980a, Liposomes directed to specific cellular targets by
    vocalently-coupled monoclonal antibody, protein A, and avidin,
    Nature 288: 602.
Leserman, L.D., Weinstein, J.M., Blumenthal, R., and Terry, W.D.,
    1980b, Receptor-mediated endocytosis of antibody-opsonized
    liposomes by tumor cells, Proc. Natl. Acad. Sci. 77: 4089.
Magee, W.E., Cronenberger, J.H. and Thor, D.E., 1978, Marked
    stimulation of lymphocyte-mediated attach on tumor cells by
    target-directed liposomes containing immune RNA, Cancer Res.
    38:1173.
Magin, R.L., 1979, A microwave system for the controlled production
    of local tumor hyperthermia in animals, IEEE Trans. Microwave
    Theory Tech. 27:78.
Magin, R.L. and Johnson, R.K., 1979, Effects of local tumor hyper-
    thermia on the growth of solid mouse tumors, Cancer Res. 39:
    4534.
Schabel, F.M., 1977, Quantitative evaluation of anticancer agent
    activity in experimental animals, Pharmacology and Therapeutics
    (Part A) 1:411.
Scherphof, G., Morselt, H., Regts, J. and Wilschut, J.C., 1979, The
    involvement of the lipid phase transition in the plasma-induced
    dissolution of multilamellar phosphatidylcholine vesicles,
    Biochim. Biophys. Acta 56: 196.
Streffer, C., 1978, "Cancer Therapy by Hyperthermia and Radiation",
    Urban and Schwarzenberg, Baltimore.
Suurkuusk, J., Lentz, B.R., Barenholz, Y., Biltonen, R.L., and
    Thompson, T.E., 1976, A calorimetric and fluorescent probe
    study of the gel-liquid crystalline phase transition in small
    single-lamellar dipalmitoylphosphatidylcholine vesicles,
    Biochemistry, 15: 1393.
Szoka, F., Jr., and Papahadjopoulos, D., 1978, Procedure for pre-
    paration of liposomes with large internal aqueous space and
    high capture by reverse-phase evaporation, Proc. Natl. Acad.
    Sci. USA. 75: 4194.
Weinstein, J.N. Blumenthal, R., Sharrow, S.O. and Henkart, P.A.,
    1978, Antibody-mediated targeting of liposomes: Binding to
    lymphocytes does not ensure incorporation of vesicle contents
    into the cells, Biochim. Biophys. Acta 509: 272.
Weinstein, J.N., Magin, R.L., Cysyk, R.L. and Zaharko, D.S., 1980,
    Treatment of solid L1210 murine tumors with local hyperthermia
    and temperature-sensitive liposomes containing methotrexate.

Cancer Res. 40: 1388

Weinstein, J.N., Magin, R.L., Yatvin, M.B., and Zaharko, D.S., 1979, Liposomes and local hyperthermia: Selective delivery of methotrexate to heated tumors, Science 204: 188.

Weinstein, J.N., Yoshikami, S., Henkart, P.A., Blumenthal, R. and Hagins, W.A., 1977, Liposome-cell interaction: Transfer and intracellular release of a trapped fluorescent marker, Science 195: 489.

Weinstein, J.N., Klausner, R.D., Innerarity, T.L., Ralston, E., and Blumenthal, R., 1981, "Phase transition release" (PTR), a new approach to the interaction of proteins with lipid vesicles: Application to lipoproteins, Biochim. Biophys, Acta, in press.

Weissmann, G., Bloomgarden, D., Kaplan, R., Cohen, C., Hoffstein, S., Collins, T., Gotlieb, A. and Nagle, D., 1975, A general method for the introduction of enzymes, by means of immunoglobulin-coated liposomes, into lysosomes of deficient cells, Proc. Natl. Acad. Sci. USA. 72: 88.

Yatvin, M.B., Weinstein, J.N., Dennis, W.H., and Blumenthal, R., 1978, Design of liposomes for enhanced local release of drugs by hyperthermia, Science 202: 1290.

Yatvin, M.B., Kreutz, W., Florwitz, B.A. and Shinitzky, B., 1980, Ph-Sensitive liposomes: Possible clinical implications, Science 210: 1253.

Yatvin, M.B., Muhlensiepen, H., Porschen, W., Weinstein, J.N., and Feinendegen, L.E., 1981, Selective delivery of liposome encapsulated cis-dichlorodiammineplatinum (II) by heat: Influence on tumor drug uptake and growth, Cancer Res. 41: 1602

Zaharko, D.S., Dedrick, R.L., Peale, A.L., Drake, J.C. and Lutz, R.J., 1974, Relative toxicity of methotrexate in several tissues of mice bearing Lewis lung carcinoma, JPET 189: 585.

HYPERTHERMIA-MEDIATED TARGETING OF LIPOSOME-ASSOCIATED

ANTI-NEOPLASTIC DRUGS[a]

Milton B. Yatvin, Theodore C. Cree[b], Jerry J. Gipp

University of Wisconsin
Department of Human Oncology, WCCC
Madison, WI 53792

INTRODUCTION

One of the major obstacles limiting the effectiveness of chemo-therapeutic programmes is the inability of the present drug inventory to discriminate normal from malignant neoplastic tissue. As the search for selective anticancer drugs has been largely ineffective to date, considerable research effort has been directed toward the development of drug carrier systems[1]. One of the systems being investigated are closed vesicles composed primarily of phospholipids [2,3]. Liposomes have been extensively used as models[3,4] for biological membrane research and have contributed to understanding the physico-chemical properties of biological membranes[6,7]. They have also advanced our understanding of cell-cell recognition[8,9], fusion [10,11] and protein-lipid interaction[12,13]. The self-assembly properties of phospholipid amphiphiles make possible the entrapment of water soluble compounds within the aqueous lumen of the liposome[14]. It became evident that entrapment of enzymes within liposomes might provide a therapeutic vehicle useful in treatment of diseases of enzyme deficiency[15,16].

Major efforts have been directed toward the application of liposome technology as drug-carrier and delivery systems. One of the goals presently being explored is the targeting of liposomal drugs to specific sites in vivo. In vitro application of immuno-logical technology appeared promising at first. However, the capillary endothelial system severely limits cell-liposome interactions, particularly in peripheral tissues. The purpose of this paper is to discuss another major limitation; that is, the consequence of interaction of the liposome bilayer with blood components and the reticuloendothelial system.

223

HYPERTHERMIA MEDIATED DRUG RELEASE

At present, the successful application of liposome–drug technology has been limited to localised delivery (e.g. subcutaneous or intramuscular injection, aerosol delivery into the trachea or infusion into the lymphatic system) or exploitation of the natural fate of liposomes in vivo (uptake by reticuloendothelial macrophages). Recently, Yatvin et al.[17] have suggested that by exploiting the biophysical and physiological characteristics of liposomes and the target area, preferential drug release and localised uptake might be realised in response to local hyperthermia. It was envisioned that liposomes which have a transition temperature that was slightly above physiological would release entrapped drugs as the circulating liposomes passed through the heated area. Repeated passage by the liposomes through the heated area would ensure continued release and local concentration of the drug. This protocol is based on the prediction that liposomes retain their designed physical properties and remain in the circulatory system long enough for the hyperthermic treatment to affect maximal drug release.

Liposomes composed of 70–75% dipalmitoylphosphatidylcholine (DPPC) and 25–30% distearoylphosphatidylcholine (DSPC) exhibit a maximum rate of release of water soluble compound in vitro at 42–43° C^{18}. When ^3H-Methotrexate (MTX) entrapped in such liposomes was injected i.v. into mice bearing Lewis lung tumors, an approximate four-fold increase in tumor ^3H activity was realised in tumors heated to 42°C compared to unheated tumors[18]. Similar studies employing solid L1210 murine tumors resulted in a 14:1 ratio of tumor associated drug in heated versus unheated tumors[19]. The differences between the two studies could be attributed to inherent biochemical and physiological differences in the tumors as well as their anatomical location. These results were attributed to local release of drug in response to local hyperthermia. Analysis of tumor associated ^{14}C-DPPC activity by these investigators led to the conclusion that sequestering of intact liposomes in the tumor capillary bed in response to hyperthermia was not responsible for the observed concentration of ^3H activity.

We also studied the distribution of dual–labelled liposomes containing ^{14}C-DPPC and ^3H-MTX in blood and tumor tissue and preliminary results are presented. C3H mice hearing MTGB tumors in their flank were subjected to local hyperthermia by submersion of the tumor-bearing leg in a water bath. Three different liposome preparations composed of phosphatidylcholines were used. The DPPC:DSPC (3:1, w/w) preparation exhibits a sharp transition temperature (as defined by maximal rate of release of entrapped water soluble compounds) in vitro of 42°C. Liposomes composed of DPPC:DSPC (1:1, w/w) were also tested. It was presumed that these liposomes would possess a transition temperature well above that achieved by local hyperthermia in vivo and would thus exhibit minimal response to local hyperthermia. The

final liposome preparation was composed of 88% diheptadodecylphospha-
tidylcholine (DHPC), 12% N-palmitoyl homocysteine (PHC) and tracer
quantities of ^{14}C-DPPC. These liposomes are a modification of the pH
sensitive liposomes described by Yatvin et al.[20]. The inclusion of
the latter liposome preparation in these experiments was fortuitous
and not originally by design.

Liposomes were prepared by sonication in the presence of 270 μM
^{3}H-MTX in PBS (pH7.4). Free drug was removed by exclusion chromatography. Animals were injected with liposomes i.v. via the tail vein,
anesthetized with chloral hydrate, and placed into the water bath 10
minutes following liposome administration for a period of one hour.
Blood samples were taken at 30, 60 and 90 minutes following liposome
administration and prepared for liquid scintillation counting. At
90 minutes, the animals were sacrificed, tumors removed, digested in
Protosol (New England Nuclear) and prepared for liquid scintillation
counting.

Clearance of liposomal ^{3}H-MTX from blood is presented in Fig. 1.
With all three liposome preparations, there was a significant decrease
in the circulating ^{3}H label by 30 minutes in animals subjected to
local hyperthermia compared to unheated controls. Note that a significant loss of ^{3}H label occurs in control animals i.e. only 20 (DPPC:
DSPC, 3:1) to 40% (DPPC:DSPC, 1:1) of the injected ^{3}H remains in the
blood at 30 minutes and that the rate of loss is greatest for the
first 30 minutes. These results are similar to those reported by
Weinstein et al[18] but are at variance with those more recently reported by the same investigators for subsequent analogous experiments[19]. The possible significance of these observations will be
discussed below.

For the purpose of this discussion, we will assume that the
^{14}C-DPPC label reasonably approximates a circulating liposomal marker
for the relatively short duration of these experiments, especially
the first 30 minutes. Clearance of ^{14}C-DPPC label from blood is shown
in Fig. 2. Data from all three liposome preparations were not significantly different from each other (not shown) and are therefore
presented as the pooled means of experiments with or without local
hyperthermia. Local hyperthermia had little or no effect on the
clearance of ^{14}C label from blood. Also, the rate of clearance was
far less than those observed for the ^{3}H label, 70% of the injected
label remaining by 30 minutes. Given our assumption, the decrease
in the ^{3}H/^{14}C ratio at 30 minutes compared to the injected ratio
mitigates against sequesterisation of liposomes by the reticuloendothelial system as the major cause of ^{3}H label loss and supports the
concept of removal of free circulating MTX lost from liposomes due to
leakage.

If the ^{3}H/^{14}C ratio in blood is expressed relative to the

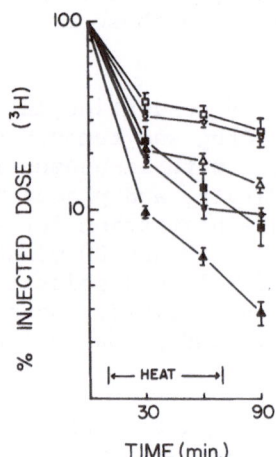

Fig. 1. Clearance of ^{3}H-methotrexate from whole blood. A 5 μl
        sample of blood was withdrawn from a tail vein in heparinised
        micropipettes, digested in Protosol (New England Nuclear)
        and prepared for liquid scintillation counting. Open figures,
        unheated controls; closed figures, local hyperthermia. pH
        sensitive liposomes (O ●), DPPC:DSPC, 3:1 w/w liposomes (∆ ▲),
        DPPC:DSPC, 1:1 w/w liposomes (□ ■). Means ± S.D. (n=4) are
        presented.

injected ratio, i.e. $\dfrac{^3\text{H}/^{14}\text{C (blood)}}{^3\text{H}/^{14}\text{C (injected)}}$, the percent ^{3}H-MTX that remains associated with circulating liposomes can be calculated. Hence,
38, 27, and 44% of the original encapsulated ^{3}H-MTX remained with the
circulating liposomes at 90 minutes repsectively for the pH sensitive
DPPC:DSPC (3:1) and DPPC:DSPC (1:1) liposomes in control animals.
The corresponding values for animals receiving local hyperthermia
are 17, 5 and 16%.

     If selective uptake of ^{3}H label or sequesterisation of intact
liposomes does not occur in the tumor tissue, the ^{3}H/^{14}C ratio of the
tumor tissue should approximately reflect the ratio found in the
blood at 90 minutes i.e. liposomes "caught" in the tumor circulatory
system at sacrifice. Table I presents the ^{3}H/^{14}C ratio found in
tumors at 90 minutes compared to the injected ratio. The ratios

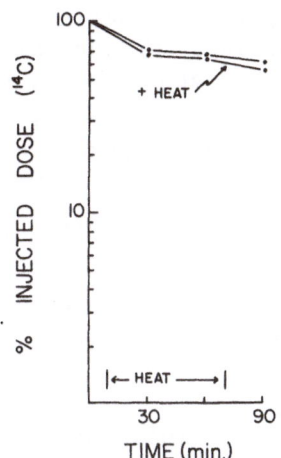

Fig. 2. Clearance of ^{14}C-dipalmitoyl phosphatidylcholine from whole blood. Procedure was as described in Figure 1. Data from the three liposome preparations were not statistically different and is presented as pooled means. Separate data for controls and local hyperthermia is presented.

presented are clearly greater than those found in the blood at 90 minutes (see above). Significantly, the ratios obtained with the pH sensitive and DPPC:DSPC (3:1) liposomes are greater for control animals than for animals in which the tumors were heated. Interpretation of this data is not straightforward and could be interpreted as selective uptake ^{3}H-MTX, mechanical sequesterisation of liposomes or both. Nevertheless, we feel that if local heating caused increased ^{3}H release and concomitant local uptake of the released ^{3}H, and if mecahnical sequestering of ^{14}C label is insignificant, the ratios obtained in the heated tumors should be greater compared to unheated tumors.

The effect of tumor heating is presented in Table II. An enhancement in ^{3}H retention was obtained for all three liposome preparations but did not approach the 4:1 ratio obtained previously[18]. This could be due in part to the different animals and tumors used and probably more importantly, the application of heat 10 minutes after liposome administration rather than before or at the time of administration. Enhancement of ^{14}C entrapment was also observed.

Table 1. Tumor $^3H/^{14}C$ Ratio Relative to Injected $^3H/^{14}C$ Ratio
(tumor ratio/injected ratio)

Tumors were removed 90 minutes following liposome administration,
digested in Protosol (New England Nuclear) and prepared for
liquid scintillation counting. Median values were used to
calculate ratios which were normalised/mg tissue (n=4).

	Liposome Preparation		
	pH sens.	3:1 DPPC:DSPC	1:1 DPPC:DSPC
no heat	0.91	0.64	0.78
+ heat	0.67	0.50	0.89

This could reflect an expanded fluid space of the tissue or a stag-
nated blood flow in response to hyperthermia. At present, the data
does not allow differentiating significant differences in entrapment
of the ^3H label from the ^{14}C label.

DEFINING A PROBLEM

From analysis of the data presented here and elsewhere[18], we
feel that a major obstacle to hyperthermia mediated liposomal delivery
of water soluble drugs in vivo exists and should be addressed. That
is, it would appear that liposomes optimised for maximal leakage at
temperatures slightly above physiological, lose this critical property
rapidly upon being mixed with blood components in vivo. As shown
by Kimelberg[21], the circulating half-life of liposomal ^3H-MTX app-
roached 10 hrs. when the liposomes contained 32% cholesterol. However, as such liposomes do not possess a discrete phase transition,
they would not be sensitive to the hyperthermic mode for local release. It is quite likely that activity by the reticuloendothelial
system is partly responsible for the initial rapid drop in circulating ^3H activity. It could explain the initial drop in SUV associated
^3H -MTX reported by Kimelberg[21]. However, the magnitude of the drop
observed in this and other studies[18], plus the low $^3H/^{14}C$ ratios
found in tumors compared to the injected ratio suggest leakage of
^3H-MTX from liposomes whether or not local hyperthermia is present.

Recent work by Scherphof et al. has shown that small unilamellar
vesicles composed only of phosphatidylcholine lose phosphatidylcholine
(PC) residues to high density lipoproteins resulting in liposome
dissolution and concomitant loss of internalised markers to the
surrounding media[22]. Further, these investigators have shown that

Table II.   Tumor Heat Enhancement Ratio for ^{3}H and ^{14}C Labels
(dpm with heat/dpm no heat)

Procedure was as described in Table I.

	^{3}H	^{14}C
pH sens. 3:1	1.99	2.71
DPPC:DSPC 1:1	2.33	2.94
DPPC:DSPC	2.18	1.77

the rate of such reactions is greatly enhanced when discrete phase boundaries exist in the bilayer (as is required to achieve maximal rate of release of internalised MTX)[23]. Additions of 33% cholesterol to liposomes appeared to abolish these interactions. They have also shown that liposomes composed of monotectic mixtures of phosphatidylcholines appear to interact more slowly than those composed of a pure PC. However, it appeared that coexistence of phase boundaries in these liposomes was not required for liposome–lipoprotein interaction[23].

From the foregoing discussion, it would appear likely that small unilamellar vesicles composed of pure phosphatidylcholines undergo relatively rapid interactions with plasma components which render them more permeable to entrapped species. It would also appear that such changes are, for practical considerations, irreversible. Hence the enhanced release of internalised markers at the transition temperature from liposomes incubated in vitro in the presence of plasma components probably reflects increased bilayer disorder caused lipoproteins interaction[18]. The reversibility or irreversibility of such interactions was not determined from these experiments.

TOWARDS A SOLUTION

It appears the present state of the art is not sufficiently advanced to allow us to engineer liposomes possessing the desired physical properties to optimize hyperthermic mediated release with reasonable retention of these properties in vivo for a reasonable period of time (1-2 hours). However, inclusion of other membrane stabilising components such as sphingomyelin have not been tested, especially in regard to hyperthermic sensitive liposomes. Inclusion of a significant amount of sphingomyelin possessing specific hydrocarbon chains might be possible resulting in liposomes with greater resistance to change in vivo but still retaining the precise physical properties desired. Recent evidence presented by Scherphof indicates that substitutions of lecithin by sphingomyelin appears to prolong

the half-lives of small as well as large unilamellar liposomes in
vivo[24].

The data presented in Table II and by others[18,19] suggests that
some sequestering of liposomes in response to local hyperthermia
occurs.   Electron microscopic examination of tumors obtained 30 minutes after initiation of local hyperthermia shows considerable breakdown of the capillary endothelium manifested by inclusion of red
cells in the interstitial spaces (unpublished data).   This raises
the possibility that liposome-cell contact could occur making previously mentioned targeting modalities (e.g. antibody-antigen, lec-
ithin-glycoprotein or membrane fusion with liposomes and red cells)
more feasible.

Another factor of great importance is the relative time of heat
application, and liposome administration.   Unlike the previous reports[18,19,25], local hyperthermia was applied 10 minutes after liposome administration.   This is probably why a greater heat enhancement ratio (Table II) for ^{3}H was not realised.   If the liposomes used
in these studies suffer rapid irreversible modification by plasma
components, it is obvious that the first few moments of the liposomes'
life in vivo are the most important.   Therefore, optimisation of the
heating regime with respect to time and temperature are probably
more important than previously thought.   Along this line, it is
possible that the enhanced rate of ^{3}H clearance from blood as a
result local hyperthermia (see Figure 1) might result from a more
rapid rate of interaction of liposomes with blood components as the
liposomes pass through the heated region.   Hence, one pass through
the heated region results in a greater population of irreversibly
damaged liposomes resulting in a greater rate of ^{3}H loss from blood.
It should be noted that this interpretation is not equivalent to that
of increased loss of ^{3}H label as the liposomes repeatedly traverse
the heated region as postulated previously[18,19].   The former interpretation is also supported by the data presented in Table I which
shows that for 2 of the 3 liposome preparations, application of heat
was actually detrimental with respect to the entrapped ^{3}H/^{14}C ratio
suggesting accelerated loss ^{3}H label to areas other than the tumor.

If one examines the clearance profiles for small or large liposomes from blood, a curve that approaches a biphasic nature is nearly
always obtained.   The eventual reduced rate of clearance of large
liposomes could represent clearance of a contaminating population of
smaller liposomes whereas the initial rapid rate of clearance of small
liposomes might represent a small contaminating fraction of larger
liposomes.   An alternate explanation reviewed by Kimelberg[10] is that
opsonization of liposomes may be required for phagocytosis of the
liposomes by the reticuloendothelial system.   The biphasic nature
of liposomal clearance may be due to titration of serum components
required to opsonize the liposomes.   Similarly, if one were to pre-
load the circulatory system with "empty" liposomes, it might be

possible to titrate or otherwise saturate serum lipoproteins with substrate and thus reduce the rate of interaction with subseqently administered "loaded" hyperthermic sensitive liposomes. Such an approach might be more effective if preloading were done with fatty acid micelles rather than liposomes as there should be a much greater number of particles/mg lipid.

The above discussion has been addressed to hyperthermia mediated delivery of water soluble compounds such as MTX. The possibility of hyperthermia mediated delivery of drugs that partition into the lipid bilayer has been addressed by Yatvin et al[25]. They have demonstrated in vitro that heat sensitive liposomes containing the antineoplastic drug cis-dichlorodiammineplatinum(II) (PDD) can be designed to exhibit a maximum rate of release of PDD at 42°C. Furthermore the temperature dependent release profile of these liposomes was unaltered whether in the presence of 10% mouse serum or Sarcoma 180 tumor cells. The final phase of clearance from blood of PDD contained in small unilamellar vesicles exhibits a half-life of about two hours, nearly identical to that of the ^{14}C-DPPC label of MTX containing liposomes. The amount of drug associated with the liposome fraction following exclusion chromatography was about 20 fold greater than that which could have theoretically been entrapped within the aqueous compartment of the liposome. The above observations support the concept that during sonication, the PDD favourably partitions into the lipid bilayer from the aqueous phase.

Two major differences obtained from in vivo studies with PDD containing liposomes compared MTX containing liposomes are: (1) the clearance profile of the PDD marker from the blood of animals subjected to local hyperthermia was not statistically different from unheated controls; (2) the ratio of tumor associated PDD (heated/unheated) after 4 hours was only 1.86. The behaviour of the PDD marker strongly resembles that of the ^{14}C-DPPC marker presented here.

An amphiphile has been described as a molecule that is sufficiently large for different regions of the molecule to behave in a discrete fashion[2]. PDD does not really fit this description being a relatively compact neutral molecule. Given the proper conditions, it appears that PDD favourably partitions into the hydrophobic portion of the bilayer. In a static setting, an equilibrium should be reached as the PDD partitions between the aqueous and lipid phases. If PDD were removed from the aqueous phase, it follows that somePDD must partition out of the bilayer to re-establish the equilibrium. It is possible that the partition coefficient and/or the rate of partitioning is affected by the phase state of the bilayer. Thus, when empty liposomes (DPPC:DSPC, 7:1 w/w) are incubated with PDD (1 mg/ml)in PBS buffer (pH 7.4) for one hour at 25,42, or 55°C, the amount of PDD associated with the reisolated liposomes were respectively, (ng PDD/mg lipid) 93, 300 and 792 (unpublished results).

In the study reported by Yatvin et al[25], a therapeutic enhancement expressed as tumor growth delay was obtained for animals receiving PDD liposomes plus heat (5.25 days/μg PDD/g mouse) compared to those receiving PDD liposomes without heat or free PDD (0.8 days/μg PDD/g mouse) or heat alone (little or no growth delay observed over a period of 13 days). It is reasonable to assume that PDD was transferred from the liposomes to the tumor (as evidenced by growth delays) and that such a transfer would cause minimal or undetectable changes in blood PDD content. That is, uptake of PDD by 200 mg of tumor might have little effect on the total PDD distributed in the 2 ml volume of blood of a mouse.

If hyperthermia mediated transfer of drugs that partition into the lipid bilayer can be realised, the original concept of local hyperthermia mediated targeting of drugs can be greatly expanded. It appears that loss of such drugs due to interaction of liposomes with serum components is greatly reduced while the amount of drug associated/mg lipid can be greatly enhanced. If the previously discussed problems associated with the aqueous drug carrying liposomes can be overcome, the possibility of targeted multiple drug modalities exists. It may also be possible to construct drug carrying micelles from fatty acids or lysophospholipids. As the micelles are much smaller than small unilamellar liposomes and can obtain ellipsoidal or rod-like shapes[15,26], the circulating half-life of drugs packaged in this manner might be greatly enhanced. Also, the small size of such particles opens up other avenues for targeting previously discussed.

The strategy of using local heating to induce preferential release of drugs from liposomes does not, however, effectively address the major problem in human cancer: the metastatic lesions. An alternative would be the release of drugs from pH sensitive vesicles in tumors whose interstitial fluids have ambient pH's considerably below that of normal tissue[27]. If metastases also have a lower pH, such vesicles could be of particular value in chemotherapy. We have described such pH-sensitive vesicles[20] and anticipate using them in conjunction with local heating in an attempt to improve the therapeutic potential of heat sensitive liposomes.

The problems facing both hyperthermia and pH mediated targeting of drug bearing liposomes need to be more accurately defined before they can be resolved. However, we feel that the concept of selective drug release that we have introduced and developed hold great promise for tumor therapy and should be pursued actively.

ACKNOWLEDGEMENTS

a.   These studies were supported in part by NIG Grant GM-91846.
b.   This investigation was supported by Grant S T32 CA 09206 awarded by the NCI, DHEW.

REFERENCES

1.   G. Gregoriadis, ed., "Drug carriers in biology and medicine",
     Academic Press, London, New York and San Francisco (1979).
2.   D. Papahadjopoulos, ed., "Liposomes and their use in biology
     and medicine", Ann. NY Acad. Sci. (1978).
3.   A.C. Allison and G. Gregoriadis, eds., "Liposomes in biological
     systems", John Wiley and Sons Ltd., New York (1980).
4.   A.D. Bangham, H.W. Hill, and N.G.A. Miller in: "Methods in
     membrane biology" 1, E.D. Korn, ed., Plenum Press, New York
     (1974).
5.   D. Papahadjopoulos and H.K. Kimelberg, in: "Progress in surface
     science", S.G. Davison, ed., Pergamon Press, Oxford (1974).
6.   A.D. Bangham, M.M. Standish, and J.C. Watkins, The action of
     steroids and streptolysin S on the permeability of phospholipid
     structures to cations, J. Mol. Biol., 13: 138 (1965).
7.   G. Gregoriadis, The carrier potential of liposomes in biology
     and medicine, (part I), New Engl. J. Med., 295: 704 (1976).
8.   H.K. Kimelberg and E.G. Mayhew, Properties and biological
     effects of liposomes and their uses in pharmacology and toxi-
     cology, CRC Crit. Rev. Toxicol., 6: 25 (1978).
9.   M. Finkelstein and G. Weissmann, The introduction of enzymes
     into cells by means of liposomes, J. Lipid Res., 19: 289 (1978).
10. R.E. Pagano and J.N. Weinstein, Interactions of liposomes with
     mammalian cells, Ann. Rev. Biophys. Bioeng., 7: 435 (1978).
11. F. Szoka, and D. Papahadjopoulos, Comparative properties and
     methods of preparation of lipid vesicles (Liposomes), Ann. Rev.
     Biophys. Bioeng., 9: 467 (1980).
12. G. Gregoriadis, The carrier potential of liposomes in biology
     and medicine (part II), New Engl. J. Med., 295: 765 (1976).
13. D.A. Tyrell, D. Heath, G.M. Colley and B.R. Ryman, New aspects
     of liposomes, Biochim. Biophys. Acta, 457: 259 (1976).
14. G. Tanford, "The hydrophobic effect: formation of micelles and
     biological membranes", Wiley-Interscience, New York (1980).
15. J.N. Israelachvili, D.J. Mitchell and B.W. Ninham, Theory of
     self-assembly of hydrocarbon amphiphiles into micelles and
     bilayers, J. Chem. Soc. Faraday Trans., 72: 1525 (1976).
16. A.D. Bangham, Lipid bilayers and biomembranes, Ann. Rev.
     Biochem., 41: 753 (1972).
17. M.B. Yatvin, J.N. Weinstein, W.H. Dennis, and R. Blumenthal,
     Design of liposomes for enhanced local release of drugs by
     hyperthermia, Science, 202: 1290 (1978).
18. J.N. Weinstein, R.L. Magin, M.B. Yatvin, and D.S. Zaharko,
     Liposomes and local hyperthermia: selective delivery of metho-
     trexate to heated tumors, Science, 204: 188 (1979).
19. J.N. Weinstein, R.L. Magin, R.L. Cysyk, and D.S. Zaharko,
     Treatment of solid L1210 murine tumors with local hyperthermia
     and temperature-sensitive liposomes containing methotrexate,
     Cancer Res., 40: 1388 (1980).
20. M .B. Yatvin, W. Kreutz, B.A. Horwitz and M. Shinitzky, pH-

Sensitive liposomes: possible clinical implications, Science
210: 1253 (1980).

21. H.K. Kimelberg, Differential distribution of liposome-entrapped
    ^{3}H–methotrexate and labelled lipids after intravenous injection
    in a primate, Biochim. Biophys. Acta, 448: 531 (1976).

22. G. Scherphof, F. Roerdink, M. Waite, and J. Parks, Disintegra-
    tion of phosphatidylcholine liposomes in plasma as a result of
    interaction with high–density lipoproteins, Biochim. Biophys.
    Acta, 542: 196 (1978).

23. G. Scherphof, H. Morselt, J. Regts, and J.C. Wilschut, The
    involvement of the lipid phase transition in the plasma-induced
    dissolution of multilamellar phosphatidylcholine vesicles,
    Biochim. Biophys. Acta, 556: 196 (1979).

24. G. Scherphof, The role of the liver in the clearance of lipo-
    somes from the blood, second WCCC international workshop on
    experimental oncology, Madison, Wisconsin (1981), Abs. 22.

25. M.B. Yatvin, H. Muhlensiepen, W. Porshcen, J.N. Weinstein, and
    L.E. Feinendegen, Selective delivery of liposome-associated
    cis-dichlorodiammineplatinum (II) by heat and its influence on
    tumor drug uptake and growth, Cancer Res., 41: 1602 (1981).

26. A. Watts, D. Marsh, and P.F. Knowles, Characterization of
    dimyristoyl phosphatidylcholine vesicles and their dimensional
    changes through the phase transition: molecular control of
    membrane morphology, Biochemistry, 17: 1792 (1978).

27. P.M. Gullino, H. Grantham, S.H. Smith, and A.C. Haggerty,
    Modification of the acid-base status of the internal milieu of
    tumors, J. Natl. Cancer Inst., 34: 857 (1965).

LIPOSOMES - FURTHER CONSIDERATIONS OF THEIR POSSIBLE ROLE AS CARRIERS OF THERAPEUTIC AGENTS

Brenda E. Ryman and Gillian M. Barratt

Department of Biochemistry,
Charing Cross Hospital Medical School
(University of London)
Hammersmith, London, W6 8RF, U.K.

Liposomes, for many years a tool of the membranologists, have over the last 12 years been used in many other areas of research. Apart from their continuing use in membrane research, including immunological investigations, these phospholipid vesicles have found themselves the centre of attraction as possible carriers of materials of therapeutic interest.

Enzyme entrapment (for enzyme replacement therapy), drug delivery (particularly those drugs used in anticancer therapy where enhanced specificity and tumour targeting would be especially desirable), hormone delivery, e.g. oral administration of insulin or intra-articular delivery of cortisol derivatives, are all areas under investigation. In addition entrapment of informational molecules such as DNA and RNA (including plasmids and viruses), the possible uses of liposomes in the treatment of tropical diseases, heavy metal poisoning, myocardial infarction and of dried phospholipids in respiratory distress, in the preparation of adjuvants and vaccines are all fields where liposome research is yielding interesting results. However, despite a plethora of ideas for utilising liposomes in delivery and targeting of material of therapeutic interest, it must be emphasised that the original concept of a biodegradable carrier whose properties could be manipulated to induce tissue or cell specificity has not as yet been achieved, although in some areas of the research the potential may become a reality.

Several review articles have been written, e.g. Tyrrell et al. (1976); Ryman et al. (1978); Ryman and Tyrrell (1979); Ryman and Tyrrell (1980); Gregoriadis (1979), where more detailed references to earlier work will be available.

It is intended only to discuss work from our laboratory carried out over the last two years, and in two specific areas.

1. Liposomal drug delivery in anticancer chemotherapy and in the early detection of metastases.

2. Liposomally entrapped antibodies in (a) digoxin overload and (b) detection of tumours.

LIPOSOMAL DRUG DELIVERY IN ANTICANCER CHEMOTHERAPY AND IN THE EARLY DETECTION OF METASTASES

Does entrapment change therapeutic index?

There is no doubt that entrapment of anticancer drugs in liposomes changes their pharmacokinetics upon administration, e.g. daunomycin given in the free state has a half life of $<$ 5 min and this is extended to 150 min when the drug is administered in a liposomally entrapped form. However, despite the earlier evidence that many tumour cell lines are penetrated by liposomes in vitro, there is less clear-cut evidence in vivo. While several workers, including our own laboratory, have shown that small negatively charged liposomes appear to gain access to certain tumours in animals, we have been unable to detect any such uptake into a wide variety of human tumours (Ryman et al., 1978; Richardson et al., 1978a, 1979).

It will be appreciated that if liposomally entrapped drugs in anticancer chemotherapy are to be regarded as superior to treatment employing free drug then a change in the therapeutic index of that drug must be observable. The therapeutic index (TI) is a measure of the ratio of LD_{50} to the minimal effective dose (MED) and clearly if both parameters change simultaneously there is no change in TI and hence no advantage in the formulation. If only one aspect of TI is measured no conclusion can be reached regarding the superiority or otherwise of the entrapped drug. While there are many claims in the literature (see Ryman and Tyrrell, 1980) that entrapment of anti-tumour drugs in liposomes results in a lowering of toxicity of the drug and increased survival time of tumour bearing animals, it must be hastened to add that in most studies only one of these parameters has been studied.

In an attempt to clarify the effect of entrapment in liposomes of a commonly used antitumour drug on TI over a wide dose range, Kaye et al. (1981) have used in AKR mice the highly actinomycin D-sensitive mouse Ridgway osteosarcoma which exhibits an orderly dose-response curve for the drug (Schwartz et al., 1966). Tissue distribution of the free and entrapped drug was also followed and confirmed other work in which, using a variety of antitumour drugs, it has been shown that entrapment results in reduced peak concentrations in many organs. Of particular interest in this respect are the small intestine and bone marrow, which are normally unwanted targets for the drug. Liver and spleen, as was to be expected (since liposomes are taken up avidly by reticuloendothelial elements in these organs) exhibited high levels of the drug when administered in the entrapped form. As was predictable the liposome associated drug persisted much longer in the circulation.

The data on survival time of animals and drug effectiveness against the tumour are shown in Fig. 1a. The mean tumour weight at

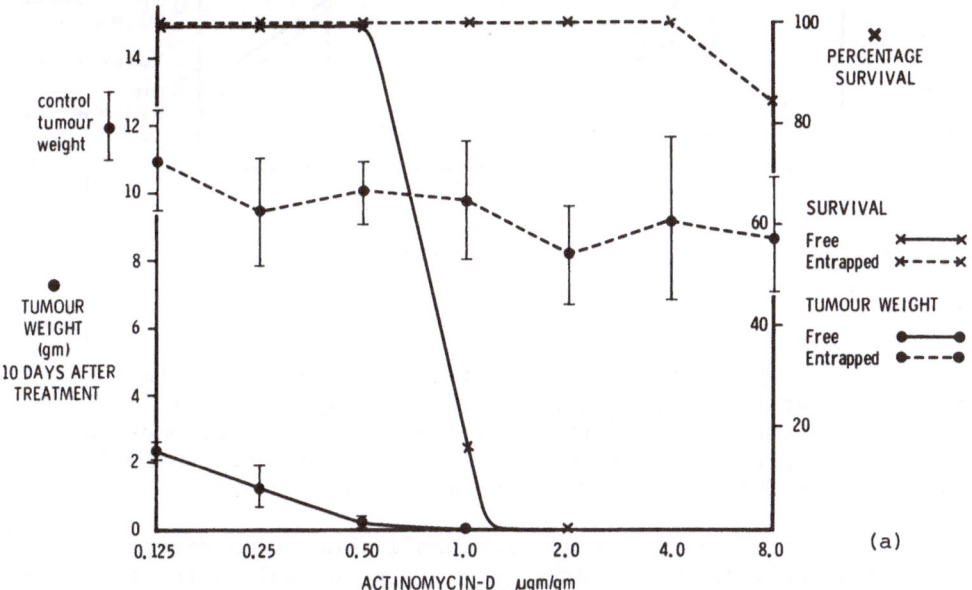

Fig. 1. Therapeutic-toxicity data on the treatment of Ridgway osteogenic sarcoma-bearing AKR mice with actinomycin D (a) and methotrexate (b) in the free and (cationic) liposome-entrapped form. Liposome composition was phosphatidyl-choline:cholesterol:stearylamine in the molar ratio 18:4:5. Each point refers to mean for six mice with standard error shown. Untreated control tumour weight at 10 days (11.8± 1.0 g) is also shown. For actinomycin D in the free form, the LD_{50} is 0.8 μg/g and the MED_{10} (dose inhibiting tumour growth to 10% of control) is 0.3 μg/g. Neither LD_{50} nor MED_{10} is reached using liposome-entrapped actinomycin D in doeses up to 8 μg/g. In contrast, for methotrexate in the free form the LD_{50} is 80 μg/g and the MED_{20} (20% control tumour growth inhibition) is 160 μg/g, whereas for methotrexate in the liposome-entrapped form, the LD_{50} is 12 μg/g and the MED_{20} is 20 μg/g, i.e. there is no significant improvement in the therapeutic index.

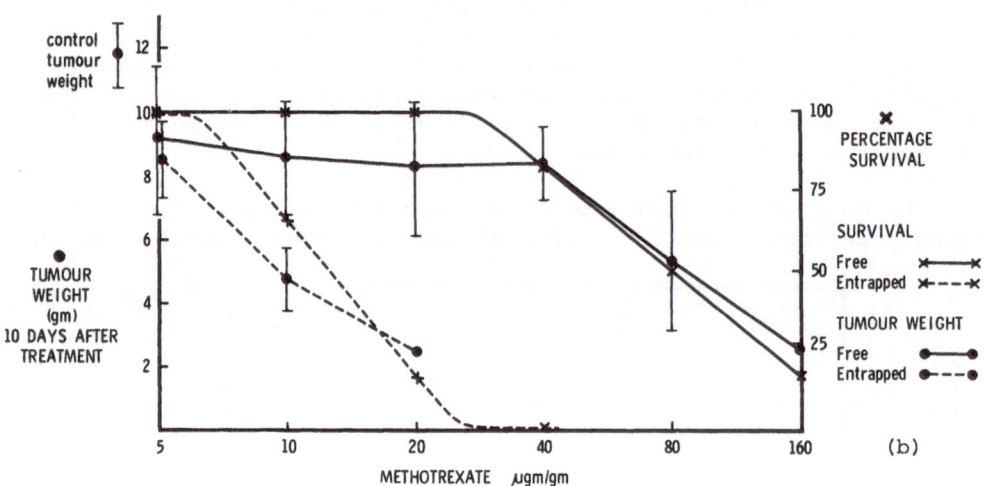

Fig. 1 (cont.).   (Ryman and Tyrrell, 1980).

10 days of 9 control untreated mice is shown, together with tumour
weight at 10 days over a dose range of actinomycin D (0.125–8.0 μg/g).
All control animals were given empty liposomes and liposomes for
control and experimental animals were composed of phosphatidylcholine:
cholesterol:stearylamine in 18:4:5 molar ratio.

Fig. 1a shows that whereas liposomally entrapped drug, x----x,
is far less toxic than free drug, x——x, nevertheless the efficacy
of the drug is greatly diminished. Thus the antitumour activity,
expressed as the minimum effective dose (inhibition to 10% of control
tumour weight) of free, ●——●, drug is 0.3 μg/g, whereas the
entrapped actinomycin D in doses up to 8 μg/g fails to inhibit tumour
growth to less than 68% of the untreated tumours, ●----●. While the
LD_{50} for free actinomycin D is 0.8 μg/g even at the highest dose of
entrapped drug (8 μg/g) survival of the animals is 83%.

The treatment with empty liposomes alone showed some fall in
tumour weight which can probably be explained on the inhibitory
effect on the tumour of the cationic (stearylamine containing)
liposomes.

Similar experiments were performed again using the AKR mice
bearing the Ridgway osteosarcoma (Kaye et al., 1981) but using methotrexate as the drug. The results are shown in Fig. 1b and are somewhat different in that entrapped methotrexate, x----x, was more toxic
than free drug, x——x, and was more effective against the tumour as

assessed by the drop in tumour weight in the entrapped form, ●----●, compared with the free drug, ●——●, but in neither of the experiments described, i.e. using actinomycin D or methotrexate, is there any change in TI and thus no evidence of advantageous properties of administering the drugs in liposomes.

Does entrapment overcome drug resistance?

An actinomycin D resistant Ridgway osteosarcoma was derived by successive passages of tumour fragments in the phase of regrowth after repeated treatments of the animals with actinomycin D commencing at a dose of 0.25 μg/g (given 4 times at 14 day intervals and progressively increasing the dose in successive generations). After passaging tumours through seven generations of treated mice the tumours grew despite treatment with 0.8 μg/g of i.v. actinomycin D (the LD$_{50}$ for the free drug). When animals bearing the resistant tumour were treated with liposomally entrapped actinomycin D it was clear that the drug was ineffective (Table 1).

Table 1. Therapeutic-toxicity study using liposome-entrapped actinomycin D in the treatment of resistant Ridgway osteosarcoma subline.

Dose (μg/g body wt)	Mean tumour wt (g) on day of treatment (SEM)	Mean tumour wt (g) 10 days after treatment (SEM)	No. of survivors at 10 days / No. of treated animals
*	1.31 (0.09)	9.77 (0.64)	6/6
0.125	1.21 (0.20)	10.19 (1.35)	6/6
0.25	1.10 (0.19)	10.75 (2.54)	6/6
0.5	1.22 (0.18)	10.77 (2.54)	6/6
1.0	1.38 (0.18)	9.33 (1.85)	6/6
2.0	1.17 (0.24)	10.10 (2.81)	6/6
4.0	1.21 (0.28)	9.53 (2.59)	5/5
8.0	1.39 (0.37)	9.39 (3.43)	5/5

*Empty liposomes equivalent to 12.5 mg of lipid.

The distribution of free and entrapped drug remained similar to that observed with the actinomycin D sensitive tumour, implying a similar method of drug handling. However, a major difference is seen in tumour drug concentration following injection of free actinomycin D in the sensitive and resistant tumour, Fig. 2. Whereas the initial

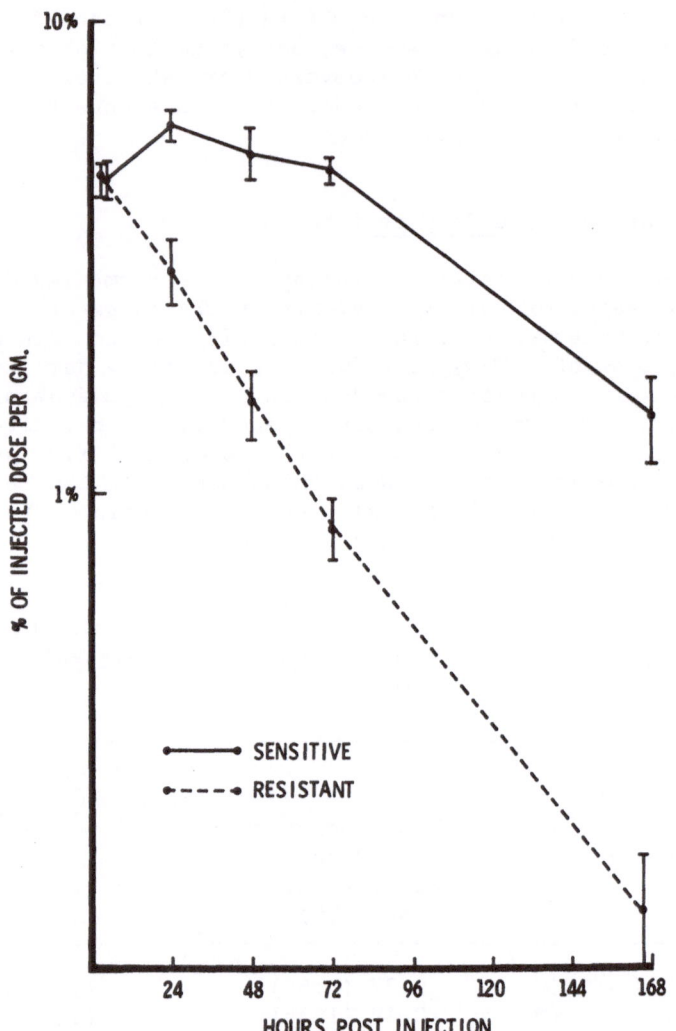

Fig. 2.   Concentration of ^{3}H-actinomycin D (AD) in the sensitive
          and resistant Ridgway osteosarcoma from 3 hours to 7 days
          following injection of free AD (500 μg/kg).   (Kaye et al.
          1981).

levels are similar there is a difference between the sensitive and
resistant sublines of the tumours in that the resistant one shows
a rapid and consistent fall in the actinomycin D, whereas in the
sensitive line the drug is retained efficiently.

The claims that drug resistance can be overcome by entrapment
of the drug in liposomes (Papahadjopoulos et al., 1976; Kosloski

et al., 1978) perhaps emphasise the difficulties of translating the
in vitro to the in vivo situation and furthermore the method of
inducing the resistance may be very important if one is attempting
to mimick the situation which exists in drug resistance in man (Kaye
et al., 1981). While liposomes may fulfil a role in transporting a
drug into resistant cells where there is a defect in the entry process of the drug, in our model this appears not to be the case.

In summary therefore from our work we must conclude that in the
case of actinomycin D, a non-phase-specific drug, we can find no
evidence that entrapment in liposomes changes the TI of the drug.
In a resistant subline no evidence could be found that liposomally
entrapped actinomycin D overcomes the resistance.

No change in TI could be observed when methotrexate was examined
in the free and entrapped form in the Ridgway osteogenic sarcoma in
mice. The reported work by Rustum et al. (1979) on cytosine arabinoside (another phase-specific drug) has also suggested that the
apparent increased efficacy of this drug in the entrapped form may
reflect the slow release due to its leakage from the liposome in the
body, and it will be necessary to compare the performance of such
drugs given in this way with the currently used form of administration, namely slow infusion in cancer chemotherapy.

Detection of metastases in lymph nodes

In earlier work from our laboratory we reported animal studies
which showed that ^{99m}Tc-labelled liposomes could be used for regional
lymph node imaging (Osborne et al., 1979; Ryman et al., 1978) and
that nodes involved in metastatic spread showed a suppression of
uptake of labelled liposomes made from phosphatidylcholine and
cholesterol (Richardson et al., 1978b). It was also demonstrated
that regional lymph nodes draining an area infected with irradiated
tumour cells showed enhanced uptake of the labelled liposomes while
the presence of inflammation did not alter uptake patterns compared
with normal animals (Osborne et al., 1981a).

This study was part of a larger project to assess the possibility of using lymphoscintigraphy of internal and axillary lymph
node chains to improve the pre-operative staging of breast cancer,
and 40 patients with breast cancer have now been assessed. Forty-
five per cent of these patients had abnormal scintigrams (suppression
of uptake), suggesting the presence of lymph node metastases, 35%
had normal images and 20% were technically unsatisfactory, usually
due to poor technetium labelling efficiency. Twenty-two of the 32
interpretable images were correlated with the results of histopatho-
logical examinations of lymph node removed by radical mastectomy.
Twelve of these had abnormal patterns, of which one had histologically normal nodes and constituted a false positive. Ten had normal

patterns, of which two with enhanced uptake were found to have
minimal lymph node metastases in the lower nodes with reactive hyper-
plasia of the nodes above (Osborne et al., 1981a).

These findings support our animal experiments and suggest that
labelled liposomes may be a useful means of assessing in vivo
activity of lymph nodes in response to the presence of a tumour and
thus yield valuable information pre-operatively on which lymph nodes
have cancer deposits and maybe identify lymph nodes draining a tumour
which has not yet metastasized. Further work is continuing in this
area (Osborne et al., 1981b).

LIPOSOMALLY ENTRAPPED ANTIBODIES

Attachment of antibodies to liposomes either co- or non covalently has mainly been aimed at targeting of the vesicles to
tissues other than liver and spleen - the natural homing sites of
liposomes (Gregoriadis and Ryman, 1972a,b). In the two aspects to
be considered this natural homing has been exploited for two specific
purposes.

Antibody to digoxin

Life-threatening toxicity continues to be observed in patients
treated with digoxin, probably because adequate digitalization in
some patients requires a plasma level in the commonly accepted toxic
range, and conversely concentrations which are usually considered
safe may be toxic to some individuals. Antibody specific for this
cardiac glycoside not only neutralises the drug, but removes it from
mammalian cells and reverses certain of its pharmacological properties. While such an approach to overcoming toxicity appears very
attractive, the possibility of hypersensitivity reactions to digoxin-
specific antibodies and an uncertain accumulation of antigen-antibody
complexes cannot be ignored. We have shown that liposomally-bound
antibodies to digoxin bind digoxin in vivo and remove the digoxin to
the liver and spleen and thereby reduce the intravascular level of
the drug compared to treatment with free antibody (Campbell et al.,
1980; Tyrrell et al., 1978). Enhanced removal of the digoxin following liposome-antibody administration via the kidney compared with free
antibody was also observed (Campbell et al., 1980) and it has been
suggested that the rationale of antibody administration in liposomes
suggested in this digoxin study may be applicable to chemically-toxic
compounds such as paraquat and compounds active on the CNS.

Antibody (Secondary) to Antibody (Primary) to Tumour Products

Radiolabelled antibodies (primary) to tumour products may be

used to detect tumour sites by external scintigraphy (Goldenberg et
al., 1978; Begent et al., 1980; Barratt et al., 1981). Such an
approach is not, however, entirely satisfactory due to the high background radioactivity in the circulation and other compartments and
a computerised subtraction technique using ^{99m}Tc-albumin and labelled
pertechnetate is currently employed in an attempt to overcome these
difficulties and increase the clarity of the scan. We have carried
out preliminary investigations to ascertain the feasibility of
entrapment in liposomes of antibody (secondary) to this primary antibody to allow removal of the radiolabelled primary antibody to the
liver and spleen. Primary antibody to the human colonic tumour product carcinoembryonic antigen (CEA) was raised in goats, purified and
labelled with ^{125}I by the chloramine T method (Hunter and Greenwood,
1962). Secondary antibody raised in horse was fractionated to yield
IgG for entrapment in liposomes. The liposomes used for entrapment
of this IgG were labelled with either ^{3}H-cholesterol or ^{99m}Tc and
were composed of phosphatidylcholine:cholesterol:phosphatidic acid

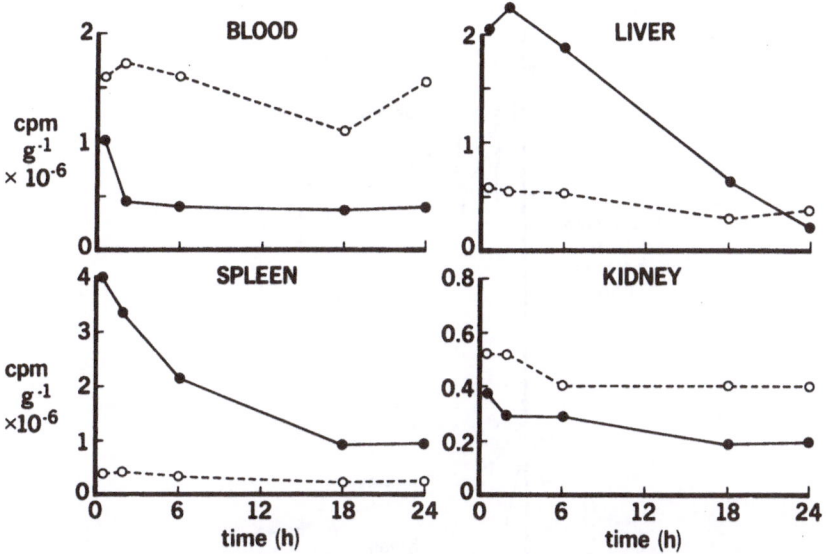

Fig. 3.   (^{125}I)-Anti-CEA distribution in normal mice after treatment
          with liposomes containing secondary antibody. All points
          are the mean of three animals. All animals were given i.v.
          injections of 15 μCi of (^{125}I)-anti-CEA (primary antibody)
          24 h before the start of the experiment. Liposome-treated
          animals (●——●) were given sonicated, negatively-charged
          liposomes containing secondary antibody (approximately 10
          μmoles lipid per mouse) i.v. at 0 h. Control mice (o----o)
          received no further treatment. (Ryman et al., 1981, Alfred
          Benzon Symposium 17, Optimization of Drug Delivery; in press).

(9:9:2 molar ratio) (Barratt et al., 1981). Despite the fact that
the majority of the secondary antibody entrapped was not exposed at
the liposome surface, it was possible to demonstrate that liposomally
entrapped secondary antibody, when given to AKR mice pretreated with
^{125}I primary antibody, led to a lowering of blood level of the primary
antibody and an enhanced accumulation of label in liver and spleen
compared with control animals, who received no secondary antibody in
liposomes. These results are presented in Fig. 3. Similar results
were obtained when ^{99m}Tc-labelled liposomes were used (Fig. 4).

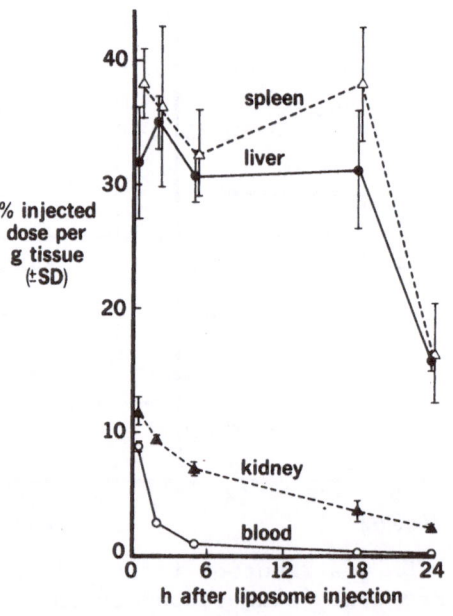

Fig. 4.   Distribution of ^{99m}Tc-labelled liposomes containing
          secondary antibody in normal mice pretreated with primary
          antibody. Each point is the mean of counts from 3 animals.
          Mice were given ^{125}I-primary antibody 24 h prior to the
          start of the experiment, and, at 0 h, 9 μmoles of lipids
          as liposomes containing entrapped secondary antibody and
          externally labelled with ^{99m}Tc.

Similar experiments were performed in nude mice bearing xeno-grafts of human colonic tumours. Two different tumour lines were used, P116, which is a poor secretor of CEA, and TAF, a good secretor. Again, injection of ^{125}I-labelled primary antibody was followed in the experimental group by liposomally entrapped secondary antibody, and in the controls by no further treatment. ^{125}I was determined in tissues including the tumours. In all experiments the ^{125}I primary antibody remaining in the blood of animals treated with liposomes containing secondary antibody was reduced compared to controls, and the reduction was related to the amount of lipid administered as liposomes (Table 2). Up to 6 h after liposome injection the tumour radioactivity in treated animals was not different from the controls, as shown in Fig. 5. Twenty-four hours after liposome treatment tumour-associated ^{125}I-labelled primary antibody was reduced relative to controls; however, the tumour to blood ratio of primary antibody was still increased in treated animals (Table 2).

These results indicate that the liposomes containing secondary antibody cause a redistribution of blood borne primary antibody to the liver and spleen. The fact that radioactivity in the tumours liposome-secondary antibody-treated rats remained similar to the controls up to 6 h after treatment and the clearance of primary

Table 2. (^{125}I)-Anti-CEA distribution in nude mice bearing human tumour xenografts after treatment with liposomally-entrapped secondary antibody.

Tumour line	Dose of liposomes (μmoles lipids)	Time after injec-tion	Tissue radio-activity as a % that in untreated controls		Ratio of tumour radioactivity to blood radioactivity	
			Blood	Tumour	Control	Liposomes
P116	3	6 h	30	122	0.30	1.22
		24 h	39	64	0.20	0.32
TAF	10	½ h	56	92	0.50	0.73
		2 h	34	140	0.40	1.69
		6 h	30	107	0.54	1.92
	27	24 h	5	51	0.53	5.57

Values are means for 2-3 mice. All mice were given an i.v. injection of (^{125}I)-primary antibody 24 h prior to the start of the experiment. Treated mice were given liposomes (PC:CH:PA. 9:9:2, 10 min sonication) containing secondary antibody at 0 h.

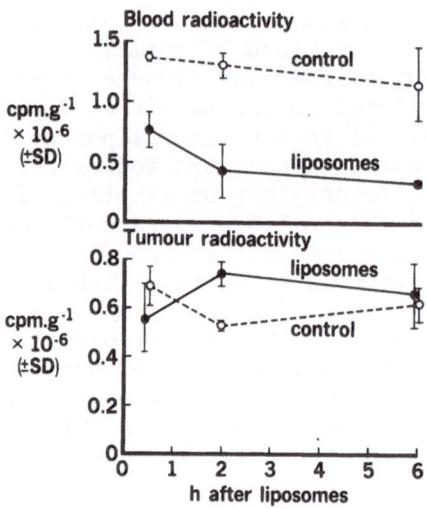

Fig. 5.   (^{125}I)-Anti-CEA distribution in tumour-bearing mice after
          treatment with liposomes containing secondary antibody.
          Values are means for 3 nude mice bearing TAF tumour xeno-
          grafts. All mice were given an i.v. injection of (^{125}I)-
          primary antibody 24 h prior to the start of the experiment.
          Treated mice were given 10 moles of lipid as liposomes at
          0 h. (Ryman et al., Alfred Benson Symposium 17, 1981; in
          press).

antibody by the liposome-secondary antibody was rapid with a plateau
after 2 h adds support to the idea that these strategies may be useful in increasing the clarity of scans designed to seek out tumours,
and we are currently planning such investigations in man.

     It is our pleasure to acknowledge collaborators in the work
described - Drs. Begent, Campbell, Harding, Kaye, Keep, McCready,
Searle, Tyrrell, Miss J. Boden, Miss J. Payne, Mr. M.P. Osborne and
Professor K.D. Bagshawe. The skilled assistance of Miss Linda
Readings in the preparation of the manuscript is appreciated.

References

Barratt, G.M., Ryman, B.E., Boden, J.A., Keep, P.A., Searle, F., Begent, R.H. and Bagshawe, K.D., 1981, Liposomal clearance of antibodies to tumour products: Possible improvement of tumour detection. Biochem. Soc. Trans. 9: in press.

Begent, R.H., Stanway, G., Jones, B.E., Bagshawe, K.D., Searle, F., Jewkes, R.F. and Vernon, P., 1980, Radioimmunolocalization of tumours by external scintigraphy after administration of ^{131}I antibody to human chorionic gonadotrophin: preliminary communication, J. R. Soc. Med. 73: 624.

Campbell, P.I., Harding, N.G.L., Ryman, B.E. and Tyrrell, D.A., 1980, Redistribution and altered excretion of digoxin in rats receiving digoxin antibodies incorporated in liposomes, Eur. J. Biochem., 109: 87.

Goldenberg, D.M., Deland, F., Kim, E., Bennett, S., Primus, F.J., van Nagell, J.R., Estes, N., De Simone, P. and Rayburn, P., 1978, Use of radiolabelled antibodies to carcinoembryonic antigen for the detection and localization of diverse cancers by external photoscanning, New Engl. J. Med., 298: 1384.

Gregoriadis, G., 1979, in: "Drug Carriers in Biology and Medicine," G. Gregoriadis, ed., Academic Press, London and New York.

Gregoriadis, G. and Ryman, B.E., 1972a, Fate of protein-containing liposomes injected into rats. An approach to the treatment of storage diseases, Eur. J. Biochem., 24: 485.

Gregoriadis, G. and Ryman, B.E., 1972b, Lysosomal localization of β-fructofuranosidase-containing liposomes injected into rats: some implications in the treatment of genetic disorders. Biochem. J., 129: 123.

Hunter, W.M. and Greenwood, F.C., 1962, Preparation of iodine-131 labelled human growth hormone of high specific activity, Nature, 194: 495.

Kaye, S.B., Boden, J.A. and Ryman, B.E., 1981, The effect of liposome (phospholipid vesicle) entrapment of actinomycin D and methotrexate on the in vivo treatment of sensitive and resistant solid murine tumours, Eur. J. Cancer, 17: 279.

Kosloski, M.J., Rosen, F., Milholland, R.J. and Papahadjopoulos, D., 1978, Effect of lipid vesicle (liposome) encapsulation of methotrexate on its chemotherapeutic efficacy in solid rodent tumors, Cancer Res., 38:2848.

Osborne, M.P., Ryman, B.E., Payne, J.H. and McCready, V.R., 1981a, The use of ^{99m}Tc-labelled neutral liposomes in lymphoscintigraphy: A comparison of scintigram interpretations with node histology in a series of breast cancer patients, in "Progress in Radiopharmacology" vol. 2, P.H. Cox, ed., Elsevier/North-Holland Biomedical Press, Amsterdam.

Osborne, M.P., Richardson, V.J., Jeyasingh, K. and Ryman, B.E., 1981b, Potential applications of radionuclide-labelled liposomes in the detection of the lymphatic spread of cancer, Int. J. Nucl. Med. Biol., submitted.

Papahadjopoulos, D., Poste, G., Vail, W.J. and Biedler, J.L., 1976, Use of lipid vesicles as carriers to introduce actinomycin D into resistant tumour cells, Cancer Res., 36: 2988.

Richardson, V.J., Jeyasingh, K., Jewkes, R.F., Ryman, B.E. and Tattersall, M.H.N., 1978a, Possible localization of ^{99m}Tc-labelled liposomes: Effects of lipid composition, charge and liposome size, J. Nucl. Med., 19: 1049.

Richardson, V.J., Osborne, M.P., Jeyasingh, K., Ryman, B.E. and Burn, J.I., 1978b, Differential localization of (^{99m}Tc)tech-netium labelled liposomes in normal and tumour-bearing lymph nodes of the rat, Br. J. Cancer, 38: 177.

Richardson, V.J., Ryman, B.E., Jewkes, R.F., Jeyasingh, K., Tattersall, M.H.N., Newlands, E.S. and Kaye, S.B., 1979, Tissue distribution and tumour localization of 99m-technetium-labelled liposomes in cancer patients. Br. J. Cancer, 40: 35.

Rustum, Y.M., Dave, C., Mayhew, E. and Papahadjopoulos, D., 1979, Role of liposome type and route of adminsitration in the anti-tumor activity of liposome-entrapped 1-β-D-arabinofuranosyl-cytosine against mouse L1210 leukaemia, Cancer Res., 39: 1390.

Ryman, B.E., Jewkes, R.F., Jeyasingh, K., Osborne, M.P., Patel, H.M., Richardson, V.J., Tattersall, M.H.N. and Tyrrell, D.A., 1978, Potential applications of liposomes to therapy, Ann. N.Y. Acad. Sci., 308: 281.

Ryman, B.E. and Tyrrell, D.A., 1979, Liposomes - Methodology and Applications, in "Lysosomes in Biology and Pathology", vol. 6, J.T. Dingle, P.J. Jacques and I.H. Shaw, eds., Elsevier/North-Holland Biomedical Press, Amsterdam.

Ryman, B.E. and Tyrrell, D.A., 1980, Liposomes - Bags of Potential, in: "Essays in Biochemistry" vol. 16, P.N. Campbell and R.D. Marshall, eds., Academic Press, London.

Schwartz, H.S., Sodergren, J.E., Sternberg, S.S. and Philips, P.S., 1966, Actinomycin D: Effects of Ridgway osteogenic sarcoma in mice, Cancer Res., 26: 1873.

Tyrrell, D.A., Campbell, P.I., Harding, N.G.L., Munroe, A. and Ryman, B.E., 1978, Antidigoxin antibody incorporation into liposomes - a potential therapy for digoxin toxicity, Biochem. Soc. Trans., 6: 1239.

Tyrrell, D.A., Heath, T.D., Colley, C.M. and Ryman, B.E., 1976, New aspects of liposomes, Biochem. Biophys. Acta., 457: 259.

THERAPEUTIC EFFICACY OF CYTOSINE ARABINOSIDE TRAPPED IN LIPOSOMES

E. Mayhew[1], Y.M. Rustum[2] and F. Szoka[1,3]

1. Department of Experimental Pathology
   Roswell Park Memorial Institute
   Buffalo, New York 14263, USA

2. Department of Experimental Therapeutics and
   Grace Cancer Drug Center
   Roswell Park Memorial Institute
   Buffalo, New York 14263, USA

3. Present Address: Department of Pharmacy
   University of California
   San Francisco, California, USA

INTRODUCTION

A number of cancer chemotherapeutic agents have been encapsulated in liposomes and tested for their therapeutic effects (Kimelberg and Mayhew, 1978; Gregoriadis, 1979). However there have been few reports where direct comparisons of the therapeutic index of the liposome-entrapped drug and the free drug, administered under optimal conditions, have been made. There have been reports which indicate no increase in therapeutic effect for methotrexate (Kimelberg and Atchison, 1978; Kaye et al., 1980) or Actinomycin D (Kaye et al., 1979; Kaye and Ryman, 1980; Kedar et al., 1981) whereas increases in therapeutic index have been reported for adriamycin (Forssen and Tokes, 1979, 1981; Rahman et al., 1980, Olson et al., in press) after entrapment of these clinically useful drugs in liposomes.

Cytosine arabinoside (ara-c) has been the most widely investigated drug trapped in liposomes and all results confirm the markedly altered therapeutic responses of this drug after entrapment in liposomes (review Kimelberg and Mayhew, 1978; Kataoka and Kobayashi, 1978; Mayhew, et al., 1978, Rustum, et al., 1979; Ganapathi et al.,

1980). However in most of these reports the free drug was not
administered optimally.

Here we compare the therapeutic efficacies of free and liposome-
entrapped ara-c against mouse leukemia L1210. In addition, we report
attempts to increase the therapeutic effectiveness of ara-c liposomes
by pretreatment of mice with non-drug containing liposomes before
treatment with ara-c liposomes. A preliminary report of some of
these observations has been published (Mayhew et al., 1980).

MATERIALS AND METHODS

Liposomes

Dipalmitoylphosphatidylcholine (DPPC) was synthesized from
glycerophosphorylcholine-cadmium chloride complex and palmitic
anhydride with N,N-dimethyl-4-amino- pyridine as a catalyst, essentially by the procedure of Gupta et al. (1977). Final purification
was done on a Waters HPLC using a prepak silica 500 column and chloro-
form:methanol (9:1, V/V) as solvent to remove all fatty acids,
followed by chloroform:methanol:water (60:30:4 V/V/V) to recover
pure DPPC. Cholesterol (chol) obtained from Fluka A.B. was recrystal-
lized twice from methanol as described previously (Mayhew et al.,
1979). Liposomes were prepared by the reverse phase evaporation
procedure (Szoka and Papahadjopoulos, 1978). Two types of liposomes
were made using a molar ratio of DPPC:chol, 1:1; those containing
ara-c and plain non-drug containing liposomes. All liposomes were
extruded through 0.4 μnucleopore filters as described previously
(Szoka et al., 1980) to obtain a more homogenous population as
regards size distribution. The final liposome preparations had a
mean liposomal diameter of 0.4 μm and in those containing ara-c the
ara-c concentration was 0.3mg ara-c/μmole total lipid, or 20mg ara-
c/ml aqueous space. The permeability properties of these liposomes
was determined as described previously (Mayhew et al., 1979) and the
T$\frac{1}{2}$ (time for half the entrapped ara-c to leak out of the liposomes
was approximately 1 year in phosphate buffered saline (PBS) at 4°C,
600 hours at 37°C in PBS and 45 hours at 37°C in 80% calf serum.

Ara-c and liposome administration

Liposome entrapped ara-c or plain liposomes were administered
to DBA 2J female mice intraperitoneally (i.p.) or intravenously
(i.v.) by bolus injection. The volume was kept below 0.5ml per
mouse. Free drug was administered i.p. or i.v. by bolus injection
as described for liposome administration. In addition, free drug
was administered by slow infusion using Harvard infusion pumps
delivering 0.2ml/hour i.v. into the tail veins of mice (Semon and
Grindey, 1978). Mice were set-up individually in modified cages
so that they could move around freely. All doses were administered
on a mg/kg basis for each mouse.

Toxicity studies

Groups of non-tumor-bearing 6-8 week old female DBA 2J mice weighing 17-20 gms were injected with free ara-c or liposome ara-c as described above. The doses used were liposome ara-c 5 to 150 mg/kg single injection, free ara-c 6 injections at 4 hour intervals at 10 to 500 mg/kg per injection. Continuous i.v. infusion was done at 1-20 mg/kg/day for 5 days. The number of mice varied from 3 to 10 mice per group. Animals were also injected with non-drug containing liposomes at doses of 50 μMole/kg to 12.5 mMole/kg (about 10 gms/kg) total lipid by i.v. or i.p. routes. At doses above 1.5 mMole/kg more than one injection of plain ara-c was used. The day of death of the animals was recorded and the LD_{50} calculated.

L1210 Leukemia

L1210 leukemia maintained at RPMI in DBA 2J mice was used throughout. 1 x 10^5 or 1 x 10^6 cells from animals bearing 4 day i.p. tumor were injected i.p. or i.v. in DBA 2J female mice. Treatments usually commenced 24 hours later (day 1). The ara-c liposomes (single injection) or free ara-c (Multiple injection i.p. or i.v. or i.v. infusion) were administered. Day of death was observed. Experiments were normally terminated at 30 days. Mice surviving more than 30 days normally did not succumb to L1210 leukemia.

RESULTS

Toxicity

Table 1 shows the comparative toxicity of free or liposome-entrapped ara-c. It can be seen that liposome ara-c has a similar toxicity by i.p. or i.v. routes. On a total ara-c mg/kg basis, liposome ara-c is much more toxic than free ara-c injected by multiple doses but the total doses are somewhat similar comparing i.v. infusion of free drug and liposome single dose.

The LD_{50} of non-drug containing DPPC:chol liposomes was approximately 5 gms/kg i.v.

Effects on L1210 leukemia

(a) i.p. tumor, i.p. treatment

Table 2 shows that single doses of liposome-ara-c result in significant numbers of long-term survivors, whereas no long-term survivors were found after a single multiple dose treatment of free ara-c. 15 mg/kg free ara-c x 6 is approximately 1/8 of the LD_{50} dose and this is approximately equivalent to 7.5 mg/kg lip-ara-c single dose in terms of toxicity. It can be seen that at 5 or 10 mg/kg single dose of lip-ara-c long-term survivors were found.

Table 1. Toxicity (LD_{50}) of cytosine arabinoside administered in
          liposomes or in the free form in non-tumor-bearing DBA
          2J mice

Dosage Form	Mode of Administration	LD_{50}
Liposome	1 x i.p.	80 mg/kg
Liposome	1 x i.v.	80 mg/kg
Free	6 doses at 4 hour intervals	120 mg/kg (720 mg total)
Free	5 day i.v. infusion	10 mg/kg/day

Table 2. Effects of free ara-c and liposome entrapped ara-c on
          L1210 tumor (i.p. tumor, i.p. treatment)

Treatment	Mean Survival Time ± S.D. (days)	Median Survival Time	Long Term Survivors
Free ara-c 30 mg/kg x 6	16.1 ± 7.5	17	0/7
" " 15 " x 6	20.7 ± 4.7	18	0/7
" " 7.5 " x 6	21.1 ± 4.3	20	0/7
REV-ara-c 30 mg/kg x 1	17.9 ± 3.2	> 30	4/7
" " 15 " x 1	21.5 ± 2.9	24	2/7
" " 7.5 " x 1	21.5 ± 6.1	30	3/7
" " 3.75 " x 1	22.0 ± 7.0	25	1/7
Buffer 0	7.4 ± 0.5	7	0/7

Thus, in terms of therapeutic index, lip-ara-c is superior to free
ara-c. In order to "cure" mice with free ara-c by multiple injections,
several courses of treatment, e.g. days 1, 6, 10, are needed (Skipper
et al., 1967). Studies to compare multiple courses of treatment of
free drug with multiple spaced single injections of lip-ara-c have
not been done.

Table 3. Effect of i.v. infused free ara-c compared with a single
          dose of REV-ara-c against i.p. L1210 tumor

Treatment	Mean Survival Time(a)± S.D.	Median Survival Time (b)	Long Term Survivors(c)
Infusion 2.0 mg/kg/day x 5 days	11.6 ± 4.1	10	0/18
REV-ara-c 10 mg/kg x 1	10.9 ± 6.6	14	13/34
20 mg/kg x 1	13.9 ± 6.9	17	9/45
Controls (infusion)	7.2 ± 0.6	7	0/14
Controls (REV)	7.4 ± 0.5	7	0/14

(a) in days of mice dying on or before 30 days
(b) in days
(c) mice surviving more than 30 days out of total number of mice

(b) i.p. tumor, i.v. treatment

Table 3 shows that at approximately equivalent doses in terms
of LD_{50} a single dose of liposome-ara-c was more effective than a
5 day infusion of free drug in terms of long-term survivors. Thus,
in this situation, liposome ara-c has a greater therapeutic efficacy
than infused free ara-c.

(c) i.v. tumor, i.v. treatment

Table 4 shows that at approximately equivalent doses in terms
of LD_{50}, there was no difference in the therapeutic efficacy comparing a single dose of lip-ara-c with a 5 day infusion of free
ara-c.

It is of interest to note that prolonged infusion of free ara-c
does not cure mice bearing i.p. L1210 tumor indicating that a sufficiently cytotoxic level sufficient to kill all tumor cells (mainly in
the peritoneal cavity) is not able to be attained at the maximum
tolerated dose. A question arises as to how i.v. administered liposome entrapped ara-c may act in this situation as there is no reason

Table 4. Effect of i.v. infused free ara-c compared with a single
          dose of REV-ara-c against i.v. L1210 tumor

Treatment	Mean Survival Time (a)± S.D.	Median Survival Time (b)	Long Term Survivors (c)
Infusion 2.0 mg/kg/day x 5.0 days	12.5 ± 6.0	14	1/15
REV-ara-c 10 mg/kg x 1	11.9 ± 5.6	15	0/28
20 mg/kg x 1	12.3 ± 6.2	13	0/31
Control (infusion)	5.8 ± 0.4	6	0/8
Control (REV)	5.2 ± 0.6	5	0/24

(a) in days of mice dying on or before 30 days
(b) in days
(c) mice surviving more than 30 days out of total number of mice

to suppose that the drug is better able to be transported from liposomes into the peritoneal cavity from the circulation. If liposomes
were acting simply as a circulating slow release system, then the
therapeutic index should be similar. It can be suggested that rather
than lip-ara-c being transported into the peritoneal cavity well,
free ara-c is transported particularly poorly into and/or is rapidly
metabolized before reaching the peritoneal cavity.

    This suggestion is supported by the observation that when i.v.
L1210 is treated by i.v. lips-ara-c or i.v. infusion, the comparative
therapeutic efficacy is similar, supporting the conclusion that ara-c-
liposomes act by slowly releasing ara-c into the circulation.

    Although the therapeutic efficacy in the i.v./i.v. situation is
similar for free and entrapped drug as far as the case of administration is concerned, a single injection is equivalent to 5 days infusion.
If sufficient control over toxicity could be maintained, a single
injection of drug would be much simpler for administration purposes
than prolonged infusions.

Again, though the question arises as to why infused free ara-c does not cure a significant number of mice i.v./i.v. or i.v./i.p. There are several possible explanations including:

(a)   rapid development of drug resistance;
(b)   mouse death resulting from tumor in areas where ara-c may be poorly transported (e.g. brain); or
(c)   that a high initial level of ara-c may be required in addition to prolonged relatively low plasma concentration of ara-c.

Thus, in conclusion we can state that liposome entrapped ara-c can increase the therapeutic index of this drug against i.p. inoculated L1210 by single i.p. or i.v. injections compared with an i.p. multiple dose schedule of free ara-c or i.v. infused ara-c. No increase in therapeutic index was found when the effects of liposome ara-c were compared with infused free ara-c against i.v. L1210 tumor. In order to attempt to potentiate the effects of liposome ara-c the following experiments were done.

Use of non-drug containing liposomes to enhance the effects of drug containing liposomes against i.v. L1210 tumor

One suggestion for altering the effects of substances entrapped in liposomes has been to treat animals with non-drug containing (NDC) liposomes prior to, or concurrent with, treatment with drug containing liposomes (Gregoriadis and Neerunjun, 1974, Gregoriadis et al., 1977, Haynes and Kang, 1978). Such a strategy is based on the premise that pretreatment may saturate liposome binding sites in non-target cells and tissues such as reticuloendothelial-system cells in various organs (e.g. liver) so that a subsequent treatment with drug containing liposomes can be potentiated.

Female DBA 2J mice weighing 20-25 gms were injected (i.v.) with 10^6 L1210 cells from mice bearing 5 day old intraperitoneal L1210 tumor. 24 and/or 48 hours later mice were injected i.v. with non-drug-containing liposomes (250 μmoles total lipid/kg). At 25 or 49 hours the mice were injected i.v. with ara-c liposomes to give a dose of ara-c of 10 or 5 mg/kg and lipid dose of 40 or 20 μmole/kg respectively. The effects of pretreatment with non-drug containing liposomes on the subsequent effects of ara-c liposomes are shown in Table 5.

This table shows (a) treatment of mice with non-drug-containing liposomes alone did not increase mean survival time (MST) of tumor bearing mice. (b) A single injection of free ara-c with or without pretreatment with non-drug containing liposomes did not increase MST. (c) Treatment with ara-c liposomes at 10 mg/kg single dose (no pretreatment) at 25 or 49 hours increased MST compared to control mice (treated with free ara-c) about 66% ($p < 0.01$, Students t-test).

Table 5. Effect of i.v. pretreatment of mice bearing i.v. L1210 tumor with non-drug containing liposomes on survival time of drug treated mice.

Ara-C Treatment	Non-drug Containing Liposome Treatment			
	None	DPPC:chol REV 24 hr	DPPC:chol REV 24,48 hr	DPPC:chol REV 48 hr
None	6.0 ± 0.7 (0/43)*	6.2 ± 0.5 (0/19)	6.3 ± 0.5 (0/7)	–
Free Ara-C (100 mg/Kg) 25 hr	7.5 ± 0.8 (0/19)	7.4 ± 0.9 (0/5)	–	–
Free Ara-C (100 mg/Kg) 49 hr	6.8 ± 0.6 (0/17)	7.2 ± 0.7 (0/5)	7.5 ± 0.5 (0/13)	6.9 ± 0.8 (0/9)
DPPC:chol REV Ara-C 25 hr				
10 mg/Kg	12.2 ± 1.9 (0/22)	18.0 ± 6.4 (8/20)	–	–
5 mg/Kg	9.5 ± 2.4 (0/24)	11.3 ± 2.0 (0/14)	–	–
DPPC:chol REV Ara-C 49 hr				
10 mg/Kg	11.3 ± 3.3 (0/26)	–	15.3 ± 5.0 (5/20)	16.1 ± 6.6 (2/17)
5 mg/Kg	8.4 ± 1.5 (0/26)	–	16.1 ± 6.4 (5/21)	15.2 ± 5.1 (1/17)

* Mean survival time (not including long-term survivors) ± standard deviation. Number of mice surviving more than 30 days out of total number of mice in group given in parentheses. The results shown in the table are the pooled results from 6 experiments (not all groups were done in each experiment).

The slight increase in survival at 5 mg/Kg was not statistically significant (p > 0.2), indicating the minimally effective single dose of ara-c liposomes against i.v. L1210 tumor is between 5 and 10 mg/Kg. (d) Non-drug containing liposome treatment at 24 hours, 1 hour before injection with ara-c liposomes (10 mg/Kg) increased the mean survival time compared with mice treated with ara-c liposomes only (p < 0.01) resulted in some long term survivors. The survival time of mice treated with 5 mg/Kg ara-c liposomes 1 hour after non-drug containing liposome treatment was significantly increased compared with controls and mice treated with ara-c liposomes 5 mg/Kg only (p < 0.02). This indicates that after pretreatment, a previously ineffective dose of ara-C liposomes can be potentiated to give significant anti-L1210 activity. (e) Similar increases in MST were found when mice were treated with ara-c liposomes 10 mg/Kg at 49 hours after pretreatment with non-drug containing REV either 1 or both 1 and 25 hours previously. These results clearly show that pretreatment of tumor bearing animals with non-drug containing liposomes can significantly potentiate the therapeutic effects of a subsequent treatment with non-drug containing liposomes.

Although the purpose of the investigations reported here was to determine the therapeutic effects of NDC liposome pretreatment, a few comments can be made regarding the mechanism of the observed effects. The simplest explanation is that pretreatment saturates liposome binding sites, thereby increasing the circulation time of the drug-liposomes. Recent evidence (Ellens et al., in press) shows that pretreatment of mice with REV liposomes reduces tissue uptake and prolongs the circulation time of a second dose of similar liposomes. This may facilitate delivery of the drug-liposomes by altering the tissue distribution to the target tumor cells or prolonging slow release of the drug into the circulation. Although it is probable that the binding sites of liposomes include cells of the reticulo-endothelial system (RES) (Rahman and Wright, 1975, Wisse et al., 1976) in organs such as the liver, it is by no means proven that these sites constitute all or even the majority of the liposome binding sites after liposome injection. An alternative possibility is that the blocking dose depletes serum factors that destabilize liposomes.

If non-drug liposomes are taken up by RES cells, then the results suggest that these cells are not involved in the cytotoxicity of Ara-C liposomes against L1210 tumor. If this were the case, reduction in liposome cytotoxicity could have been found after pretreatment with empty liposomes. Since mice die of L1210 tumor at a constant tumor load (Skipper et al., 1967) the similarity in survival times after treatment at 25 or 49 hours, where comparisons can be made, probably indicates that ara-C liposomes kill a constant fraction of the tumor load at either time of injection. The increases in survival time of pretreated mice indicate a significant improvement in tumor cell kill which is attributable to the pretreatment procedure. It is possible that the size and composition of the lipo-

somes used in the pretreatment scheduling may modulate the pharmacologic effects of the drug—containing liposomes. Although the best
type of "blocking" liposome might be the same as the therapeutic
liposome, in some applications this would perhaps not be so. For
example, it has been shown that uptake of liposomes by the lung is
enhanced by increases in liposome diameter (Hunt et al., 1979). Thus,
for therapeutic applications in the lung the best non-lung binding
liposomes should be used as the pretreatment NDC liposome.

As the doses of empty liposomes used in the present experiments
were less than 1/20 of the L.D.$_{50}$ dose and were without overt toxic
effects, it is probable that further improvement of the anti-L1210
effects could be achieved by optimization of both non-drug containing
and drug-liposome scheduling, dose and type. It is possible that
similar effects may be found in certain other therapeutic applications
of liposomes.

ACKNOWLEDGMENTS

Supported in part by grants CA-28494 (E.M.), CA-13038 (Y.R.)
and contract CM-77118 (E.M.) and CA-16056. We thank R. Lazo, T. Isac,
D. Milholland and J. Goranson for technical assistance.

REFERENCES

Ellens, H., Mayhew, E. and Rustum, Y., Reversible depression of the
    reticulo—endothelial system by liposomes, Biochim. Biophys.
    Acta. (submitted).
Forssen, E.A. and Tokes, Z.A., 1979, In vitro and in vivo studies
    with adriamycin-liposomes, Biochem. Biophys. Res. Comm. 91:
    1295.
Forssen, E.A. and Tokes, Z.A., 1981, Use of anionic liposomes for
    the reduction of chronic doxorubicin induced cardiotoxicity,
    Proc. Nat. Acad. Sci. U.S.A., 78: 1873.
Ganapathi, R., Krishan, A., Wodinsky, I., Zubrod, C.G. and Lesko,
    L.J., 1980, Effect of cholesterol content on antitumor activity
    and toxicity of liposome-encapsulated 1-β-D-arabinofuranosyl-
    cytosine in vivo, Cancer Res., 40: 630.
Gregoriadis, G., 1979, Liposomes in: "Drug Carriers in Biology and
    Medicine", G. Gregoriadis, ed., Academic Press, London.
Gregoriadis, G. and Neerunjun, D.E., 1974, Control of the rate of
    hepatic uptake and catabolism of liposome-entrapped proteins
    injected into rats, Possible therapeutic applications, Eur.
    J. Biochem., 47: 179.
Gregoriadis, G., Neerunjun, D.E. and Hunt, R., 1977, Fate of a
    liposome-associated agent injected with normal and tumour-
    bearing rodents, Attempts to improve localization in tumour
    tissues, Life Sciences, 31: 357.
Gupta, C.M., Radhakrishnan, R. and Khorana, H.G., 1977, Glycero-
    phospholipid syntheses: Improved general method and new analogs

    containing photoactivable groups, Proc. Nat. Acad. Sci. USA,
    74: 4315.
Haynes, D.H. and Kang, C.H., 1978, Saturation of uptake of liposomes
    by the reticulo-endothelial system: possible use for increased
    tumor specificity, Ann. N.Y. Acad. Sci., 308: 440.
Hunt, C.A., Rustum, Y.M., Mayhew, E. and Papahadjopoulos, D., 1979,
    Retention of cytosine arabinoside in mouse lung following intra-
    venous administration in liposomes of different size, Drug
    Metabolism and Disposition, 7: 124.
Kataoka, T. and Kobayaski, T., 1978, Enhancement of chemotherapeutic
    effect by entrapping 1-β-D-arabinofuranosylcytosine in lipid
    vesicles and its mode of action, Ann. N.Y. Acad. Sci., 308:
    387.
Kaye, S.B., Boden, J.A., Bagshaw, K.D. and Ryman, B.E., 1979, Effect
    of liposome encapsulation of actinomycin D on its therapeutic
    efficacy, Brit. J. Cancer, 40: 818.
Kaye, S.B., Boden, J.A. and Ryman, B.E., 1980, Application of lipo-
    some entrapped cytotoxic drugs to the treatment in vivo of drug
    resistant solid murine tumors, Proc. Am. Assoc. Cancer Res.,
    21: 254.
Kaye, S.B. and Ryman, B.E., 1980, The fate of liposome-entrapped
    actinomycin D in vivo and its therapeutic effect in a solid
    murine tumor, Biochem. Soc. Trans., 8: 107.
Kedar, A., Mayhew, E., Moore, R.H. and Murphy, G.P., 1981, Failure
    of Actinomycin D entrapped in liposome to prolong survival in
    renal cell adenocarcinoma-bearing mice, Oncology, 38: 311.
Kimelberg, H.K. and Atchison, M.L., 1978, Effects of entrapment in
    liposomes on the distribution degradation and effectiveness of
    methotrexate in vivo, Ann. N.Y. Acad. Sci., 308: 395.
Kimelberg, H.K. and Mayhew, E., 1978, Properties and Biological
    effects of liposomes and their uses in pharmacology and toxi-
    cology in: "CRC Critical Reviews in Toxicology," L. Goldberg,
    ed., CRC Press Inc., Florida.
Mayhew, E., Papahadjopoulos, D., Rustum, Y.M. and Dave, C., 1978,
    Use of liposomes for the enhancement of the cytotoxic effects
    of cytosine arabinoside, Ann. N.Y. Acad. Sci., 308: 371.
Mayhew, E., Rustum, Y. and Szoka, F., 1980, Efficacy of liposome-
    entrapped cytosine arabinoside compared with infused free Ara-C
    against L1210 tumor, Proc. Am. Assoc. Cancer Res., 21: 293.
Mayhew, E., Rustum, Y.M., Szoka, F. and Papahadjopoulos, D., 1979,
    Role of cholesterol in enhancing the antitumor activity of
    cytosine arabinoside entrapped in liposomes, Cancer Treatment
    Reports, 63: 1923.
Olson, F., Mayhew, E., Maslow, D., Rustum, Y. and Szoka, F., 1982,
    Characterization, toxicity and therapeutic efficacy of adriamycin
    encapsulated in liposomes, Eur. J. Cancer. (in press).
Rahman, A., Kessler, A., More, N., Silkie, B., Rowden, G., Woolley, P.
    and Schein, P.S., 1980, Liposomal protection of adriamycin-
    induced cardiotoxocity in mice, Cancer Res., 40: 1532.
Rahman, Y.E. and Wright, B.J., 1975, Liposomes containing chelating

agents, Cellular penetration and a possible mechanism of metal
    removal, J. Cell. Biol., 65: 112.
Rustum, Y.M., Dave, D., Mayhew, E. and Papahadjopoulos, D., 1979,
    Role of liposome type and route of administration in the anti-
    tumor activity of liposome-entrapped 1-β-D-arabinofuranosyl-
    cytosine against mouse L1210 leukemia, Cancer Res., 39: 1390.
Semon, J.H. and Grindey, G.B., 1978, Potentiation of the Anti-tumor
    activity of Methotrexate by Concurrent Infusion ofThymidine,
    Cancer Res., 38: 2405.
Skipper, H.E., Schabel, F.M., Jr. and Wilcox, W.S., 1967, Experimental
    evaluation of potential anticancer agents, XXI. Scheduling of
    arabinosylcytosine to take advantage of its S-phase specificity
    against leukemia cells, Cancer Chemotherapy Reports, 51: 125.
Szoka, F. and Papahadjopoulos, D., 1978, Procedure for preparation
    of liposomes with large internal aqueous space and high capture
    by reverse-phase evaporation, Proc. Nat. Acad. Sci. U.S.A.,
    75: 4194.
Szoka, F., Olson, F., Heath, T., Vail, W., Mayhew, E. and Papahadjo-
    poulos, D., 1980, Preparation of unilamellar liposomes of inter-
    mediate size by a combination of reverse phase evaporation and
    extrusion through poly-carbonate membranes, Biochim. Biophys.
    Acta, 601: 559.
Wisse, E., Gregoriadis, G. and Deams, W.Th., 1976, Electron micro-
    scopic cytochemical localization of intravenously injected
    liposome-encapsulated horseradish peroxidase in rat liver cells,
    Adv. Exp. Med. Biol., 73: 237.

STIMULATION OF HOST RESPONSE AGAINST METASTATIC TUMORS

BY LIPOSOME-ENCAPSULATED IMMUNOMODULATORS

George Poste[a], Corazon Bucana[b] and Isaiah J. Fidler[b]

[a]Smith Kline and French Laboratories, Philadelphia, PA
19101 and Department of Pathology and Laboratory
Medicine, University of Pennsylvania, Philadelphia, PA
19104; [b]Cancer Metastasis and Treatment Laboratory
NCI-Frederick Cancer Research Center, Frederick, MD
21701, USA

INTRODUCTION

The metastatic spread of malignant tumors to form metastases
at other sites in the body remains the principal cause of failure
in the treatment of neoplastic disease[1]. Several factors are
responsible for this unfortunate situation. First, metastases are
frequently too small to be detected at the time the primary tumor
is removed. Second, widespread dissemination of metastases often
takes place before symptoms of metastatic disease occur. Third,
the anatomic location of many metastatic lesions renders them
inaccessible to surgical removal and/or limits the effective dose
of therapeutic agents that reach metastases. The final, and most
formidable, problem concerns emergence of metastatic lesions that
are resistant to conventional therapy. Recent work suggests that
metastases arise from non-random spread of specialized subpopulations
of cells within the primary tumor and that the responsiveness of
these metastatic subpopulations to therapy may not only differ from
that of non-metastatic tumor cells in the primary tumor but may
also vary significantly between the tumor cell subpopulations
present in individual metastases within the same patient (review, 2).
The depressing implication of this marked heterogeneity in the
response of malignant cells to chemotherapy and other therapeutic
modalities is that the only successful approach to the therapy of
metastases will be one that circumvents the problem of cellular
diversity between tumor cells in primary and metastatic lesions, and
between different metastatic foci.

There is increasing evidence that this demanding requirement could perhaps be fulfilled by activated macrophages. Activated macrophages kill tumor cells by an immunologically non-specific mechanism and will kill tumor cells of syngeneic, allogeneic or xenogeneic origin while leaving normal cells unharmed (review, 3). Although the mechanism of macrophage-mediated killing is not known, it is independent of such tumor cell characteristics as antigenicity, invasiveness and metastatic potential (see, 3). Unlike the action of many chemotherapeutic agents, killing of tumor cells by activated macrophages is not limited to a specific phase of the tumor cell cycle. Activated macrophages are also capable of killing tumor cells that are resistant to various anticancer drugs. Another intriguing aspect of macrophage-mediated tumoricidal activity is that the frequency of tumor cell resistance to killing appears to be extremely low. In contrast to the relative ease with which tumor cell variants resistant to cytotoxic drugs, antibodies, cytotoxic lymphocytes or NK cells can be selected, efforts to select tumor cells that are resistant to activated macrophages have so far been unsuccessful (see, 4). Evidence that activated macrophages are capable of contributing to host defense against tumors in vivo comes from studies showing that i.v. injection of activated syngeneic macrophages restricts tumor growth at both primary sites[5] and metastatic lesions[6-9]. Conversely, administration of agents which impair macrophage function enhance metastatic spread of malignant tumors (see, 9). Collectively these observations suggest that methods for augmenting macrophage-mediated tumoricidal activity in vivo might be of value in the therapy of metastatic disease.

As mentioned, intravenous transfusion of activated macrophages augments host resistance to metastatic tumors. For clinical use, however, this approach has several shortcomings. Foremost is the need to transfuse large numbers of autologous or histocompatible macrophages. The alternative approach is to develop efficient methods for activation of macrophages in situ. This strategy is considered feasible because even though intratumoral macrophages isolated from progressively growing tumors often lack tumoricidal activity, they are still able to respond to exogenous activating stimuli (review, 10).

Macrophage activation can be induced by a wide variety of materials (review, 11). These fall into two general categories. The first embraces a diverse range of microorganisms and parasites and surface components isolated from these organisms. These stimuli induce activation by interacting directly with macrophages (see, 11). The other major pathway for macrophage activation involves an indirect mechanism in which a lymphokine, macrophage activation factor (MAF), released by antigen- or mitogen-stimulated T lymphocytes binds to a surface receptor on macrophages to elicit activation (review, 12).

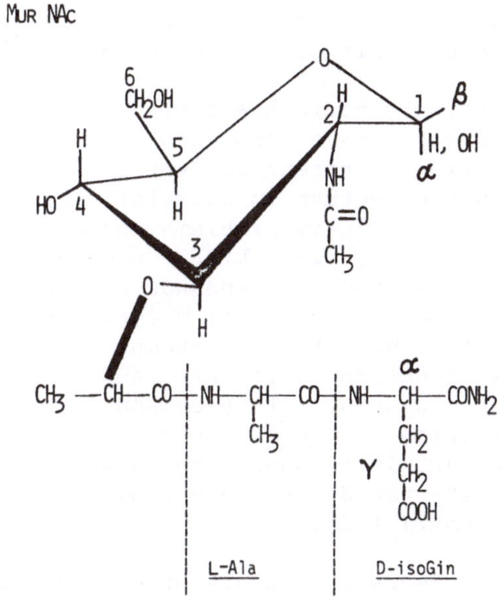

Figure 1. Muramyl Dipeptide

Attempts to use macrophage activators as therapeutic agents
to augment host defense against tumors have been largely unsuccessful. Direct injection of lymphokine preparations containing MAF
has been reported to induce regression of skin tumors and cutaneous
metastases[13,14] but similar preparations administered systemically
fail to limit the growth of distant metastases. After injection
into the circulation, MAF is inactivated rapidly by binding to serum
proteins[15] and biologically effective concentrations do not reach
macrophages in distant tumor foci. A further obstacle to macrophage
activation in situ by passive immunotherapy with lymphokines is
that macrophages are only susceptible to activation by MAF for 3-4
days after their emigration from the circulation[16]. In addition,
once activated, their tumoricidal activity persists for only 3-4
days and with decay of the tumoricidal phenotype they become
refractory to a second cycle of activation by MAF[16].

Attempts to activate macrophages with agents which interact
directly with macrophages have also encountered significant problems.
Systemic administration of potent activators such as BCG or C.
parvum, though highly effective in stimulating macrophages, is
accompanied by serious toxicity problems, granuloma formation and
allergic reactions (review, 11). Little progress has been made in
developing non-toxic, synthetic compounds with immunopotentiating
activity. Muramyl dipeptide (Fig. 1; N-acetylmuramyl-L-alanyl-D-
isoglutamine; MDP) is a prototypic compound for this class of agent.
MDP is the minimal structural unit that can replace Mycobacteria
in Freund's complete adjuvant. This compound stimulates a variety
of macrophage activities in vitro, including tumoricidal activity
(review, 17). However, it is unable to induce macrophage activation
in vivo because of its rapid clearance from the body after systemic
administration (<1 hour) (see,17).

In the last few years our laboratories have examined the
feasibility of using liposomes as carrier vehicles to deliver
activators to macrophages in situ in an effort to overcome some of
the problems that limit the effectiveness of these materials when
administered in conventional fashion as free molecules. Liposomes
offer several attractive features as carriers for macrophage
activators.

First, when injected i.v., the majority of liposomes localize
in macrophages of the reticuloendothelial (RE) system and circulating
blood monocytes (review, 18). This localization pattern reflects
the well-documented role of these cells in clearance of particulate
materials from the circulation (see, 18). Unlike ambitious efforts
to actively "target" liposomes to specific cell types in situ by
incorporating ligands into the liposomal membrance which "recognize"
the desired target cell[19-21], the natural tendancy of i.v. injected
liposomes to localize in macrophages can be exploited to achieve
"targeting" of liposomes, albeit passively, to macrophages.

Second, encapsulation of activators within liposomes prevents their inactivation by serum components and reduces the risk of immunological sensitization of the recipient to the activator.

Third, unlike activation by free MAF which requires binding of MAF to a fucoglycolipid receptor on the macrophage surface[22], liposome-encapsulated MAF can activate macrophages which lack the surface receptor and are unresponsive to free MAF[16-23]. This observation is important in relation to the failure of macrophages that have undergone one cycle of activation elicited by free MAF to be reactivated by MAF[16]. This phenomenon poses a potential problem for therapeutic efforts to activate macrophages in vivo. Agents that act indirectly by stimulating lymphocytes to produce MAF will probably prove ineffective because a significant fraction of macrophages within a tumor may be unresponsive to free MAF. In contrast, liposome-encapsulated MAF, by eliciting activation via a mechanism that does not require participation of the surface receptor[23], is not subject to this problem. Finally, for activators such as muramyl dipeptide, which are ordinarily cleared from the body too rapidly to be active in vivo, administration as a liposome-encapsulated preparation extends the active half-life within the body sufficiently to enable it to induce macrophage activation in situ[24].

In this paper we present a brief review of our studies on the use of liposome-encapsulated macrophage activators to stimulate host defense against established lung metastases.

TECHNIQUES

Full details of the origin and properties of the tumor systems, preparation of liposome-encapsulated macrophage activators, macrophage isolation, assay of macrophage-mediated tumoricidal activity and methods for evaluating metastatic tumor growth are given in references cited in the following sections. Unless stated otherwise, all references to liposomes made in the remainder of this paper refer to multilamellar (MLV) liposomes prepared from phosphatidyl-serine (PS) and phosphatidylcholine (PC) (3:7 mole ratio).

ACTIVATION OF TUMORICIDAL LUNG MACROPHAGES BY LIPOSOMES CONTAINING MACROPHAGE ACTIVATORS

In evaluating the ability of liposome-associated macrophage activators to augment host defense against metastases, we have given particular attention to the therapy of lung metastases. The lung is a major site for metastatic disease and a major objective in our studies has been to devise a method for augmenting the tumoricidal properties of alveolar macrophages.

Table 1. Activation of Tumoricidal Properties in Murine Alveolar Macrophages (AM) by I.V. Injection of Liposomes Containing Lymphokines

Treatment of AM Donors[a]	Radioactivity (cpm ± S.D.) in live B16-BL6 cells on day 3[b]
no AM, tumor cells alone	2561 ± 149
HBSS	2347 ± 116
free lymphokines (200 l)	2170 ± 123
PC liposomes (lymphokines)	2416 ± 139
PC liposomes (HBSS) + free lymphokines (12.5 l)[c]	2293 ± 84
PS/PC liposomes (lymphokines)	1319 ± 102 (44%)[e]
PS/PC liposomes (HBSS) + free lymphokines (12.5 l)[c]	2274 ± 133

[a]Groups of five mice were injected i.v. with the indicated materials 24 hours before harvesting AM by pulmonary lavage. Liposomes (5μmoles lipid/mouse) were suspended in either HBSS or HBSS supplemented with the indicated volume of free lymphokines and 0.2 ml aliquots injected i.v.

[b]Five thousand target B16–BL6 cells labelled with (^{125}I)IdUrd were plated onto AM macrophages in culture dishes with 38 mm^2 culture wells at a macrophage to target cell ratio of 10:1. Cultures were maintained in CMEM refed 24 hours after addition of target cells and cell-associated radioactivity measured after 72 hours. The results are mean values ± S.D. from triplicate cultures.

[c]Corresponds to volume of lymphokines encapsulated within MLV liposomes.

[d]Number in parenthesis = percentage cytotoxicity compared with control AM treated with HBSS.

[e]Statistically significant (P <.001).

Table 2. Activation of Tumoricidal Properties in Murine Alveolar Macrophages by I.V. Injection of Liposomes Containing MDP

Treatment of AM Donors[a]	Radioactivity (cpm ± S.D.) in live B16-BL6 cells on day 3[b]
no AM, tumor cells alone	1894 ± 60
HBSS	1840 ± 18
free MDP (200 μg)	1774 ± 66
PC liposomes (MDP:2.5 μg)	1809 ± 43
PS/PC liposomes (MDP:2.5 μg)	1085 ± 79 (41%)[c]
PS/PC liposomes (HBSS) + free MDP (2.5 μg)	1784 ± 121

a-b As in footnotes a and b in Table 1.
c As in footnote d in Table 1 ($P < 0.001$).

As reported in detail elsewhere[25], comparison of a variety
of liposomes of differing size, surface charge and lipid composition
has established that negatively-charged MLV liposomes (1-2 μm
diameter) prepared from PS and PC (3:7 mole ratio) represent the
optimal type of liposome for efficient localization in the lung
capillary bed after i.v. injection. Liposomes of this composition
containing either MDP or lymphokines rich in MAF activity produce
significant activation of tumoricidal properties in alveolar macrophages in both mice (Tables 1 and 2; refs. 9, 24-26) and rats[27].
In contrast, neutral MLV liposomes prepared from PC alone show
limited arrest in the lung[25] and liposomes of this composition
containing MDP or lymphokines fail to activate lung macrophages
(Tables 1 and 2).

Two lines of evidence suggest that the activated macrophages
recovered by pulmonary lavage from animals injected i.v. with PS/PC
liposomes containing macrophage activators are in fact blood
monocytes that engulf liposomes in lung capillaries and then migrate
into the alveoli[28].

Electronmicroscopic studies reveal significant uptake of MLV
liposomes by blood monocytes within pulmonary capillaries within 1
hour after i.v. injection of liposomes (Fig. 2; ref. 28). By
4 hours after injection, macrophages containing liposomes are
found in the alveoli (Fig. 2) and can be recovered by lavage of
the alveoli[25-28]. However, no evidence has been obtained to
suggest that liposomes are capable of crossing the capillary wall
to reach macrophages in the alveoli. No examples have been found
of liposomes either in transit across the capillary wall or free
within the alveoli. These ultrastructural observations suggest
that liposomes are first engulfed by blood monocytes within the
lung capillaries and that these cells then migrate to the alveoli.

Additional support for this interpretation comes from studies
on the recruitment of macrophages to the lung[28].

Alveolar macrophages originate from blood monocytes[29-32].
Whole body irradiation suppresses circulating blood monocytes and
by damaging monocyte precursors in the marrow prevents recruitment
of alveolar macrophages to the lung[29]. Reconstitution of the
bone marrow in irradiated animals results in reappearance of
alveolar macrophages in lavage fluids in 7-10 days [29]. In
contrast, local irradiation of the chest damages preexisting
alveolar macrophages but this is rapidly compensated by recruitment
of blood monocytes into the alveoli[29]. We have exploited these
properties to determine the origin of tumoricidal alveolar macrophages recovered from mice injected i.v. with liposomes containing
encapsulated lymphokines. Whole body irradiation of mice 24 hours
before injection of liposome-encapsulated lymphokines abolishes
activation of alveolar macrophages by liposome-encapsulated

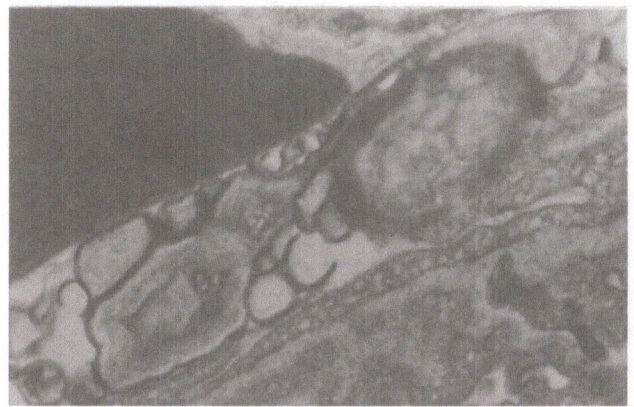

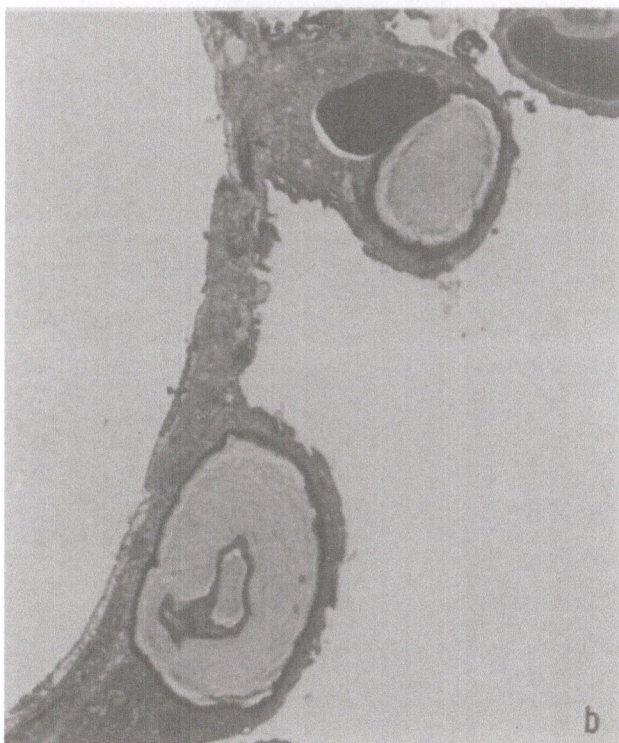

Fig. 2. Electronmicrographs of mouse lung following i.v. injection
of 5 μmoles of multilamellar liposomes (PS/PC, 3:7 mole ratio).
   a.   Ten min. after injection showing liposomes of various
        sizes free within pulmonary capillaries. (X400)
   b.   One hour after injection showing free liposomes within
        capillaries. (X200)

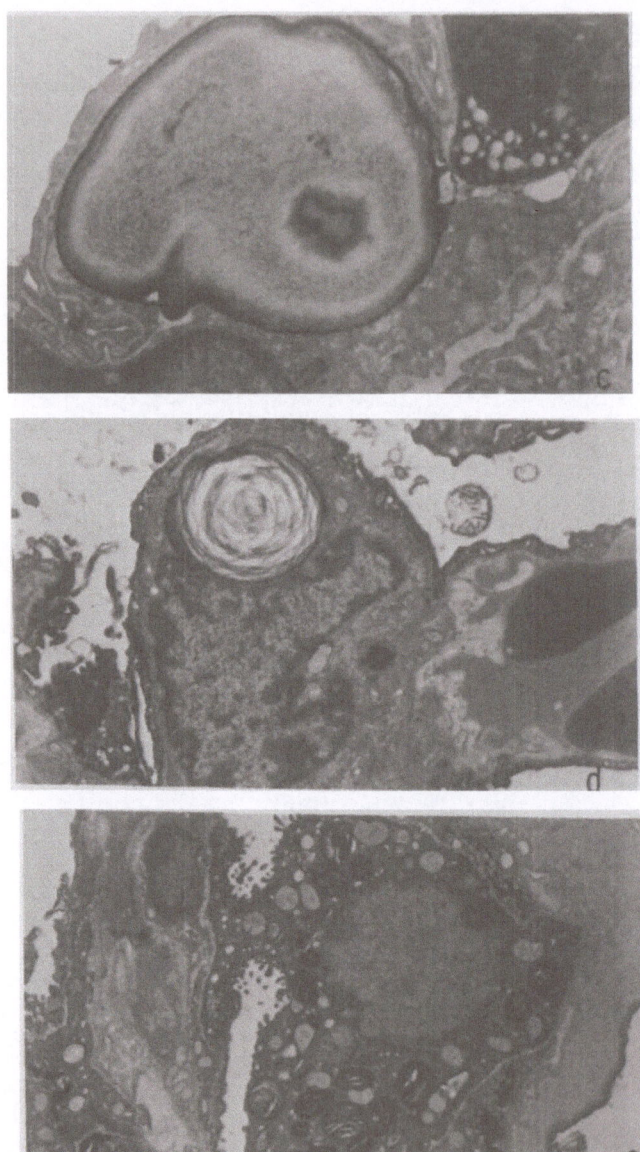

Fig. 2. c.   Higher power field showing free liposome adjacent to PMN
(cont.)   leukocyte (top right) and monocyte (lower left) 1 hour
             after injection. (X400)

       d.   Monocyte containing internalized liposome within a lung
             capillary 1 hour after injection. (X200)

       e.   Type II pneumocyte. The arrangement of stacked lamellae
             in the surfactant inclusions can be distinguished from
             the "whorled" lamellae of liposomes shown in a-d.(X200)

lymphokines (Table 3). This experiment is complicated, however, by the problem that very few viable cells can be recovered from the lung. Lavage fluids from these animals contain primarily dead cells and debris. However, similar loss of responsiveness to liposome-encapsulated lymphokines is seen in animals in which the thorax is protected during irradiation (Table 3). These animals yield comparable numbers of alveolar macrophages to untreated controls[28]. The alveolar macrophages recovered from these animals can be activated, however, by incubation in vitro with liposomes containing lymphokines (Table 3). Shielding of the thorax during irradiation protects alveolar macrophages which are already in the alveoli but damages circulating monocytes and macrophage precursors in the bone marrow[29]. The failure of the protected alveolar macrophages to respond to liposome-encapsulated lymphokines in vivo, while fully responsive in vitro, suggests that liposomes are not reaching these cells in vivo. In contrast, mice subjected to local irradiation of the chest before injection with liposome-encapsulated lymphokines yield alveolar macrophages with significant tumoricidal activity (Table 3). This procedure destroys macrophages in the alveoli but has no effect on circulating monocytes and their recruitment to the lung. These data again indicate that tumoricidal macrophages are derived from blood monocytes which interact with liposomes within the microcirculation and migrate into the alveoli.

Recovery of the response of alveolar macrophages to liposome-encapsulated lymphokines in irradiated mice after bone marrow reconstitution also supports this interpretation. Irradiated mice are unresponsive to liposome-encapsulated lymphokines injected 1 day after irradiation and bone marrow reconstitution but show a significant tumoricidal response when tested 7 days after reconstitution when normal levels of circulating monocytes have been restored (Table 3).

THERAPY OF ESTABLISHED LUNG METASTASES BY INTRAVENOUS INJECTION OF LIPOSOMES CONTAINING MACROPHAGE ACTIVATORS

The ability of liposome- associated macrophage activators to augment host response to established lung metastases has been tested using the murine B16 melanoma. C57BL/6 mice are injected in the footpad with 5×10^4 melanoma cells from the highly metastatic B16-B16 line[33]. Four weeks later when the tumor implants have reached a size of 10-12 mm, the leg bearing the tumor and the popliteal lymph node are amputated. Three days later, animals are injected intravenously with 5 μmoles of liposomes containing a macrophage activator. Control animals are injected either with free (unencapsulated) activator or liposomes containing encapsulated saline but suspended in free activator. Both test and control groups are treated twice weekly for 4 weeks. Two weeks after the final treatment, the animals are killed and necropsied. The presence of metastases is determined microscopically and all suspected

Table 3. Tumoricidal Activity of Alveolar Cells Recovered by Pulmonary
Lavage After Whole- and Partial-Body Irradiation and I.V.
Injection of MLV Liposomes (PS/PC 3:7 mole ration) Containing
Encapsulated Lymphokines*

In vivo treatment	% Destruction of B16 melanoma cells by alveolar cells	
	no additional treatment	incubation in vitro with liposome-encapsulated lymphokines
untreated controls	6 ± 2	44 ± 13
liposome-lymphokines	39 ± 14	53 ± 16
whole body irradiation + liposome-lymphokines (24 hr post-irradiation)	0**	N.D.
whole body irradiation (thorax protected) + liposome-lymphokines (24 hr post-irradiation)	8 ± 3	47 ± 12
thorax irradiated + liposome-lymphokines (24 hr post-irradiation)	32 ± 14	49 ± 15

whole body irradiation + bone marrow reconstitution + liposome-lymphokines (24 hr post-reconstitution)	0**	N.D.
whole body irradiation + bone marrow reconstitution + liposome-lymphokines (7 days post-reconstitution)	30 ± 18	42 ± 11

*Methods described in (28).
**No viable cells recovered.
N.D. + not done.

lesions confirmed histologically. Spontaneous pulmonary and lymph
node metastases are well established in animals at the time liposome
therapy is started and several individual lung metastases are visible
macroscopically[24,25]. As shown in Table 4, i.v. injection of such
rapidly into lesions exceeding 2-3 mm in diameter and by 40 days at
least 70% of the inoculated animals will be dead.

    Our initial experiments were done using liposomes containing
lymphokines rich in MAF activity harvested from mitogen-stimulated
lymphocytes[23].   As shown in Table 4, i.v. injection of such
preparations produced a significant reduction in the number of lung
metastases. No significant reduction in metastatic burden was
detected in control groups.

    The use of crude, unfractionated lymphokine preparations has a
number of shortcomings. First, the lack of a quantitative assay for
the specific lymphokine(s) responsible for macrophage activation
frustrates accurate measurement of dose-response relationships.
Second, many other potent biological mediators are present in such
preparations. This not only complicates interpretation of the
mechanism of the host response but the presence of other mediators
with mitogenic, angiogenic and vascular permeabilizing activities
might even enhance tumor growth under certain conditions. It is
therefore desirable, and probably mandatory for clinical trials
in man, that efforts to augment host resistance to tumors employ
agents of defined composition and purity. For this reason, our
current reasearch is now directed to assessing the efficacy of
muramyl dipeptide (MDP) and structurally related compounds as
macrophage activating agents.

    MDP (N-acetyl-L-alanyl-D-isoglutamine; Fig. 1) is the minimal
structural unit (mol wt 492) with immunopotenitator activity that
can replace Mycobacteria in Freund's complete adjuvant (FCA)
(review, 35). Although MDP has potent effects on macrophage
function in vitro (see, 35) its effectiveness in vivo is limited
by its extremely rapid clearance from the body (90% of MDP injected
i.v. is excreted in the urine within 1-2 hours; see, 35). Even
when MDP is injected i.v. at very high doses (500 μg) it fails to
stimulate significant macrophage-mediated antitumor activity[24].
We have shown recently, however, that i.v. injection of MDP encapsulated in MLV liposomes is highly effective in activating rodent
macrophage populations in vitro and in vivo (Table 2; refs. 9,24)
and in enhancing destruction of metastases in tumor-bearing animals
(Table 4).

    In the experiments described in Table 3 the tumor burden in the
lung at the start of therapy exceeds 10^7 cells[24]. In addition to
reducing the number of metastases, parallel experiments revealed
that 65% of mice treated with liposome-encapsulated MDP survived at
least 120 days after the final treatment. This indicates that the

Table 4. Therapy of Established Lung Metastases by Intravenous Injection of MLV Liposomes Containing Muramyl Dipeptide (MDP) or Lymphokines

| Treatment[a] | | | Metastatic Burden[b] | |
Liposome composition	Encapsulated agent	Unencapsulated suspension	Median number of pulmonary metastases (range)	Number of mice with metastasis/total
none	none	HBSS	36 (0-94)	25/29
none	none	200 μg MDP	29 (0-66)	10/12
PC	2.5 μg MDP	--	22 (0-73)	10/13
PC	HBSS	2.5 μg MDP	17 (0-59)	13/15
PC/PS	2.5 μg MDP	--	0 (0-6)[c]	3/14[c]
PC/PS	HBSS	2.5 μg MDP	26 (0-84)	13/14
none	none	200 μl lymphokines	30 (0-51)	8/10
PC	HBSS	6.25 μl lymphokines	34 (0-108)	12/14
PC	6.25 μl lymphokines	--	24 (0-83)	12/15
PC/PS	HBSS	6.25 μl lymphokines	30 (0-78)	12/15
PC/PS	6.25 μl lymphokines	--	5 (0-42)[c]	4/15[c]

[a]Groups of 5 mice were injected i.v. with liposomes containing the indicated encapsulated materials suspended in 0.2 ml HBSS or in 0.2 ml HBSS containing either 6.25 μl free lymphokine or 2.5 μg free MDP. Mice received injections (2.5 moles lipid/mouse) twice weekly for 4 weeks.

[b]Spontaneous metastases arising from B16-BL6 cells implanted s.c. Mice were killed 2 weeks after completion of treatment and necropsied. Lung metastases were counted under a microscope and confirmed histologically.

[c]Significant reduction in the incidence of metastasis (P < 0.001, chi square test) compared to other treatment protocols and untreated control animals.

tumor burden in these animals was probably reduced to fewer than
10 viable cells because they survived longer than 40-50 days which
is the median life span of mice implanted with 10 viable B16
cells[24,36].

STIMULATION OF HOST RESISTANCE TO METASTASES BY LIPOSOMES CONTAINING MACROPHAGE ACTIVATORS IS MEDIATED BY ACTIVATED MACROPHAGES

To test whether tumoricidal macrophages are responsible for
the enhanced destruction of metastases produced by treatment with
PS/PC liposomes containing encapsulated lymphokines or MDP, agents
that impair macrophages in situ were administered to animals
immediately before and after liposome therapy[9].

If macrophages are important in the destruction of metastases,
then their impairment by treatment with antimacrophage agents such
as silica, carrageenan, or hyperchlorinated drinking water should
abrogate the therapeutic benefits observed following the systemic
administration of liposomes containing macrophage activators. Such
was the case (Table 5). These results indicate that experimental
depletion of macrophage populations in situ by treatment with
antimacrophage agents abolishes the ability of tumor-bearing mice
to respond to liposome-encapsulated lymphokines or MDP. Although
the agents used to impair macrophage function are selective for
macrophages[37-43], the selectivity is not absolute. Both silica and
carrageenan have previously been reported to alter functions mediated
by lymphocytes [42,44] and natural killer cells[45,46].   There is
evidence to suggest, however, that the effects of silica and
carrageenan shown in Table 5 result primarily from their action
on macrophages rather than T lymphocytes or natural killer cells.
Firstly, mice depleted of natural killer cell by chronic administration of 17 - estradiol resemble normal mice in that they show increased antitumor resistance after treatment with liposome-encapsulated
lymphokines or MDP[46]. Secondly, the systemic activation of macrophages to the tumoricidal state by liposome-entrapped MDP appears to
be independent of the thymus, since it can be accomplished in adult
thymectomized and X-irradiated mice as well as athymic nude mice[47].
These data suggest that macrophages are the essential effector cell
in the destruction of metastases. The data do not, however, rule
out the possibility that macrophages do not function alone or that
tumor destruction is accomplished by macrophage recruitment of other
host effector cells or factors.

Additional evidence that macrophages activated by liposome-
encapsualted lymphokines or MDP can act directly as cytotoxic
effecotr cells comes from the adoptive transfer experiments [9].
In these experiments tumor-bearing mice were not injected with
liposomes containing macrophage activators. Rather, mice were
injected i.v. with macrophages that had been incubated in vitro with
liposomes containing either MDP (activated) or saline (non-activated).

Table 5. The In Situ Activation of Tumoricidal Properties in Alveolar Macrophages (AM) and Destruction of Pulmonary Metastases by I.V. Injection of Liposomes Containing Lymphokines or MDP in Mice Pretreated with Antimacrophag Agents

Pretreatment of mice with anti-macrophage agent[a]	Liposome[b,c] treatment	% Destruction of B16-BL6 melanoma cells in vitro	Number of mice with metastasis/total	Median number of pulmonary metastases (range)
none, controls	none	2	12/15	39[f] (0-102)
none, controls	PC/PS (lymphokines)	34	9/14	7[f] (0-51)
none, controls	PC/PS (MDP)	48	4/14	1[f] (0-12)
silica	PC/PS (lymphokines)	14[e]	12/14	65[g] (0-171)
silica	PC/PS (HBSS)	4[e]	13/14	85[g] (3-214)
carrageenan	PC/PS (lymphokines	3[e]	12/14	39[g] (0-123)
carrageenan	PC/PS (HBSS)	9	12/14	67[g] (1-153)
hyperchlorinated water	PC/PS (MDP)	21[e]	9/12	56[g] (0-202)
hyperchlorinated water	PC/PS (HBSS)	2[e]	11/14	95[g] (0-209)

[a] Groups of mice were treated with the indicated agents prior to liposome therapy as described in (9).
[b] For the assays of in vitro mediated cytotoxicity by AM, control and test groups were injected with PC/PS (7:3 mole ratio) liposomes containing the indicated encapsulated materials as a single i.v. injection (5 μmole lipid/mouse) in 0.2 ml HBSS. Additional groups of control animals injected with 0.2 ml HBSS alone or liposomes containing encapsulated HBSS suspended in HBSS containing free lympho-kines (12.5 μl) or MDP (2.5 μg) in a total volume of 0.2 ml HBSS did not differ significantly from control animals injected with liposome-encapsulated HBSS (data not shown).
[c] For treatment of spontaneous metastases arising from B16-BL6 cells implanted s.c., mice were injected i.v. with the indicated liposomes containing HBSS, lymphokines or MDP twice weekly for 4 weeks. AM were harvested from animals 24 hr after injection with liposomes and assayed for their ability to destroy (^{125}I) iododeoxyuridine-labeled B16-BL6 melanoma cells using the 3-day cytotoxicity described in footnote b in Table 1. The results represent mean values from two separate experiments. Deviations from the mean did not exceed 15%.
[e] Statistically significant reduction in cytotoxicity compared to corresponding controls (P < 0.001).
[f] Statistically significant reduction in metastasis as compared to untreated controls (P < 0.001).
[g] Statistically significant increase in metastatic burden compared to untreated control animals (P < 0.01).

Table 6. Destruction of Pulmonary Metastases by Intravenous Injection of Macrophages Activated in vitro by Liposome-Encapsulated MDP

In vitro treatment of macrophages[a]	In vitro macrophage-mediated cytotoxicity[b]	Pulmonary metastasis in mice injected i.v. with macrophages[c]		
		Number of metastases		Number of mice with metastasis/total
		median	range	
untreated	2	14	0– 95	12/15
liposome MDP	69[d]	4	0– 90	12/20[e]
liposome HBSS + free MDP (1 μg)	13	19	0–112	13/18

[a]Peritoneal macrophages were incubated for 16 hours in supplemented media at 37°C with PC/PS (7:3 mole ratio) liposomes containing either MDP or HBSS. Macrophages were then washed three times with HBSS. A small aliquot was used to assess in vitro cytotoxicity and the remainder injected i.v. into tumor-bearing mice.

[b]Determined as described in footnote b in Table 1.

[c]Mice injected i.v. with 3 X 10^6 macrophages 3, 5 and 7 days after i.v. injection of 2 X 10^4 B16–BL6 melanoma cells. Lung metastases were determined 4 weeks after the last injection.

[d]Statistically significant (P <0.001) increase in cytotoxicity.

[e]Statistically significant (P <0.01 Mann Whitney U test) reduction in metastases as compared to the other treatment groups.

Macrophages rendered tumoricidal by incubation in vitro with liposome-encapsulated MDP produced a significant reduction in the metastatic burden when injected i.v. into tumor-bearing animals (Table 6). This is consistent with previous reports in which adoptive transfer of macrophages activated in vitro reduced tumor growth in syngeneic mice[5-8].

CONCLUSIONS

The disappointing results obtained in experimental and clinical efforts to devise effective specific active immunotherapy procedures for the treatment of cancer have stimulated renewed interest in mechanisms of non-specific "natural" antitumor surveillance mediated by macrophages and NK cells. A significant effort is now underway in many laboratories to develop effective agents that will stimulate the antitumor activities of these cells. Data presented here, and in our previous publications[9,23-28,34,47-49], indicates that systemic administration of lymphokines or MDP encapsulated in MLV liposomes activates macrophages in vivo and augments host antitumor defenses. Dose-response measurements reveal that liposome-encapsulated lymphokines or MDP are significantly more effective in activating macrophages and stimulating host resistance to tumors than the same materials administered in unencapsulated form. Horeover, MDP is ordinarily cleared from the body in less than 1 hour after parenteral administration. This is too short to evoke the activated state and free MDP injected i.v. at high doses (200-500 μg) does not render macrophages tumoricidal. The encapsulation of MDP within liposomes leads to retention of MDP within the macrophage where it is released over 2-3 days and maintains the tumoricidal state.

The findings described in this chapter suggest that amplification of host defense systems by liposome-encapsulated immunomodulators could be useful in the therapy of metastatic disease. Activated macrophages appear to be able to recognize and destroy neoplastic cells without regard to their phenotypic diversity and macrophage-mediated cytotoxicity appears to be devoid of the problem of cellular resistance to killing which is routinely encountered in efforts to destroy tumor cells by cytotoxic drugs.

The demonstration that the augmented antitumor response produced by liposome-encapsulated lymphokines or MDP is mediated by activated macrophages is also important for development of an effective therapeutic modality for treating cancer. There is a growing body of evidence that activated macrophages are major effector cells in host resistance to tumors (review, 5). Recent data also suggest that the progressive growth of neoplasms may be caused, in part, by host immune deficiencies that frustrate macrophage involvement in tumor rejection[2,51]. One such example is the decreased ability of lymphocytes in animals bearing large tumors

to interact with tumor cells and release lymphokines that recruit
and activate macrophages[10]. If such a defect is common in the tumor-
bearing host, administration of agents that attempt to augment anti-
tumor responses by stimulating lymphokine production in situ may prove
of little value because of a preexisting functional lesion in "target"
lymphocytes. In contrast, agents that act directly on macrophages
would not be expected to encounter this problem. Furthermore, recent
findings showing that the tumoricidal phenotype in activated macrophages persists for only a few days[16,52] before macrophages become
refractory to "reactivation" by physiologic mediators such as
lymphokines[16], no agent should be considered as a therapeutic
candidate unless it is capable of overcoming this refractory state.
In this respect, it should be noted that phagocytic uptake of
lymphokines or MDP encapsulated in liposomes can successfully
activate previously activated macrophages that are unresponsive to
free lymphokines[16].

MDP offers significant advantages over lymphokines as a
potential modality for non-specific active immunotherapy of cancer
in man. Limitation in current technology for the isolation and
purification of lymphokines dicate that lymphokine preparations
are presently of variable composition and biological potency. In
contrast, MDP is a synthetic molecule of known composition, thus
permitting reliable dose-response relationships to be determined
for antitumor activity in a variety of experimental tumors. Finally,
the availability of a large range of structural analogs of MDP
offers opportunities for correlating antitumor activity with
molecular structure and detailed analysis of the biochemical
mechanisms by which these molecules elicit tumoricidal activity
in macrophages.

The optimal conditions for systemic therapy with liposome-
encapsulated immunomodulators, and the efficacy of this modality
alone, or in combination, in treating large metastatic tumor
burdens has still to be defined. Although the initial results
reported here are encouraging, it is considered unlikely that this
therapeutic approach could serve as the sole treatment for advanced
metastatic disease. Even if the activated macrophage proves to be
consistently effective in circumventing the problem of tumor cell
heterogeneity, macrophage-mediated destruction of large tumor
burdens may not be feasible. In many neoplastic lesions, the
number of macrophages is too low to destroy all tumor cells, even
under conditions of optimal macrophage activation and expression
of cytotoxic activity. It thus seems likely that the potential
application of liposome-encapsulated macrophage-activating agents
will not be in the destruction of massive tumor burdens but rather
in the destruction of micrometastases and residual tumor cell
burdens that remain after the elimination of the majority of tumor
cells by other means such as chemotherapy.

ACKNOWLEDGEMENTS

The personal research cited in this article was sponsored by the National Cancer Institute, DHHS, under contract No. N01-CO-75380 with Litton Bionetics Inc. (I.J.F.) and USPHS Grants CA18260 and CA30192 (G.P.). The contents of this publication do not necessarily reflect the views or policies of the Department of Health and Human Services, nor does mention of trade names, commercial products, or organizations imply endorsement by the U.S. Government.

REFERENCES

1. G. Poste and I.J. Fidler, The pathogenesis of cancer metastases, Nature, 283: 139 (1980).
2. I.J. Fidler and M.L. Kripke, Biological variability within murine neoplasms, Antibiot. Chemother. 28: 123 (1980).
3. I.J. Fidler, Recognition and destruction of target cells by tumoricidal macrophages, Isr. J. Med. Sci. 14: 177 (1978).
4. R.S. Kerbel, Implications of immunological heterogeneity of tumours, Nature 280: 358 (1979).
5. E. Den Otter, F.J. Dullens Hub, H. Van Lovern and E. Pels, Antitumor effects of macrophages injected into animals: a review, in: "The Macrophage and Cancer," K. James, B. McBride and A. Stuart, eds., Econoprint, Edinburgh, (1977).
6. I.J. Fidler, Inhibition of pulmonary metastasis by intravenous injection of specifically activated macrophages, Cancer Res. 34: 1074 (1977).
7. L.A. Liotta, C. Gattozzi, J. Kleinerman and G. Saidel, Reduction of tumor-cell entry into vessels by BCG-activated macrophages, Brit. J. Cancer 36: 639 (1977).
8. I.J. Fidler and G. Poste, Macrophage destruction of micro-metastases, in: "Manual of Macrophage Methodology," H.B. Herscowitz, H.J. Holden, J.A. Bellanti and A. Ghaffar, eds., Marcel Dekker, New York (1981).
9. I.J. Fidler, Z. Barnes, W.E. Fogler, R. Kirsh, P. Bugelski and G. Poste, Evidence for the involvement of macrophages in the eradication of established metastases following intravenous injection of liposomes containing macrophage activators, Cancer Res. - submitted.
10. S.W. Russell, G.Y. Gillespie and J.L. Pace, Evidence for mono-nuclear phagocytes in solid neoplasms and appraisal of the nonspecific cytotoxic capabilities, in: "In Situ Expression of Tumor Immunity," I. P. Witz and M.G. Hanna, eds., Plenum, New York (1980).
11. A.C. Allison, Mode of action of immunological adjuvants, J. Reticuloendothel. Soc. 26: 619 (1979).
12. I.J. Fidler and A. Raz, The induction of tumoricidal capacities in mouse and rat macrophages by lymphokines, in: "Lymphokines," E. Pick, ed., Vol. 3, Academic Press, New York, (1981).
13. B.W. Papermaster, O.A. Holterman, E. Klein, I. Djerassi,

D. Rosner, T. Dao and J.J. Costanzi, Preliminary observations
on tumor regressions induced by local administration of a
lymphoid-cell culture supernatant fraction in patients with
cutaneous metastatic lesions, Clin. Immunol. Immunopathol.
5: 31 (1976).

14. S.B. Slavin, J.S. Youngner, J. Nishio and R. Neta, Brief
communication: tumor suppression by a lymphokine released
into the circulation of mice with delayed hypersensitivity,
J. Nat. Cancer Inst. 55: 1233 (1975).

15. N.E. Adelman, M.G. Hammond, S. Cohen and H.F. Dvorak, Lymphokines as inflammatory mediators, in: "Biology of the Lymphokines," S. Cohen, E. Pick and J.J. Oppenheim, eds., Academic
Press, New York (1979).

16. G. Poste and R. Kirsh, Rapid decay of tumoricidal activity
and loss of responsiveness to lymphokines in inflammatory
macrophages, Cancer Res. 39: 2582 (1979).

17. L. Chedid, F. Audibert and A.G. Johnson, Biological activities
of muramyl dipeptide, a synthetic glycopeptide analogous to
bacterial immunoregulating agents, Progr. Allergy 25: 63 (1978).

18. G. Gregoriadis and A.C. Allison, eds., in: "Liposomes in Biology
and Medicine," Wiley Interscience, New York (1980).

19. T.D. Heath, R.T. Fraley and D. Papahadjopoulos, Antibody
targeting of liposomes - cell specificity obtained by conjugation of $F(AB)_2$ to vesicle surface, Science, 210:539 (1980).

20. L.D. Leserman, J.N. Weinstein, R. Blumenthal and W.D. Terry,
Receptor mediated endocytosis of antibody-opsonized liposomes
by tumor cells, Proc. Nat. Acad. Sci. USA, 77: 4089 (1980).

21. G. Gregoriadis and D. Neerunjun, Homing of liposomes to target
cells, Biochem. Biophys, Res. Commun. 65: 537 (1975).

22. G. Poste, R. Kirsh and I.J. Fidler, Cell surface receptors for
lymphokines. I. The possible role of glycolipids as receptors
for macrophage migration inhibitory factor (MIF) and macrophage
activation factor (MAF), Cell Immunol. 44: 71 (1979).

23. G. Poste, R. Kirsh, W.E. Fogler and I.J. Fidler, Activation
of tumoricidal properties in mouse macrophages by lymphokines
encapsulated in liposomes, Cancer Res. 39: 881 (1979).

24. I.J. Fidler, S. Sone, W.E. Fogler and Z. Barnes, Eradication
of spontaneous metastases and activation of alveolar macrophages by intravenous injection of liposomes containing muramyl
dipeptide, Proc. Nat. Acad. Sci. USA, 78: 1680 (1981).

25. I.J. Fidler, A. Raz, W.E. Fogler, R. Kirsh, P. Bugelski and
G. Poste, Design of liposomes to improve delivery of macrophage-
augmenting agents to alveolar macrophages, Cancer Res. 40: 4460
(1980).

26. I.J. Fidler, I.R. Hart, A. Raz, W.E. Fogler, R. Kirsh and
G. Poste, Activation of tumoricidal properties in macrophages
by liposome-encapsulated lymphokines: in vivo studies, in:
"Liposomes and Immunobiology," B.H. Tom and H. Six, eds.,
Elsevier, New York (1980).

27. S. Sone, G. Poste and I.J. Fidler, Rat alveolar macrophages

are susceptible to activation by free and liposome-encapsulated lymphokines, J. Immunol. 124: 2197 (1980).

28. G. Poste, C. Bucana, A. Raz, R. Kirsh, P. Bugelski and I.J. Fidler, The behaviour of intravenously inoculated liposomes in the microcirculation: implications for liposome targeting and drug delivery, Cancer Res. - submitted.

29. G.P. Velo and W.G. Spector, The origin and turnover of alveolar macrophages in experimental pneumonia, J. Pathol. 109: 7 (1973).

30. E.D. Thomas, R.E. Ramberg, G.E. Sale, R.S. Sparkes and D.W. Golde, Direct evidence for a bone marrow origin of the alveolar macrophage in man, Science, 192: 1016 (1976).

31. K.J. Johnson, P.A. Ward, G. Striker and R. Kunkel, A study of the origin of pulmonary macrophages using the Chediak-Higashi marker, Am. J. Pathol. 101: 365 (1980).

32. A. Blusse van Ould Alblas and R. Van Furth, Origin, kinetics and characteristics of pulmonary macrophages in the normal steady state, J. Exp. Med. 149: 1504 (1979).

33. I.R. Hart, Selection and characterization of an invasive variant of the B16 melanoma, Am. J. Pathol. 97: 587 (1979).

34. I.J. Fidler, Therapy of spontaneous metastases by intravenous injection of liposomes containing lymphokines, Science 208: 1469 (1980).

35. M. Parant, Biological properties of a new synthetic adjuvant, muramyl dipeptide (MDP), Semin. Immunopathol. 2: 101 (1979).

36. D.P. Griswold, Jr., Consideration of subcutaneously implanted B16 melanoma as a screening model for potential anticancer agents, Cancer Chemotherap. Rep. 3: 315 (1972).

37. M. Aalto, M. Potila and E. Kulonen, The effect of silica-treated macrophages on the synthesis of collagen and other proteins in vitro, Exp. Cell Res. 97: 193 (1976).

38. C.F. Brosnan, M.B. Bornstein and B.R. Bloom, The effects of macrophage depletion on the clinical and pathological expression of experimental allergic encephalomyelitis, J. Immunol. 126: 614 (1981).

39. P.J. Cantanzaro, H.J. Schwartz and R.C. Graham, Jr., Spectrum and possible mechanism of carrageenan cytotoxicity, Am. J. Pathol. 64: 387 (1971).

40. D.G. Hopper, M.V. Pimm and R.W. Baldwin, Silica abrogation of mycobacterial adjuvant contact suppression of tumor growth in rats and athymic mice, Cancer Immunol. Immunother. 1: 143 (1976).

41. R. Keller, Promotion of tumor growth in vivo by anti-macrophage agents, J. Nat. Cancer Inst. 57: 1355 (1976).

42. M.H. Levy and E.F. Wheelock, Effects of intravenous silica on immune and non-immune functions of the murine host, J. Immunol. 115: 41 (1975).

43. A.W. Thomson, N. Cruickshank and E.F. Fowler, Fc receptor-bearing and phagocytic cells in syngeneic tumors of coryne-bacterium-parvum treated and carrageenan treated mice, Brit. J. Cancer 39: 598 (1979).

44. S.D. Miller and A. Zarkower, Alterations of murine immuno-

logical responses after silica dust inhalation, J. Immunol. 113: 1533 (1974).

45. E. Lotzova, C. parvum-mediated suppression of the phenomenon of natural killing and its analysis, in: "Natural Cell-Mediated Immunity Against Tumors," R.B. Herberman, ed., Plenum, New York (1980).

46. G. Poste, unpublished observations.

47. I.J. Fidler, J. Immunol. - in press (1981).

48. S. Sone and I.J. Fidler, In vitro activation of tumoricidal properties in rat alveolar macrophages by synthetic muramyl dipeptide encapsulated in liposomes, Cell Immunol. 57: 42 (1981).

49. I.R. Hart, W.E. Fogler, G. Poste and I.J. Fidler, Toxicity studies of liposome-encapsulated immunomodulators administered intravenously to dogs and mice, Cancer Immunol Immunother. 10: 157 (1981).

50. S.A. Eccles, Macrophages and cancer, in: "Immunological Aspects of Cancer," J.E. Castro, ed., Univ. Park Press, Baltimore (1978).

51. M.J. Berendt and R.J. North, T-cell mediated suppression of anti-tumor immunity. An explanation for progressive growth of an immunogenic tumor, J. Exp. Med. 151: 69 (1980).

52. L.P. Ruco and M.S. Meltzer, Macrophage activation for tumor cytotoxicity: increased lymphokine responsiveness of peritoneal macrophages during acute inflammation, J. Immunol. 120: 1054 (1978).

LIPOSOMES AND THE RETICULOENDOTHELIAL SYSTEM: INTERACTIONS OF LIPOSOMES WITH MACROPHAGES AND BEHAVIOR OF LIPOSOMES IN VIVO

R.L. Juliano

The University of Texas Medical School at Houston
Department of Pharmacology, Houston, Texas 77025, USA

BASIC CHARACTERISTICS OF LIPOSOMES AS A DRUG DELIVERY SYSTEM

Liposomes represent an attractive approach to the problem of controlled drug delivery. Liposomes composed of natural body constituents are biodegradable, very weakly immunogenic and possess limited intrinsic toxicity. A great number of drugs and macromolecules can be readily encapsulated within liposomes of various types using relatively simple and efficient procedures. Incorporation of a drug within liposomes produces drastic but predictable changes in the pharmacodynamic behaviour of the substance. Current approaches to the exploitation of liposomal delivery systems have been reviewed elsewhere (Juliano, 1981, 1980; Ryman this volume, Mayhew this volume).

Liposomes can interact with cells in several distinct ways (review by Papahadjopoulos this volume). These include: a) endocytosis, of primary importance with professional phagocytes such as macrophages and neutrophils, b) adsorption to the cell surface which occurs with most types of cells and c) fusion which may occur to a limited degree with lymphocytes and certain tissue culture cells (Pagano and Weinstein, 1978). In this report we will describe some of the interactions of liposomes with macrophages in more detail, as well as studies of the behaviour of liposomes in vivo.

Upon injection of liposomes they are gradually cleared from the circulation and sequestered in the tissues where they may persist for long periods of times (hours to days depending on composition). The t 1/2 clearance of liposomes from the blood, which may range from minutes to hours, and the distribution of liposomes to the organs, can be controlled, in part, by altering the physical properties of the liposomes such as their size, fluidity and surface charge (Juliano and Stamp, 1975). Larger liposomes such as MLVs and REVs are avidly taken up by the phagocytic cells of the reticuloendothelial system. This plus the fact that large vesicles can only escape from the circulation where the walls of the capillaries are fenestrated, leads to a tissue distribution where organs such as liver and spleen are predominant sites of liposome uptake. Small vesicles (SUVs) seem to have a broader tissue distribution, but as we shall see are also taken up at the same sites as are the larger vesicles.

The propensity of liposomes to accumulate in reticuloendothelial cells can be an advantage in some instances. For example Alving et al. (this volume) have used liposome encapsulated antimonial drugs to treat leishmaniasis, a parasitic infection which affects macrophages. The liposomal drug accumulates preferentially in the cell which is the site of parasite infestation and thus the therapeutic index is enhanced. In a similar vein Poste, Fidler and their colleagues (this volume) have used liposome encapsulated immunomodulators to stimulate macrophages to tumoricidal capacity.

In most cases, however, accumulation of liposomal drug in the reticuloendothelial cells of liver and spleen represents an undesirable sink for the drug, diverting it from possible action at other sites. For example, one would like liposomes bearing anti-cancer drugs to persist in the circulation as a sort of sustained release system, or to interact with tumorous cells and tissues. With this goal in mind we have explored the possibility of delaying, minimizing or avoiding uptake of liposomes by the reticuloendothelial cells of liver and spleen.

LIPOSOME UPTAKE BY RETICULOENDOTHELIAL CELLS

In-Vitro Studies

The mononuclear cells of the reticuloendothelial (RE) system including monocytes, Küpffer cells, macrophages from spleen, lungs, lymph nodes, and peritoneal cavity, are all actively phagocytic with the capacity to accumulate various types of foreign particles including liposomes. We have used thioglycollate-elicited mouse peritoneal macrophages (MPMs) to study liposome interactions with reticuloendothelial cells; although the peritoneal cells are clearly not a perfect model for events which may occur in vivo, where other macrophage types are predominantly involved, they have the advantage of being readily available and susceptible to study in a tissue culture format.

Liposome uptake by MPMs appears to be via a "classic" phagocytic process. For example, as seen in Table 1, uptake is fully inhibited by the microfilament blocking agent cytochalasin B as well as by iodoacetate, which blocks glycolysis; by contrast sodium azide, which impedes oxidative phosphorylation, has little effect. This is consistent with previously observed results on particle phagocytosis by macrophages (Silverstein et al., 1977). MPMs can take up charged vesicles (either positive or negative) somewhat more avidly than neutral vesicles (Table 2); in particular, negatively charged vesicles seem to provide a strong stimulus to phagocytosis and are readily taken up at 37°C, while positive vesicles bind more strongly at 4°C. MPMs in vitro do not seem able to discriminate between SUVs and MLVs (Fig. 1); this latter is in contrast to the behaviour of liposomes in vivo where MLVs are cleared by the RE system much more rapidly than SUVs (see below).

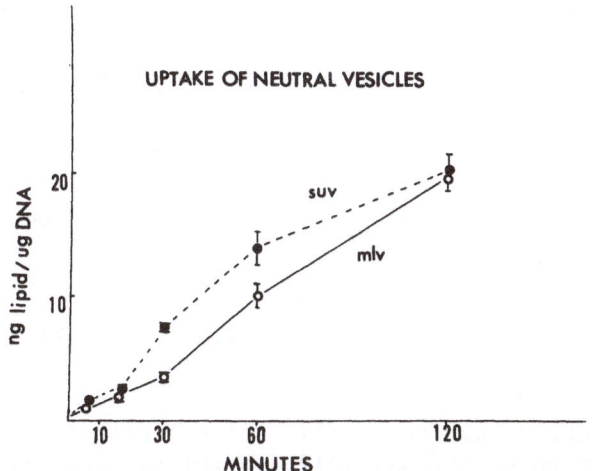

Fig. 1.   Small (SUVs) or large (MLVs) liposomes composed of DPPC/ cholesterol 1/1 molar ratio plus ^{3}H DPPC were incubated with MPMs in MEM + 1 mg/ml bovine albumin. Uptake as a function of time is given in terms of ng lipid per μg macrophage DNA. Results are the means and standard errors of quadruplicate determinations.

Table 1. Effect of Inhibitors on Liposome Uptake by Macrophages[*]

Treatment	Uptake (ng lipid/μg cell protein)
Control	6.6
Sodium azide 1 mM	5.8
Iodoacetate 5 mM	0.1
Iodoacetate + azide	0.1
Cytochalasin B 10 μg/ml	0.7
Cytochalasin B 20 μg/ml	0.6

*REV composed of DPPC and cholesterol (2/1 molar ratio) and labelled with ^{14}C-cholesteryl oleate were incubated in MEM + 1 mg/ml bovine albumin with thioglycollate elicted mouse peritoneal macrophages in 35 cm tissue culture dishes for 90 min at 37°C and 5% CO_2. The macrophage monolayers were rinsed, removed by scraping and washed 4 x in phosphate buffered saline. Aliquots of the cell pellet were assayed for protein or for radioactivity. Results are the means of triplicate determinations.

Table 2. Macrophage Uptake of Liposomes of Different Charge[*]

	Uptake (% of control)	
	4°C	37°C
Neutral REVs	15	100
Negative REVs	65	345
Positive REVs	131	215

*REV composed of DPPC/cholesterol (1/1 molar ratio) (neutral) or DPPC/ cholesterol/stearylamine (9/10/1 molar ratio) (positive), or DPPC/ cholesterol/phosphatidyl serine (9/10/1 molar ratio) (negative) and labelled with ^{14}C-cholesteryl oleate, were incubated with MPMs for 90 min at 4°C or 37°C in MEM + 1 mg/ml BSA. The amount of liposomal radioactivity taken up is expressed as % control where the 100% value is for neutral REVs at 37°C. Results are the means of tripli- cate determinations.

The uptake of liposomes by MPMs is greatly enhanced if the surface of the liposome is manipulated such that it can interact with one of the macrophage receptor systems. For example, as seen in Table 3, vesicles containing a DNP-lipid and reacted with anti-DNP antibodies can be taken up to almost a hundred fold greater degree than control vesicles; this uptake presumably takes place via the Fc receptor system of the MPMs. Table 3 also reveals that actual formulation of a liposome bound antigenantibody complex is superior to simply coating antigen free vesicles with IgG in terms of promoting uptake. Liposome uptake can also be promoted by coating the vesicles with ligands which interact with other macrophage receptor systems; for example fibronectin (Saba et al., 1978), an opsonic protein which interacts with macrophages, induces a five fold increase in vesicle uptake (Table 4). Thus simple lipid vesicles are readily taken up by macrophages in vitro via a phagocytic process. However the rate and extent of this process can be enhanced by coating the vesicles with ligands capable of interacting with macrophage surface receptors.

Table 3. Effect of IgG on Liposome Uptake by Macrophages*

Treatment	Uptake (ng lipid/μg cell protein)	
	DNP-REV	REV
Anti DNP 1/5 dil.	598.0	-
Anti DNP 1/25	243.06	45.0
Anti DNP 1/125	24.0	-
Anti DNP 1/625	16.0	16.0
Control	7.6	

*REVs were prepared with DPPC and cholesterol (2/1) either with or without the addition of 10 mol% DNP-PE (Avanti Polar Lipids) and labelled with ^{14}C-cholesteryl oleate. The vesicles were incubated with various dilutions of rabbit anti-DNP IgG (Miles for 15 min at room temperature. The REVs were then washed with MEM = bovine albumin and added to monolayers of thioglycollate elicited mouse peritoneal macrophages in 35 cm tissue culture dishes and incubated for 90 min at 37°C and 5% CO_2. The samples were processed as in Table 1. Results are the means of triplicate determinations. The antibody mediated uptake process was more than 90% inhibitable by 5 mM iodoacetate.

    Despite the fact that isolated serum components such as IgG and
fibronectin can act as opsonins and effectively promote the uptake
of liposomes by MPMs, the result of coating liposomes with whole
homologous serum is to reduce vesicle uptake. This is illustrated
in Table 5; and suggests that serum may contain anti opsonic proteins
as well as opsonins such as fibronectin and IgG. Since different
types of liposomes are known to bind different serum proteins
(Juliano and Lin, 1980), the balance between opsonic and anti-opsonic
effects may depend on the chemical and physical properties (charge,
fluidity, polar head group) of the liposome, thus possibly explaining
observed differences in the circulating lifetimes of liposomes with
similar sizes but different chemical characteristics.

In-vivo studies

    Investigators studying the behaviour of the RE system have long
known that large doses of colloidal particles are cleared more slowly
than small doses (Saba, 1970). In addition, injection of a dose of
one type of colloid can often slow the clearance of other types of
particles. This sort of behavious represents manifestations of RE
system "blockade", where the rate of clearance of a test particle is
slowed by the presence or pre-loading of a "blocking" dose of other
particles. Blockade can be due to either depletion of circulating
opsonins or to saturation of RE cell uptake capacities (Saba, 1970).

    Until recently it was not altogether clear whether liposomes
would be subject to the same types of RE system clearance phenomena
as prevail with other types of injected particles. We have now elucidated that the clearance of liposomes is subject to blockade by prior
injection of similar or by dissimilar particles, that the blockaded
state seems to be due to saturation of RE cell uptake capacity rather
than to opsonic depletion and that RE blockade can lead to an alteration of the pattern of tissue distribution of injected liposomes
(Kao and Juliano, 1981).

    As seen in Figure 2, the clearance rate of radiolabelled large
liposomes (REVs) can be markedly slowed by preloading with a dose of
"cold" liposomes of the same type. Thus the t 1/2 of clearance in
the control case was 30 min, while the t 1/2 in the case of a 63 mg
pre-load was 250 min. Similar "blockade" of REV clearance can also
be induced by preloading with unrelated particles such as latex beads
or xenogenic erythrocytes or by injecting substances such as dextran
sulfate, which are known to impair RE cell function (data not shown).
It has long been known(Juliano and Stamp, 1975) that small liposomes
(SUVs) are cleared far more slowly than large liposomes (REVs, MLVs).
However, it has been unclear whether or not SUVs accumulate in the
same RE system compartment as REVs, though at a slower rate, or
whether SUVs somehow largely escape clearance by the RE system and
accumulate at other sites in the body. We have recently shown that
preloading animals with a dose of "cold" SUVs can markedly block the

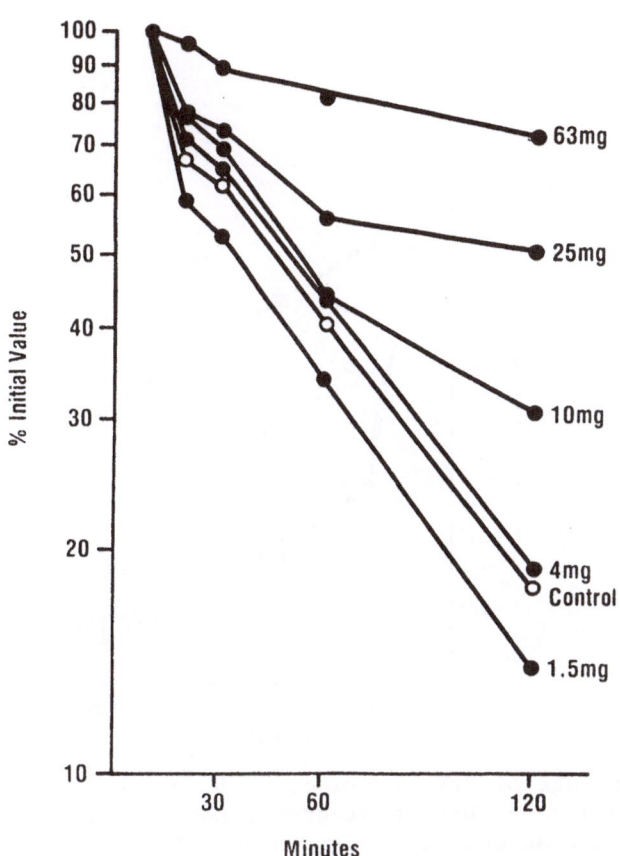

Fig. 2.   Blockade of REV clearance by REVs. Anaesthetized rats
          received a loading dose of "cold" REVs (DPPC/cholesterol-
          1/1 molar ratio) and one hour later a test dose (4 mg) of
          similar REVs labelled with ^{14}C-cholesteryl oleate. Data
          indicate the mean value for three animals. Ordinate, % ^{14}C
          remaining in circulation. Abscissa, time in minutes.

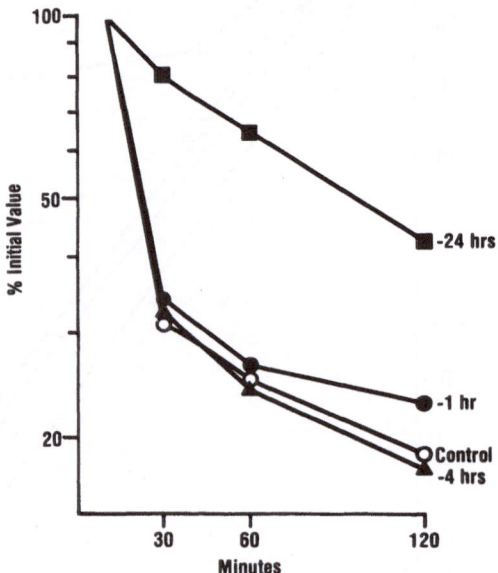

Fig. 3. Blockage of REV clearance by SUVs. Rats received a load-
         ing dose of DPPC/cholesterol SUVs at 1, 4 or 24 hr prior
         to a test dose of ^{14}C-labelled REVs. Ordinate and
         abscissa as in Figure 2.

clearance of REVs; however, the effect is delayed (24 hours) until a substantial amount of the slowly cleared SUVs can accumulate in the RE cell compartment (Figure 3). This indicates that both SUVs and REVs are taken up by the RE phagocytic system and that they can mutually interfere with each other's clearance (the experiment of using REVs to interfere with the clearance of SUVs is not practical because of the long t 1/2 of clearance of the SUV particles).

We have also investigated the question of whether the blockade of liposome clearance is due to depletion of circulating opsonins or to saturation of the uptake capacity of the mononuclear phagocytes of the RE system. In the experiment illustrated in Figure 4, the lack of involvement of opsonic factors in blockade was clearly demonstrated. Thus if the blockaded state were due to depletion of circulating factor, then preincubation of the radioactive test dose of liposomes with serum from "naive" animals should overcome the blockade caused by a loading dose of "cold" liposomes. This was clearly not the case, thus indicating that the blockade caused by preloading with liposomes is due to saturation of RE cell uptake capacities rather than to depletion of opsonic factors in the serum; this is in contrast to the situation prevailing in the clearance of gelatinized colloids where opsonin depletion is an important factor (Saba, 1978). Our results do not imply that opsonins are not involved in liposome clearance, but merely that depletion of opsonins is not involved in blockade.

RE blockade can also cause alterations in the tissue distribution pattern of injected liposomes. For example, as seen in Table 6, pre-injection of a blockading dose of latex beads results in enhanced accumulation of a test dose of liposomes in the lungs. Thus our studies suggest that both the lifetime of vesicles in the circulation, and their distribution to different tissues can be modulated _via_ blockade of the phagocytic cells of the RE system.

AVOIDANCE OF THE RE SINK VIA ALTERNATE ROUTES OF ADMINISTRATION

Another means of minimizing unwanted RE uptake of colloidal drug carrier is to avoid the intravenous route altogether. With this in mind we have explored the concept of obtaining localized or organ selective drug actions by directly depositing drug bearing liposomes at a particular site within the body. In these studies we have been mostly concerned with anti-neoplastic drugs. For example, as a possible therapy for metastatic disease of the lung, we have administered liposomes containing the anti-tumor drug cytosine arabinoside directly into the respiratory system of the rat. Using this experimental model, we have studied the pharmacokinetic and pharmacologic properties of drug given by this route, either as a bolus injection or as an aerosal spray.

Early studies (McCullough and Juliano, 1979) indicated that

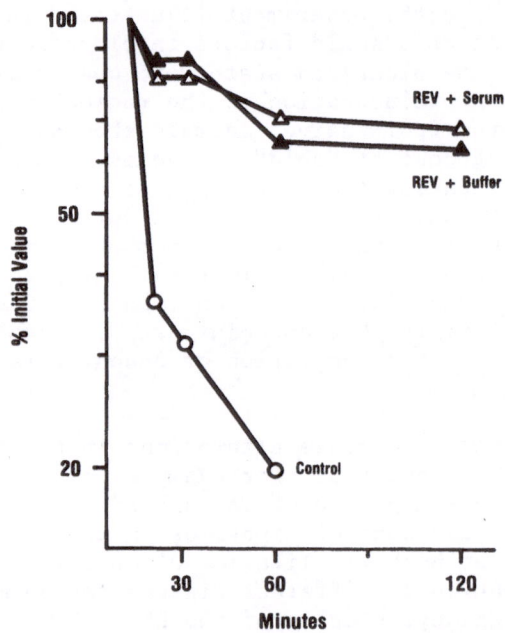

Fig. 4. Role of Opsonins in Blockade. Rats received either a
loading dose of "cold" REVs or buffered saline (controls).
One hour later the animals received a test dose of ^{14}C-
REVs preincubated either in saline or in normal rat serum.
As shown, preincubation with serum failed to reverse the
blockaded state. Ordinate and abscissa as in Figure 2.

Table 4. Effect of Fibronectin on Liposome Uptake by Macrophages*

Treatment	Uptake (ng lipid/μg cell protein)	
(μg/ml fibronectin)	− heparin	+ heparin
0	6.6	8.5
100	10.4	20.0
500	22.6	47.2

*REVs composed of DPPC/cholesterol/stearylamine (9/10/1 molar ratio) plus ^{14}C-cholesteryl oleate were incubated with affinity purified fibronectin (Harper and Juliano, 1980) for 1 hr at room temperature. The REVs were then added to monolayers of MPMs in   MEM + 1 mg/ml BSA and incubated a further 90 min at 37°C; in some cases 100 units of heparin was incubated in the incubation. Results are the means of triplicate determinations. NOTE: Fibronectin, with heparin as a co-factor, is known to mediate the clearance of certain colloids by the RE system (Saba et al., 1978).

Table 5. Effect of Homologous Serum on Liposome Uptake by Macrophages*

Treatment	Uptake (ng lipid/μg cell protein)	
	REV−DPPC/chol	REV−DPPC/chol/PS
α− MEM	10.1	11.3
α− MEM + 0.1% mouse serum	11.0	10.0
α− MEM + 1% mouse serum	7.9	6.3
α− MEM + 10% mouse serum	1.8	4.0

*Neutral (DPPC/cholesterol−1/1 molar ratio) or negative (DPPC/ cholesterol/phosphatidylserine−9/10/1 molar ratio) REVs labelled with ^{14}C-cholesteryl oleate were allowed to interact with MPMs for 90 min in the indicated media. Uptake measurements are the means of triplicate determinations.

liposomes deposited as a liquid bolus in the trachea could become
widely distributed throughout the smaller airways of the lung. We
also examined the clearance from the lung of free or liposome encapsulated cytosine arabinoside. As seen in Figure 5a, free drug was
cleared from the lung rapidly, as would be expected since the lung
mucosa are very permeable to a variety of small molecules; by contrast
liposomal drug remained within the lung for a greatly extended period
of time. This alteration in pharmacokinetics as reflected in blood
and urine levels which rose rapidly in the case of free drug but considerably more slowly in the case of encapsulated drug (Juliano and
McCullough, 1980).

The pharmacologic impact of this change in drug localization and
kinetics was examined by measuring DNA synthesis in the target organ
(the lung) and in remote organs subsequent to administration of cytosine arabinoside via the respiratory system (cytosine arabinoside is
a DNA synthesis inhibitor) (Juliano and McCullough, 1980). As seen
in Figure 5b both free and liposomal cytosine arabinoside effectively
inhibited DNA synthesis in the lung; by contrast free cytosine arabinoside also effectively inhibited DNA synthesis in remote tissues
such as intestine and bone marrow, but liposomal cytosine arabinoside
was much less effective in this regard. Thus administration of the
drug in liposomal form resulted in equal potency to free form in the
target organ (the lung) but reduced toxicity in non-target organs
where adverse side effects might occur. In this manner we have demonstrated a localized, organ-selective action of an anti-tumor drug.
Similar tissue specific actions of anti-tumor drugs have been attained
by Weinstein and his colleagues using quite different approaches
(see Weinstein, this volume).

Table 6. % Recovery of Injected ^{14}C-Cholesteryl oleate*

	Blockaded	Control
Lung	7.4 ± 0.6	0.4 ± 0.1
Heart	0.1 ± 0.1	0.2 ± 0.05
Liver	48.3 ± 4.5	41.9 ± 8.2
Spleen	8.1 ± 3.2	14.9 ± 3.7
Kidney	0.3 ± 0.1	0.2 ± 0.05

*A latex bead suspension (blockaded) or saline (controls) was injected
as in Figure 2. One hour later, the animals received approximately 4mg
of DPPC/Chol REV containing ^{14}C-cholesteryl oleate. Blood samples were
obtained at intervals, and at 2 hours postinjection the animals were
killed and the ^{14}C content of their tissues analyzed as described in
Methods. Results represent the means and standard errors for three animals.

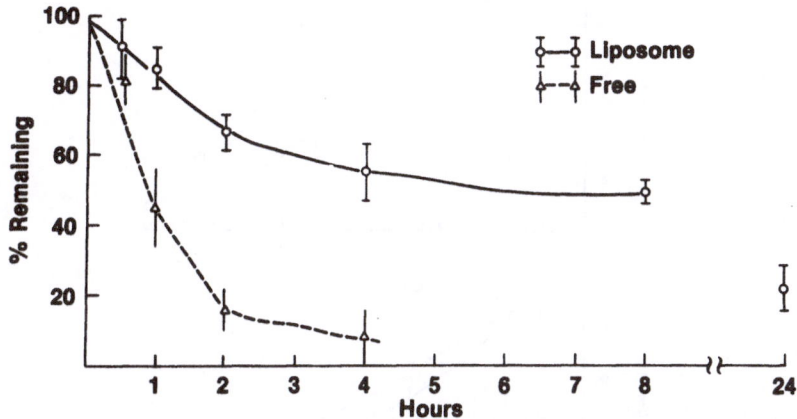

Fig. 5a.   Clearance of Ara C from the lung. Anaesthetized rats
received either free or liposomal ^{3}H-cytosine arabinoside
via tracheal instillation. Ordinate, % initial dpm
remaining in the lung. Abscissa, time in hours.
--- dotted line, free drug; ── solid line, liposomal drug.

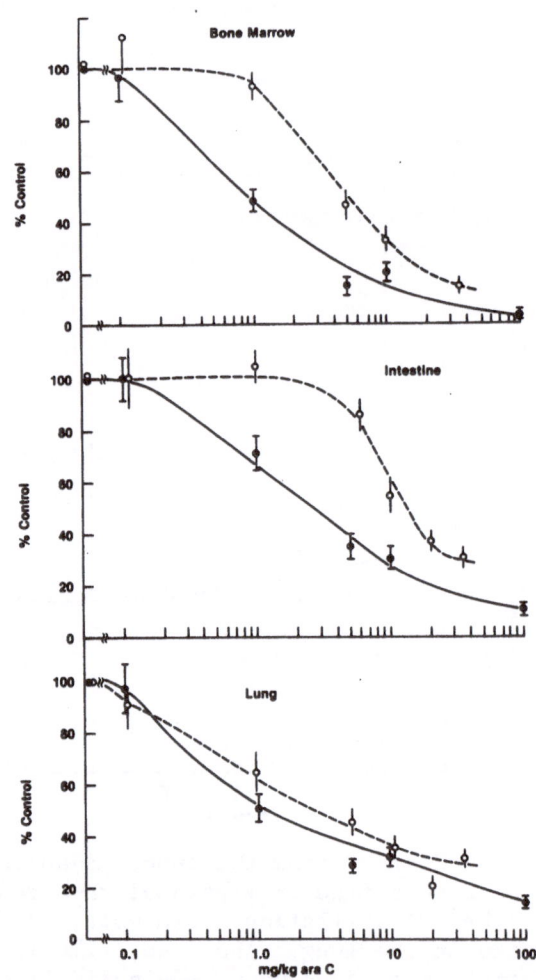

Fig. 5b. Pharmacologic effects of free or encapsulated Ara C.
Anaesthetized rats were given free or liposomal cytosine
arabinoside at various doses. One hour later the animals
received ^{14}C-thymidine and incorporation of this material
into nucleic acid was measured during a 15 minute period.
Ordinate, % of control (untreated animals). Abscissa,
dose of cytosine arabinoside (for details see Juliano and
McCullough, 1980).

dotted line, liposomal drug
solid line, free drug

SUMMARY

It is my belief that successful utilization of liposomes as a drug carrier will depend on developing means for modulating the interaction of liposomes with the phagocytic cells of the RE system. Hopefully that data presented above suggests that such modulation is possible at least to a limited degree. If there truly are antiopsonic proteins in blood, the identification and purification of these components might solve the problem of unwanted uptake of lipid vesicles by RE cells and thus add a new dimension to the utilization of the liposomal drug delivery system.

ABBREVIATIONS

SUVs — small unilamellar vesicles (20-50 nm)
MLVs — large multilamellar vesicles ($>1\mu$)
REVs — large unilamellar vesicles (0.5 - 1.0μ)
RE system — reticuloendothelial system
Ara C — cytosine arabinoside
DPPC — dipalmitoyl phosphatidylcholine
MPM — mouse peritoneal macrohpage.

ACKNOWLEDGEMENTS

The author wishes to thank Dr. Y.J. Kao, Ms. M.J. Hsu and Ms. Sandie Carter. This work was supported by a grant from the National Cancer Institute.

REFERENCES

Juliano, R.L., 1980,"Drug Delivery Systems: Characteristics and Biomedical Applications," Oxford Press, New York.
Juliano, R.L., 1981, Liposomes as a drug delivery system, Trends in Pharmacological Sciences, 2: 39.
Juliano, R.L. and Lin, G., 1980, The interaction of plasma proteins with liposomes in: "Liposomes and Immunobiology", B. Tom and H. Six, eds., Elsevier, North Holland, New York.
Juliano, R.L. and McCullough, H.N., 1980, Controlled delivery of an anti-tumor drug: localized action of liposome encapsulated cytosine arabinoside administered via the respiratory system, J. Pharmacol. Exp. Ther., 214: 381.
Juliano, R.L. and Stamp, D., 1975, Effects of particle size and charge on the clearance of liposomes and liposome encapsulated drugs, Biochem. Biophys. Res. Commun., 63: 651.
Kao, Y.J. and Juliano, R.L., 1981, Interactions of liposomes with the RE system, I. Effects of RE blockade on the clearance and tissue distribution of large unilamellar vesicles, Biochim. Biophys. Acta, in press.
McCullough, H.N. and Juliano, R.L., 1979, Organ selective action of an anti-tumor drug: pharmacologic studies of liposome encapsu-

lated β-cytosine arabinoside administered via the respiratory
system of rats, J. Natl. Cancer Inst., 63: 727.

Pagano, R.E. and Weinstein, J., 1978, Interactions of phospholipid
vesicles with mammalian cells, Ann. Rev. Biophys. Bioeng.,
7: 435.

Saba, T.M., 1970, Physiology and pathophysiology of the reticuloendothelial system, Arch. Int. Med., 126: 1031.

Saba, T.M., Blumenstock, F.A., Weber, P. and Kaplan, J.E., 1978,
α-opsonic glycoprotein, N.Y. Acad. Sci., 312: 43.

Silverstein, S.C., Steinman, R.M. and Cohn, Z.A., 1977, Endocytosis,
Ann. Rev. Biochem., 46: 669.

IMMUNOADJUVANT PROPERTIES OF LIPOSOMES

N. van Rooijen and Ria van Nieuwmegen

Medical Faculty
Free University
Postbox 7161
1007 MC Amsterdam
The Netherlands

INTRODUCTION TO LIPOSOMES

Liposomes are artificially prepared spheres of concentric phospholipid bilayers separated by aqueous compartments. They form when water insoluble phospholipids are confronted with water. The phospholipid molecules try to reach a conformation in which their hydrophobic fatty acid groups are not in direct contact with water. The formation of phospholipid bilayers in which the relatively hydrophylic head groups are localized on both outer parts of the bilayers, whereas the hydrophobic fatty acid groups are localized directly opposite to each other in the inner part of the bilayer is a logical consequence.

Liposomes may differ with respect to their dimensions, composition (different phospholipids), charge (neutral, positive or negative liposomes) and structure (multilamellar and unilamellar liposomes). Liposome-entrapped or associated compounds may be targeted to different sites in or on living cells (see recent reviews e.g. by Gregoriadis, 1980a,b,c,d; Ryman and Tyrrell, 1979, 1980). The continuously growing application of liposomes in biomedical research can be demonstrated by comparing the permuterm subject index of the Science Citation Index over the past 5 years. The occupance of liposomes in this item increased each year with about one column from 2.5 columns in 1975 to ample 6.5 columns in 1979. Immunology is one of the research areas, into which liposomes have penetrated thoroughly (Tom, 1980). Immune reactions against liposomes and associated antigens form part of the immunological applications of liposomes.

IMMUNE REACTIONS AGAINST LIPOSOMES AND ASSOCIATED ANTIGENS

When studying immune reactions against liposomes and associated antigens, it is important to consider the possible antigens against which antibodies may be elicited. Antibodies may be produced against the phospholipids, of which the liposomes have been composed (Alving, 1977; Banerji and Alving, 1981). In rabbits naturally occurring antibodies to sphingomyelin containing liposomes have been described (Strejan et al., 1979). Furthermore antibodies may be

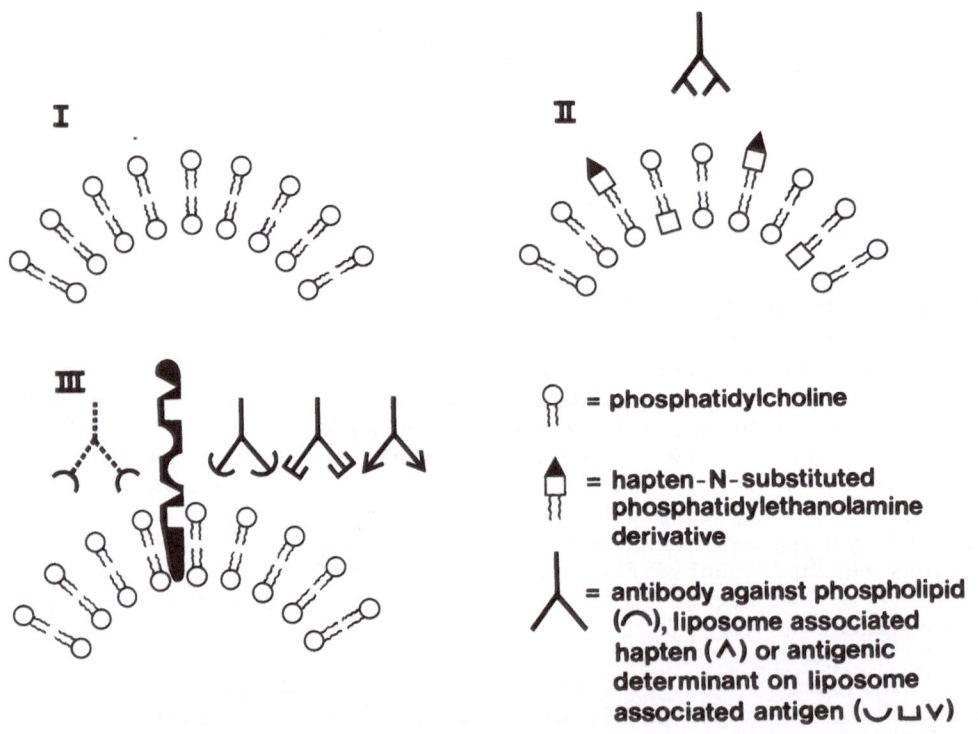

Fig. 1. Different immune reactions against liposomes and associated haptens or antigens.
I   Phosphatidylcholine liposomes without antigens do not elicit antibody production.
II   Liposomes with haptens incorporated in their bilayers may elicit anti-hapten antibody production.
III Liposomes with an antigen exposed on their surfaces may elicit the production of antibodies directed against various antigenic determinants. When lipid A is associated with liposomes, apart from antibodies against lipid A, antibodies may be elicited against the liposomal phospholipids.

formed against haptens which are fixed to liposomal membranes by incorporation of hapten -(N)- substituted phosphatidylethanolamine derivatives (Kinsky, 1980). Finally antibodies may be produced against antigen molecules (e.g. proteins) with various antigenic determinants (fig. 1), which are either coated on the liposomes in a nonspecific way (van Rooijen and van Nieuwmegen, 1980a,b), by covalent binding to one of the phospholipids, or by means of an artificially inserted receptor (Alving et al., 1980a,b).

Antibodies elicited against the liposomal phospholipids themselves may be a disadvantage, when antibody production against liposome associated haptens or antigens is intended. For the latter application of liposomes, it is advantageous that phospholipids generally are poor immunogens, especially those which are commonly used for preparation of liposomes in their role of immunoadjuvants. For instance, antibodies against phosphatidylcholine incorporated in liposomes, could only be detected after association of the immunoadjuvant lipid-A with the same bilayers (Schuster et al., 1979).

It is the purpose of the present paper to review the immunoadjuvant properties of liposomes with respect to associated antigens. This application of liposomes has been described for the first time by Allison and Gregoriadis (1974). Immune responses against haptens in which liposomes are substituted for the usual protein carriers are beyond the scope of this review. A comparison between the immune responses against hapten conjugated liposomes and antigen associated liposomes will be made only when important differences between both immune responses have been reported.

LIPOSOME ENTRAPPED ANTIGEN AND ANTIGEN
EXPOSED ON THE OUTER SURFACES OF LIPOSOMES

Two arguments have been given in earlier studies for a role of liposome entrapped antigen in generating an immune response. In immune animals, interaction of an antigen with its specific antibodies appeared to be prevented when the antigen was administered, entrapped in liposomes (Gregoriadis and Allison, 1974; Fishman and Citri, 1975). This could be caused only by the masking of antigenic determinants after entrapment. Zborowski et al. (1977) found an association between albumin and phosphatidylcholine when liposomal membranes came into contact with serum albumin. This association resulted in free albumin-phosphatidylcholine complexes but no measurable binding of albumin to the liposomes. Obviously the phosphatidylcholine molecules were removed from the liposomal bilayers, as soon as they had been associated with the albumin molecules. The adjuvant effect of the liposomes could not be attributed to such albumin-phosphatidylcholine complexes (van Rooijen and van Nieuwmegen, 1978a). That liposomes containing serum albumins did nevertheless elicit a stronger immune response than similar proteins injected free in solution (Heath et al., 1976; van Rooijen and van Nieuwmegen, 1977),

TABLE 1

Anti-BGG Titers and Anti-HSA Titers of Rabbits at Different Time Intervals after Administration of Liposome Associated BGG or HSA

Group	Amount of BGG administered (mg)	Anti-BGG titers at day:								
		0	5	6	7	8	11	14	18	21
A	4.0	0 (7)	0 (7)	0 (7)	0 (6)	4 (1/6)	4.0 ± 1.2 (4/6)	5.0 ± 2.1 (6)	5.0 ± 1.2 (5/6)	4.5 ± 2.1 (2/6)
B	0.5	0 (8)	5.6 ± 2.6 (8)	7.4 ± 2.0 (8)	8.5 ± 2.0 (8)	10.1 ± 2.2 (8)	8.6 ± 2.0 (8)	10.0 ± 1.4 (8)	11.8 ± 1.6 (8)	11.4 ± 2.3 (8)
C	2.5	0 (8)	5.5 ± 2.5 (8)	6.6 ± 2.1 (8)	7.8 ± 1.7 (8)	8.8 ± 1.8 (8)	6.9 ± 1.8 (8)	7.5 ± 1.4 (8)	9.3 ± 2.0 (8)	7.9 ± 2.2 (8)

Group	Amount of HSA administered (mg)	Anti-HSA titers at day:								
		0	5	6	7	8	11	14	18	21
A	1.0	0 (8)	0 (8)	0 (8)	0 (7)	0 (6)	0 (6)	5 (1/6)	7.7 ± 2.5 (3/6)	6.0 (3/6)
B	0.02	0 (8)	7.0 ± 2.4 (8)	10.1 ± 1.8 (8)	9.6 ± 2.1 (8)	9.3 ± 1.2 (8)	9.3 ± 2.4 (8)	8.6 ± 1.7 (8)	11.3 ± 1.0 (8)	10.6 ± 1.8 (7)
C	1.0	0 (8)	5.0 ± 1.5 (8)	5.0 ± 2.2 (8)	6.8 ± 2.3 (8)	6.3 ± 2.6 (8)	8.0 ± 3.4 (6)	9.0 ± 3.0 (6)	11.3 ± 3.4 (6)	10.8 ± 2.9 (6)

was consequently considered to support the hypothesis that liposome entrapped antigen was responsible for the immune response.

The adjuvant activity of liposomes in the immune response to gamma globulins (van Rooijen and van Nieuwmegen, 1978a) could be due, at least partly, to binding of the gamma globulins to the surfaces of liposomes (Weissmann et al., 1974; Gregoriadis and Neerunjun, 1975: Schieren et al., 1978: Huang and Kennel, 1979). Binding of immunoglobulins to liposomes is probably mediated by their Fc portions (Weissmann et al., 1974). Recently, it has been demonstrated that a very small proportion of serum albumin may also bind to liposomes, especially to the larger ones (Hoekstra and Scherphof, 1979). For that reason we have done some experiments to investigate whether either exposition of the antigens on the surfaces of liposomes, or entrapment of the antigens in their aqueous compartments, or both combinations of antigen and liposomes are responsible for the adjuvant activity of liposomes in the immune response to associated antigens (see van Rooijen and van Nieuwmegen, 1980a and table 1).

The best approach would have been to compare immune responses against 1. antigen, free in solution, 2. antigen entrapped in liposomes only, 3. antigen exposed on the surfaces of liposomes only and 4. antigen both exposed on and entrapped in liposomes. However it seems to us very difficult to produce liposomes with entrapped antigen only; there is no way to be absolutely sure that none of the antigen is exposed on the surfaces of liposomes during their preparation in the presence of antigen. Extremely small amounts of liposome exposed antigen may elicit an immune response and it may well be that this surface exposed antigen cannot be detected with the methods applied for this purpose. Moreover since e.g. albumins (Zborowski et al., 1977) and probably also other proteins may influence the liposomal membranes, it cannot be excluded that a small part of the antigen, initially entrapped, is transformed to surface exposed antigen during the experiment. For those reasons we compared the immune responses against the antigens human serum

---

TABLE 1.   Blood samples for antibody determination were obtained from the rabbits by cardiac puncture. Titers are given as $\log_2$. Way of administration: rabbits of group A received antigen free in solution; rabbits of group B received empty liposomes coated with antigen; rabbits of group C received antigen entrapped in liposomes which had also been coated with antigen after formation. For antigen coating of the empty or antigen-containing liposomes, these were brought in the same strong antigen solution which has been applied for preparation of the antigen-containing liposomes, i.e. 25 mg of antigen per ml PBS buffer. Further experimental details are given elsewhere (van Rooijen and van Nieuwmegen, 1980a).

TABLE 2

Influence of Liposome and Antigen Concentration on the Immunoadjuvant Effect of Liposomes

Exp.	Group	day: 0	4	5	6	7	8	11	14	18	21	27	Peak titers
I	100%	-----	--+++	+++++	+++++	+++++	+++++	+++++	++++	++++	++++	++++	17.2 ± 1.5
	10%	-----	-----	+++++	+++++	+++++	+++++	+++++	+++++	+++++	+++++	+++++	16.8 ± 1.5
	1%	-----	-----	-----	-+++	-+++	-+++	-++++	-++++	-++++	-++++	-+++	15.8 ± 0.5
	0.1%	----	----	----	----	----	----	----	----	----	----	----	---
	0.01%	----	----	----	----	----	----	----	----		----	----	---
II	100%	-----	---+	+++++	+++++	+++++	+++++	+++++	+++++	+++++	+++++	+++++	15.4 ± 4.2
	10%	----	----	----	-++	-+++	-+++	++++	++++		++++	++++	11.5 ± 4.0
	1%	-----	----	----	----	--+	--+	-++	-++	-+++	-+++	-+++	7.7 ± 4.0
	0.1%	----	----	----	----	----	----	----	----		----	----	---
	0.01%	----	----	----	----	----	----	----	----		----	----	---
III	100%	----	--++	++++	++++	++++		+++	+++	+++	+++	+++	14.5 ± 1.0
	10%	----	----	++++	++++	++++	++++	++++	++++	++++	++++	+++	10.8 ± 1.7
	1%	----	----	----	----	----	+++	---+	++++	++++	++++	++++	8.3 ± 4.7
	0.1%	----	----	----	----	----	----	----	----	----	----	----	---
	0.01%	---	----	----	----	----	----	----	----	----	----	----	---

Positive titers (+) and negative titers (-) are given for all rabbits at different time intervals after administration of HSA-liposomes. Log_2 peak titers of the responding rabbits are given as the mean ± S.D.

albumin (HSA) and bovine gamma globulin (BGG) in only 3 groups of
rabbits. The antigens were injected free in solution (group A)
exposed on the surfaces of empty liposomes (group B) or both exposed
on and entrapped in liposomes (group C). Further experimental
details have been given earlier (see van Rooijen and van Nieuwmegen,
1980a). The results (see table 1) show a marked adjuvant effect of
liposomes in the immune responses against both HSA and BGG. No
marked difference can be observed between the adjuvant effect of
empty liposomes coated with BGG and that of liposomes which had in
addition to the surface-associated BGG, also a relatively high amount
of BGG in their inner compartments. The adjuvant effect of empty

---

TABLE 2.   Blood samples for antibody determination were obtained
            from the rabbits by cardiac puncture. For preparation
            of the liposomes adminsitered to the rabbits in the
            100% groups of experiment I, II and III, the same
            amount of phosphatidylcholine (150 mg) and the same
            HSA concentration (25 mg HSA per ml PBS) were used.
            In experiment I, conventional phosphatidylcholine lipo-
            somes have been prepared in the presence of the antigen
            solution, in order to obtain liposomes containing HSA
            both in their inner compartments and on their surfaces.
            0.5 mg HSA associated with liposomes was given intra-
            venously to 5 rabbits of the 100% group. Rabbits of
            4 other groups (each group consisting of 5 animals)
            received 10%, 1% 0.1% and 0.01% of this dose respec-
            tively. In experiment II, empty conventional phospha-
            tidylcholine liposomes have been coated with the
            solution of 25 mg HSA per ml PBS, in order to obtain
            liposomes with surface exposed antigen only (100%
            group). The same amount of liposomes was coated with
            2.5 mg HSA per ml PBS for the 10% group, 0.25 mg HSA
            for the 1% group, 0.025 mg HSA for the 0.1% group and
            0.0025 mg HSA for the 0.01% group. Each of these HSA-
            liposome preparations was injected in 5 rabbits (intra-
            venously). In experiment III, liposomes prepared by
            ether evaporation were coated with the solution of
            25 mg HSA per ml PBS. Liposomes prepared by the ether
            evaporation method may be coated with the antigen after-
            wards, but entrapment of the antigen in the liposomes
            during their preparation is impossible since ether
            causes coagulation of protein antigens. The liposomes
            prepared for experiment III were injected in 4 rabbits
            of the 100% group (0.04 mg HSA per rabbit). Rabbits
            of 4 other groups (each group consisting of 4 animals)
            received 10%, 1%. 0.1% and 0.01% of this dose respec-
            tively, as in experiment I. Further experimental
            details are given elsewhere (van Rooijen and van
            Nieuwmegen, 1980 a,b).

liposomes coated with antigen was even a little stronger than that of liposomes which had antigen both exposed on their surfaces and entrapped in their aqueous compartments, in spite of the fact that the latter liposomes contained much more antigen totally. This phenomenon may be explained by an inhibiting effect of antigen trapped in liposomes and especially of that fixed to the inner half of the outer phospholipid double layer on the binding of antigen to the outer surface of this layer, an inhibition, which does not occur when empty liposomes are coated with the antigens. These results support the hypothesis that the surface-associated part of the antigen determines the immune response against the antigen.

TABLE 3.   Immunoadjuvant activity of liposomes

Antigen	Negatively charged liposomes with phosphatidic acid or dicetylphosphate and phosphatidylcholine	Neutral liposomes with phosphatidylcholine only	Positively charged liposomes with stearylamine and phosphatidylcholine	antigen entrapped in liposomes	antigen exposed on outer surfaces of liposomes *	adjuvant effect demonstrated by:
Diphtheria toxoid	+	not done	-	partly	partly	Allison and Gregoriadis (1974)
Bovine serum albumin (BSA)	+	+	+	partly	partly	Heath et al. (1976)
Human serum albumin (HSA)	+	+	+	partly or not	partly or only	Van Rooijen and Van Nieuwmegen (1980a, b)
Bovine gamma globulin (BGG)	+	+	not done	partly or not	partly or only	Van Rooijen and Van Nieuwmegen (1980a, b)
Bovine β-glucuronidase	+	not done	not done	yes	?	Hudson et al. (1979)
Lipid A	+	not done	not done	?	yes	Schuster et al. (1979)
Cholera toxin	+	not done	not done	no	only	Alving et al. (1980a, b)
Adenovirus proteins	+	not done	not done	yes	?	Six et al. (1980)
Hepatitis B surface antigens	+	+	+	partly	partly	Gregoriadis and Manesis (1980) Sanchez et al. (1980)
Horse radish peroxidase (HRP)	not done	+	not done	partly or not	partly or only	Van Rooijen et al. (1981)
Gross-virus associated cell-surface antigen	+	not done	not done	partly	partly	Gerlier et al. (1980)
Influenza virus haemagglutinin and Neuraminidase	+	not done	not done	partly	partly	Gregoriadis (1980b)

+ = adjuvant effect of liposomes detected; - = no adjuvant effect detected; * see table IV.

Recent experiments of Alving et al. (1980a) confirm our results that molecules that are not exposed on the liposomal surface are not immunogenic. Six et al. (1980) suggested that entrapped antigen could be responsible for the adjuvant activity of liposomes. However their liposomes with entrapped antigen probably had much more antigen exposed on their outer surfaces than the liposomes used in their mixture of empty liposomes with the adenovirus protein antigens, since only 5 μg of antigen was mixed with empty liposomes, whereas 140 μg/ml was the antigen concentration used for preparation of the liposomes with entrapped antigen. That the adjuvant activity of liposomes depends on the antigen concentration used for coating of (empty) liposomes is shown in the present study (table 2, experiment II). Six et al. (1980) further argued that when antigen is negatively charged under physiologic conditions and negatively charged liposomes are used, it is unlikely that these proteins would associate with the liposomal bilayers. Whereas we used HSA which is negatively charged under physiologic conditions and negatively charged liposomes, association of the antigen with the bilayers was nevertheless observed (van Rooijen and van Nieuwmegen, 1980a,b).

In our first studies we observed a weak adjuvant effect when empty liposomes were injected together with free antigen (van Rooijen and van Nieuwmegen, 1977). We were not surprised by this

TABLE 4. Exposition of antigens on surfaces of liposomes

Antigen	Spontaneous attachment to or incorporation in liposomal membranes demonstrated by:	Attachment to liposomes via inserted receptor or covalent attachment to liposomes via:
Serum albumins	Hoekstra and Scherphof (1979) Van Rooijen and van Nieuwmegen (1980a, b)	
Gamma globulins	Weissman et al. (1974) Gregoriadis and Neerunjun (1975) Schieren et al. (1978) Huang and Kennel (1979) Van Rooijen and van Nieuwmegen (1980a, b)	Fatty acids (Huang et al. 1980) Glycosphingolipids (Heath et al. 1981) Glutaraldehyde reaction (Torchilin et al. 1979) Heterobifunctional crosslinking reagent (Leserman et al. 1980)
Cholera toxin		Ganglioside G_{M1} (Alving et al. 1980a, b)
Hepatitis B surface antigen	Gregoriadis and Manesis (1980) Sanchez et al. (1980)	
Horse radish peroxidase	Van Rooijen et al. (1981)	Phosphatidylethanolamine (Heath et al. 1980)
Grossvirus associated cell-surface antigen	Sakai et al. (1980)	
Influenza virus haemagglutinin and neuraminidase	Almeida et al. (1975)	
Influenza virus M-protein	Buchez et al. (1980)	

finding, since Dresser showed the effectiveness of lipid and lipidophilic substances as adjuvants already in 1961. However, since we
have shown that the adjuvant effect of liposomes is due to surface
exposition of the antigens, we were interested to see whether surface
exposition could also explain these initial results mentioned above.
0.5 mg of HSA was injected together with empty liposomes in 1 ml
saline. Although 25 mg of HSA per ml liposome-suspension was used
for preparation of the antigen associated liposomes in those studies,
mixing of liposomes with antigen in a concentration of only 0.25 mg
per ml is sufficient to get some antigen coating of the liposomes
and a measurable immune response against the antigen as demonstrated
in the present study (see table 2). Obviously mixing of 0.5 mg HSA
with empty liposomes as done in our first study is sufficient to get
some extent of nonspecific adherence of the antigen to liposomes and
enough to show a weak adjuvant effect of liposomes in the immune
response against HSA for that reason. As already mentioned it is
very difficult to demonstrate whether small amounts of antigen are
associated with liposomes or not. This has been clearly demonstrated
by Hoekstra and Scherphof (1979) for serum albumins.

Apart from gamma globulin and serum albumin antigens diphtheria
toxin is also spontaneously fixed to some liposomal phospholipids
(Boquet, 1979; Alving et al., 1980c). Diphtheria toxoid was the
first antigen for which the adjuvant effect of liposomes has been
established by Allison and Gregoriadis (1974). In all probability
also in the case of diphtheria toxoid, surface associated antigen
instead of entrapped antigen explains the adjuvant effect of liposomes.
Horse radish peroxidase (HRP) is another example of an antigen
(protein with molecular weight of about 40,000) which spontaneously
binds to the surfaces of liposomes, although to a very low extent
(van Rooijen et al., 1981). It can also be bound to liposomes by
covalent attachment to phosphatidylethanolamine (Heath et al., 1980),
a method by which much higher amounts of HRP can be coupled to the
liposomes. Covalent attachment of immunoglobulins to liposomes via
glycosphingolipids has been described also by Heath et al. (1981).
several antigens for which adjuvant properties of liposomes have
been established are grouped in table 3 and their way of association with the liposomes is shown in table 4.

VARIATION IN STRUCTURE OF LIPOSOMES AND ATTACHMENT OF ANTIGENS

Comparative properties and methods of preparation of liposomes
have been reviewed recently by Szoka and Papahadjopoulos (1980).
Liposomes may differ with respect to their dimensions, charge and
phospholipid composition. These three parameters may influence the
binding of antigens to their surfaces. It would seem somewhat
surprising that relatively large multilamellar liposomes bind more
albumin than relatively small unilamellar vesicles because the
available surface area per mole lipid is much higher for the latter.
Such a difference was demonstrated by Hoekstra and Scherphof (1979)

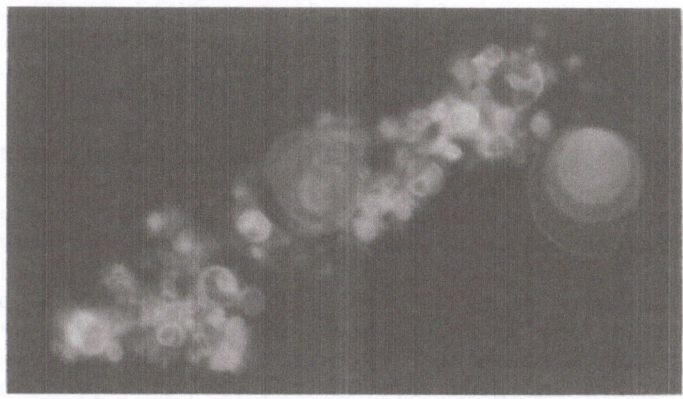

Fig. 2. A clot of multilamellar liposomes, stained with the fluoro-
         chrome acridine orange, and studied with a fluorescence
         microscope. So far as they are in focus, liposomal
         membranes (consisting of concentric phospholipid bilayers)
         can be distinguished clearly. Further experimental details
         are given in van Rooijen and van Nieuwmegen, 1978b.

and explained by differences in physical nature of the vesicles,
such as the radius of curvature. The liposomal character of various
preparations of multilamellar liposomes and their dimensions can be
studied e.g. after fluorochrome staining (van Rooijen and van
Nieuwmegen, 1978b and fig. 2).

     It is not surprising that antigens may have a different
affinity for neutral, positive or negative liposomes, since antigens
generally may be expected to have a stronger affinity for liposomes
with an opposed charge. Hepatitis-B surface antigen showed the
highest percentage of incorporation in positively charged liposomes
(Gregoriadis and Manesis, 1980). Contrary to this, diphtheria toxoid
has probably a stronger affinity for negative liposomes as we conclude from the difference in immunoadjuvant properties between
negative and positive liposomes with respect to this antigen
(Allison and Gregoriadis, 1974).

     Manipulation of the phospholipid composition however is by far
the most useful tool for preparation of liposomes with surface bound
antigens. Many of such methods for coupling of proteins to liposomes
are to be expected in future. We already mentioned that HRP can be
bound to liposomes by covalent attachment to phosphatidylethanolamine
(Heath et al., 1980). Covalent attachment of immunoglobulins to
liposomes via glycosphingolipids has been described also by Heath
et al. (1981). Immunoglobulins may also be coupled with fatty acids
covalently, followed by incorporation of these amphipathic antibodies
in liposomal membrances by a detergent-dialysis method (Huang et al.,
1980). Another method for covalent coupling of soluble proteins to

liposomes uses the heterobifunctional cross-linking reagent N-hydro-
xysuccinimidyl 3-(2-pyridyldithio) propionate (SPDP, Pharmacia)
(Leserman et al., 1980). Finally antibody can be covalently coupled
to liposomes by a glutaraldehyde reaction (Torchilin et al., 1979).

CELLS WHICH MAY BE INVOLVED IN THE LIPOSOME MEDIATED IMMUNE RESPONSE

     Interactions of liposomes with mammalian cells have been
reviewed by Pagano and Weinstein (L978). Various mechanisms of
liposome-cell interaction have been described, and both macrophages
and lymphocytes were among the cells for which some kind of interaction with liposomes has been observed. Initially it was assumed
that interaction of an antigen with its specific antibodies was
prevented when the antigens were administered entrapped in liposomes
(Gregoriadis and Allison, 1974; Fishman and Citri, 1975). That
masking of antigenic determinants did not prevent an immune reaction
pointed to a role of macrophages in the processing of liposome
entrapped antigens, because no other way than lysosomal digestion of
liposomal membranes seemed to exist for unmasking the antigenic
determinants (van Rooijen and van Nieuwmegen, 1977). Such a role of
macrophages was further supported by the negative influence of a
high proportion of liposomal cholesterol on both the immune response
against entrapped antigens (Heath et al., 1976) and the digestion of
the liposomes by macrophages (Johnson, 1975). Further arguments for
a role of macrophages came from experiments with liposomes containing
lysolecithin in their phospholipid membrances. The adjuvant effect
of liposomes was impaired after incorporation of lysolecithin in the
membranes (van Rooijen and van Nieuwmegen, 1979a). It was expected
that lysolecithin, although an adjuvant in itself would impair the
adjuvant effect of liposomes, when lysosomal digestion of liposomal
membranes would be a necessary step in the processing of liposome
entrapped antigens. In short, the mechanism by which lysolecithin
was expected to effect its adjuvant activity, i.e. inhibition of
antigen digestion, was the same which could impair the adjuvant
effect of liposomes, namely prevention of the digestion of liposomal
membranes in lysosomes, necessary for the unmasking of antigens in
the macrophages. However, our recent finding that antigen exposed
on the outer surfaces of liposomes and not the entrapped part of
antigen is responsible for the adjuvant activity of liposomes does
not support a role of macrophages in the establishment of the immunoadjuvant effect of liposomes. Unmasking of liposome entrapped
antigens is obviously not required, and the entrapped part of the
antigen rather influences the immunoadjuvant effect of the liposomes
negatively (table 1). Although a role for macrophages in mediating
the immune response against antigens exposed on the surfaces of
liposomes cannot be excluded, a direct contact between antigen
exposing liposomes and lymphocytes with surface receptors for that
antigen seems to be more likely.

     Several recent studies point to an interaction between lympho-

cytes and liposomes (e.g. Blumenthal et al., 1977; Ozato et al.,
1978; Dresdner et al., 1979; Plesser et al., 1979; Kramers et al.,
1980; Ostro et al., 1980). Cholesterol is likely to play an
important role in the interaction between lymphocytes and liposomes.
Kramers et al. (1980) found that phosphatidylcholine-cholesterol
liposomes did not bind to lymphocytes from the thymus, whereas
phosphatidylcholine liposomes, lacking cholesterol in their
membranes, bound rapidly to the cells and could not be removed by
repeated washing. During the interaction between cells and liposomes, cholesterol may be exchanged from cells to liposomes or from
liposomes to cells, dependent on the relative cholesterol contents
of both (Plesser et al., 1979; Kramers et al., 1980). That liposomes without cholesterol bind, whereas liposomes with cholesterol
do not bind to lymphocytes, may explain why various effects of
liposomes on lymphocytes are inhibited by the presence of cholesterol
in the liposomal membranes, such as liposome induced capping of
surface immunoglobulins on lymphocytes (Ostro et al., 1980), liposome induced alterations in surface architecture of lymphocytes
(Plesser et al., 1979) and the negative influence of liposomes on
the mitogenic reaction of lymphocytes (Shi-Hua Chen and Keenan, 1977;
Rivnay et al., 1978; Ng et al., 1978). Membrane cholesterol inhibits
the adjuvant effect of liposomes only when present in a relatively
high concentration (Heath et al., 1976). The affinity of liposomes
for lymphocytes may well account for the fact that two hours after
injection, a more than one hundred fold increased uptake of antigen
by the spleen was observed when liposome associated antigen was
compared with free antigen (van Rooijen and van Nieuwmegen, 1979b).
Similar results concerning the relatively high uptake of liposome
entrapped labelled compounds in the spleen have been described by
Kimelberg et al. (1976). Our results suggested that two hours after
injection only a small part of the liposome associated antigen in
the spleen had been ingested by macrophages (van Rooijen and van
Nieuwmegen, 1979b). Moreover it has been established that coating
of liposomes with protein decreases their capture by macrophages
(Torchilin et al., 1980). Adherence of liposomes to lymphocytes may
offer a good opportunity for antigens exposed on the surfaces of
liposomes to meet antigen specific receptors on the surfaces of
lymphocytes. The interaction between liposomes exposing an antigen
and lymphocytes with surface receptors for the same antigen may
result in the simultaneous recognition of several antigen molecules
by their specific receptors. It is possible that liposomes can
replace macrophages with respect to their antigen presentation
function, although macrophages are still necessary for regulation of
other lymphocyte functions (Unanue, 1978).

SUBSTANCES THAT MAY ENHANCE THE IMMUNOADJUVANT ACTIVITY OF LIPOSOMES

The influence of various adjuvants on the immune response
against an antigen may be mediated by an effect on macrophages
(Allison, 1973) or by a direct effect on T- or B-lymphocytes (Dresser

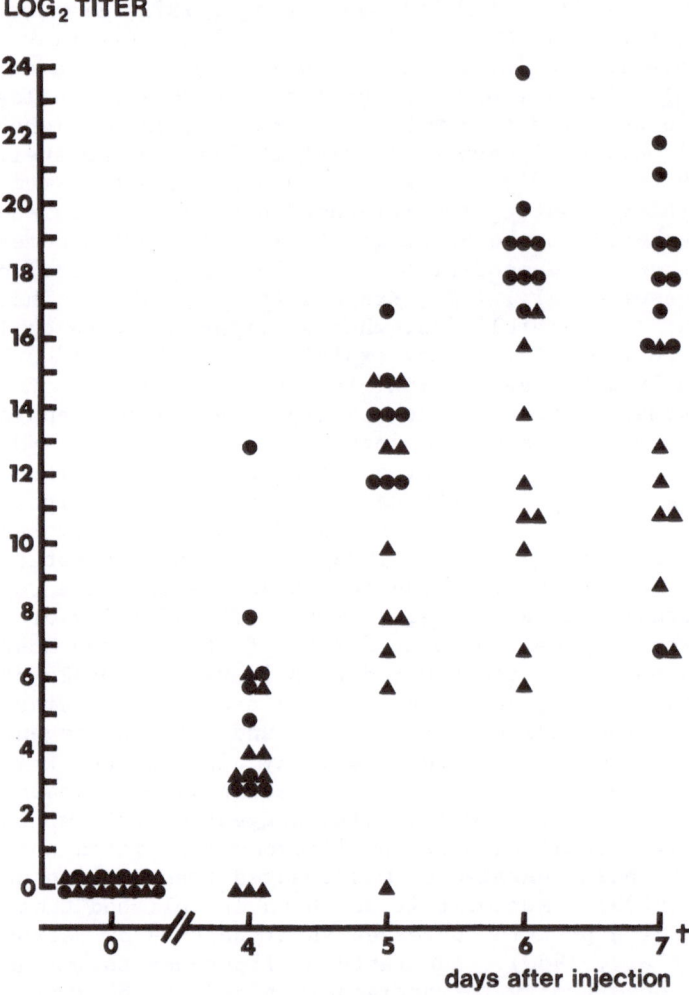

Fig. 3.   The influence of liposome associated endotoxin on the
         immune response in rabbits against HSA, that was associated
         with the same liposomes.   Anti-HSA titers were determined
         after intravenous administration of HSA-liposome (▲) or
         HSA-liposome-endotoxin (●) preparations.   Both preparations
         were injected in nine rabbits.   All rabbits received the
         same amount of liposomes and 0.5 mg HSA.   Titers are given
         as $\log_2$.   Blood samples for antibody determination were
         obtained from the rabbits by cardiac puncture immediately
         before and at 4, 5, 6 and 7 days after administration.
         Further experimental details are given elsewhere (van
         Rooijen and van Nieuwmegen, 1980c).

and Phillips, 1973). The relative potency of various adjuvants
differs markedly according to the antigen used (Bomford, 1980).
The adjuvant effect of liposomes appears to depend primarily on antigen presentation as we discussed earlier. No stimulating effect of
liposomes themselves on proliferation of lymphocytes has been observed.
On the contrary they rather inhibit the proliferation of lymphocytes
as measured by ^{3}H-thymidine incorporation into cellular DNA.
(Shi-Hua Chen and Keenan, 1977; Rivnay et al., 1978; Ng et al., 1978).
The extent of liposome mediated inhibition of ^{3}H-thymidine incorporation into DNA of L1210 cells appeared to be dependent mainly on the
phospholipid composition of the liposomes (Campbell, 1980). The fact
that different adjuvants enhance the immune response by different
effects, suggests that the adjuvant effect of liposomes, obtained
by antigen presentation, may be enhanced by combination with other
adjuvants. As discussed already earlier in this paper, lysolecithin
impairs the adjuvant effect of liposomes after incorporation in the
phospholipid bilayers (van Rooijen and van Nieuwmegen, 1979a).

     Endotoxin and the endotoxin-derived compound lipid A may enhance
the adjuvant effect of liposomes against liposome associated antigens
(Alving et al., 1980a,b; van Rooijen and van Nieuwmegen, 1980c).
When a weak albumin antigen and endotoxin were associated with the
same liposomes, antibody production in rabbits could be detected
within three days after injection of the antigen-liposome-endotoxin
preparation. When antigen and endotoxin were associated with
different liposomes and these antigen-liposome and endotoxin-liposome
preparations were injected simultaneously the adjuvant effect of the
liposomes was enhanced also, but it took one day longer before antibodies could be detected, whereas peak titers were not markedly
different. (Van Rooijen and van Nieuwmegen, 1980c). The influence
of endotoxin on the adjuvant effect of liposomes is shown in fig. 3.
Dancey et al. (1977) studied the anti-DNP (hapten) responses in mice
immunized with DNP-Cap-PE sensitized liposomes. Enhancement of
immunogenicity by lipid A was obtained only by the presence of lipid
A in the same bilayers as DNP-Cap-PE. Their results with hapten
conjugated liposomes are different from our results with antigen
associated liposomes with respect to this.

     The interaction between liposomes and endotoxin has been
suggested to be a result of the hydrophobic insertion of lipid A
subunits into the hydrocarbon region of the liposomes (Onji and Liu,
1979). In other studies it has been suggested that in phospholipid-
lipopolysaccharide mixed bilayers, the phospholipid molecules and
most probably also the lipopolysaccharide (endotoxin) molecules
exist in segregated domains, which are rather stable and persist for
long periods of time (Takeuchi and Nikaido, 1981). The structure of
liposomes is not markedly affected by endotoxin or lipid A, since
these compounds do not increase their permeability to divalent anions
(Davies et al., 1978) or non-ionic substances (Rottem, 1978).
However injection of liposomes containing lipid A produces an immune

response against lipid A as well as against the phospholipids of
which the liposomes are composed (Schuster et al., 1979) and for
this reason lipid A incorporation may be disadvantageous in some
studies. The positive influence of endotoxin (lipopolysaccharide)
on the immunoadjuvant properties of liposomes may well be caused by
its capacity to form bridges between antigen exposing liposomes and
lymphocytes with surface receptors for that antigen, since both
lipid A (Onji and Liu, 1979) and polysaccharide (Sunamoto et al.,
1980) have an affinity for liposomal and mammalian cell membranes
(Davies et al., 1978). Other lipid substances that might be incorporated into liposomes to enhance the immunogenicity of liposome-
associated antigens are e.g. acylated derivatives of muramyl
dipeptide. (Siddiqui et al., 1978).

VARIOUS ASPECTS OF LIPOSOME MEDIATED IMMUNE RESPONSES

Humoral and cellular immune responses
elicited by antigen associated liposomes

     The first studies, in which adjuvant properties of liposomes
have been described, concerned the humoral immune response (e.g.
Allison and Gregoriadis, 1974; Heath et al., 1976; van Rooijen and
van Nieuwmegen, 1977). It is shown in a recent study however, that
liposomes can be used to induce cell-mediated immunity to Herpes
simplex virus. Cytotoxic T lymphocyte responses were induced by viral
antigens incorporated into liposomes (Lawman et al., 1981). Liposomes
can also be used to induce cellular immunity to hepatitis B virus-
derived antigens (Sanchez et al., 1980).

T-cell dependent or independent immune responses

     It has been shown that hapten-conjugated liposomes produce a
primarily T-cell independent immune response (Yasuda et al., 1977;
van Houte et al., 1979). Whether protein antigens coated on the
surfaces of liposomes produce also a T-cell independent immune
response has not yet been studied. However when identical units
(haptens) arranged in a more or less linear repetitive sequence are
important for a T-cell independent immune response, analogous to the
repetitive distribution of identical haptenic groups on other T-cell
independent antigens (Katz and Benacerraf, 1972), there is no reason
to believe that protein antigens coated on liposomes produce also a
T-cell independent immune response.

Adjuvant properties of liposomes with respect
to the primary and secondary immune response

     Allison and Gregoriadis (1974) showed that both the primary
and secondary immune response against an antigen were enhanced when
the antigen had been associated with liposomes before injection.
They studied the secondary response after both priming and booster

injections with liposome associated antigen. Recently we studied
the effect of liposomes on the secondary response against the antigens HSA and HRP in rabbits. Booster injections were in all experiments given as antigen free in solution, whereas priming injections
with either free antigen or liposome associated antigen were given
in order to study the specific effect of liposomes on the generation
of immunological memory (van Rooijen et al., 1981). It appeared
that HSA-liposomes generated immunological memory to a higher extent
that the antigen did, when injected free in solution. HRP, injected
free in solution, did not generate immunological memory, contrary to
liposome associated HRP. The enhancing effect of liposomes on the
generation of immunological memory may be important, particularly
with respect to the possible application of liposomes in the preparation of human and veterinary vaccines.

ADVANTAGES OF LIPOSOMES AS AN IMMUNOADJUVANT,
PARTICULARLY WITH RESPECT TO PREPARATION OF VACCINES

The fact that liposomes, composed of phosphatidylcholine only,
can be used successfully as an immunoadjuvant (van Rooijen and van
Nieuwmegen, 1980c) increases their value for this purpose. Phosphatidylcholine is a normal ingredient of cell membranes and is biodegradable (Ferber and Resch, 1977). Moreover it is a harmless compound
when adminsitered as liposomes, although some exchange may occur with
the phospholipids of cells (Gregoriadis et al., 1977; Pagano and
Weinstein, 1978). One of the most important advantages of phosphatidylcholine liposomes as an adjuvant is that, in contrast to certain
other phospholipids such as cardiolipin, phosphatidylinositol,
phosphatidylglycerol and phosphatidic acid, phosphatidylcholine is
a very poor antigen (Alving, 1977). Schuster et al. (1979) confirmed
that liposomes by themselves do not evoke a detectable immune response
in rabbits, even in the presence of incomplete Freund's adjuvant.
They could induce an immune response against phosphatidylcholine,
when lipid A was incorporated in the injected liposomes. It may be
concluded that in multilamellar phosphatidylcholine liposomes we
have a biodegradable, harmless, easily prepared immunoadjuvant, which
has no immunogenic activity of its own and may be applied for intravenous administration. However, depending on the antigen to be
incorporated, the phospholipid composition of liposomes may be varied
in order to obtain the most efficient antigen-liposome preparation.

Edelman (1980) has composed a list of factors that are important
with respect to the safety of any adjuvanted vaccine. When one
compares the characteristics of liposomes as an immunoadjuvant, it
is clear that liposomes may be considered a promising vaccine
adjuvant. Several reports are already available, in which liposomes
are suggested as a useful vaccine adjuvant. (Siddiqui et al., 1978,
Morein et al., 1978, Alving et al., 1980b). Apart from their
application as vaccine adjuvant, liposomes may be useful as an
adjuvant in the immune response against antigens which may be harmful,

especially when they have to be injected intravenously or in a
relatively high concentration, when liposomes are omitted. Horse
radish peroxidase (HRP) is such an antigen which is frequently used
in our laboratory, since both the antigen and specific antibodies
against it can be demonstrated very easily in the cells and tissues
of the lymphoid organs (van Rooijen and Streefkerk, 1976).

NEGATIVE EFFECTS OF LIPOSOMAL IMMUNOADJUVANT ACTIVITY

Immunoadjuvant activity of liposomes may be a disadvantage when
an immune response is elicited against molecules which are entrapped
in liposomes in order to deliver these molecules to special cells in
the body. Immunoadjuvant activity of liposomes may also have a negative effect when an immune response is elicited against immunoglobulins which are coated on liposomes, containing chemotherapeutic
drugs, for targeting these liposomes to specific cells in the body.
The potential use of liposomes as carriers of enzymes for the treatment of selected inborn errors of metabolism has been extensively
studied. Liposomes are effective in delivering entrapped molecules
to the lysosomal apparatus, primarily of the liver. However since
immune responses against the entrapped enzymes may be elicited
(Hudson et al. 1979), probably because a very small part of the liposome associated enzymes is exposed on the outer surfaces of the liposomes (see discussion before), caution should be exercised in the
administration of enzymes in liposomes.

Gregoriadis and Neerunjun (1975) have suggested that liposomes,
containing chemotherapeutic drugs could be targeted to cells by
coating with immunoglobulins, specifically elicited against the target
cells. Many thereapeutic applications of such a method are possible,
when specific antibodies to the target cells are available. Recently
distinct advances have been made in targeting of liposomes by
covalent coupling with monoclonal antibody (Huang et al., 1980;
Leserman et al., 1980). Monoclonal antibodies are nowadays produced
in mice and rats mainly, but these are not the first choice for human
therapy because of the body's reaction against foreign proteins.
Efforts to develop the human equivalent of the rodent plasmacytoma
cell have been successful (Olsson and Kaplan, 1980 and Immunology
Today, no. 1, Jan. 1981) and human hybrid-forming myeloma are now
distributed to international laboratories (Immunology Today, no. 5,
Dec. 1980). An obstacle may arise, however, during the development
of therapeutic applications of liposome targeting, when immune
responses are elicited against the immunoglobulins, used for coating.
We have demonstrated that liposomes also have a very strong adjuvant
effect with respect to immunoglobulin antigens exposed on their outer
surfaces (van Rooijen and van Nieuwmegen, 1980a,b). Monoclonal antibodies from human origin may also elicit anti-idiotype antibodies,
after injection in man. Such an immune response is likely to occur
when the anti-idiotype antibody production is strongly enhanced by
liposomes, on the surfaces of which they are exposed. Such an immune

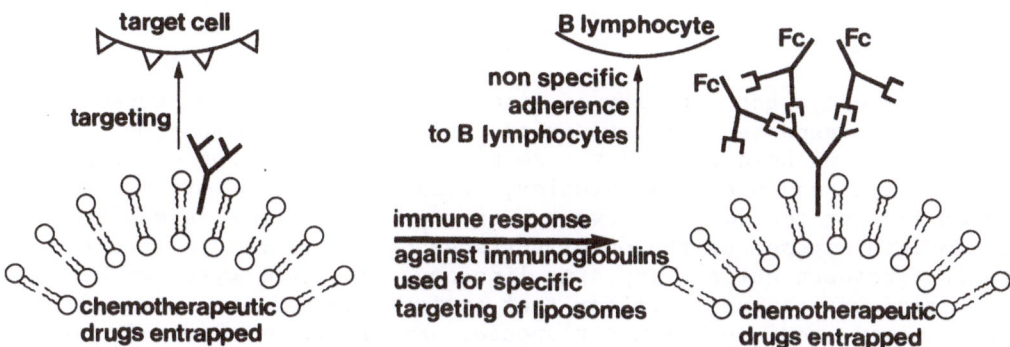

Fig. 4.   An immune response against immunoglobulins used for target-
          ing of liposomes may interfere with the results, since
          masking of the antibody combining sites of these molecules
          will occur. Fc portions of immunoglobulins elicited against
          the immunoglobulins used for targeting may cause a non-
          specific adherence to B lymphocytes.

response against the immunoglobulins, used for coating, has probably
no strong influence on targeting of the liposomes to the sites of
destination in the body when only one injection is given, since homing
of the liposomes will be finished after initiation of the antibody
response. Repeated injections will often be needed for therapeutic
application of the liposomes containing chemotherapeutic drugs. Any
further injections of the immunoglobulin coated liposomes however,
will result in complexing of these immunoglobulins with specific
antibodies elicited against them. As a consequence, masking of the
antibody combining sites which are needed for targeting of the liposomes occurs, and specific homing will no longer be achieved. To
the immunoglobulins coated on the liposomes are now other antibody
molecules attached in such a way, that Fc portions of the latter antibody molecules form the actually remaining targeting part of the anti-
body-antibody complex coating of the liposomes (see fig. 4). These
Fc portions may target the liposomes e.g. to B lymphocytes in general
(Paraskevas et al., 1972). The interference with liposome targeting
may be solved when the lymphocytes which are responsible for the
anti-immunoglobulin immune response are destroyed by the same mechanism which kills the target cells themselves. We have planned a
study to investigate whether immune reactive cells may be killed
specifically by antigen coated liposomes, containing chemotherapeutic
drugs. Such an "antigen suicide technique" has been developed originally by Basten et al. (1971). These authors used radioactively
(^{125}I) labelled antigen under conditions favouring radiation damage
to the cells carrying receptors for that antigen so that these cells
were specifically damaged. The suggested liposome mediated "antigen
suicide technique", however, may be more useful, especially for

therapeutic use in man, where high doses of radioisotopes cannot be
applied.

CONCLUSIONS

Immunoadjuvant activity of liposomes has been demonstrated in
the immune responses against various antigens. Although some
arguments have been given for a role of liposome entrapped antigen
and macrophages in earlier studies, evidence has been presented
recently that the immunoadjuvant activity of liposomes is mediated
by antigen exposed on the outer surfaces of liposomes. A direct
contact between antigen exposing liposomes and lymphocytes with
specific surface receptors for that antigen may well be involved in
the liposome mediated immune response. Endotoxin and lipid A, compounds which have adjuvant activity by themselves, may be incorporated
in the phospholipid bilayers in order to enhance the immunoadjuvant
activity of liposomes whereas lysolecithin, a phospholipid adjuvant,
inhibits their adjuvant effect. In phosphatidylcholine liposomes, we
have a biodegradable, harmless and easily prepared immunoadjuvant,
which has no immunogenic activity of its own and may be applied for
intravenous administration. Depending on the antigen to be incorporated, the phospholipid composition of liposomes may be varied in
order to obtain the most efficient antigen-liposome preparation.
Liposomes have already been suggested as promising vehicles for
vaccines. The immunoadjuvant activity of liposomes may be disadvantageous, when targeting of liposomes, containing chemotherapeutic
drugs and coated with monoclonal antibodies, is intended.

ACKNOWLEDGEMENT

The authors are indebted to Mrs. G.W.J.M. Kaizer-Verhagen for
excellent typing of the manuscript.

REFERENCES

Allison, A.C., 1973, Effects of adjuvants on different cell types
    and their interactions in immune responses, in: "Immunopotenti-
    ation," G.E.W. Wolstenholme and J. Knight, eds., Elsevier
    Amsterdam.
Allison, A.C. and Gregoriadis, G., 1974, Liposomes as immunological
    adjuvants, Nature, 252: 252.
Almeida, J.D., Brand, C.M., Edwards, D.C. and Heath, T.D., 1975,
    Formation of virosomes from influenza subunits and liposomes,
    Lancet , ii: 899.
Alving C.R., 1977, Immune reactions of lipids and lipid model
    membrances, in: "The antigens," M. Sela, ed., Academic Press,
    New York.
Alving, C.R., Banerji, B., Clements, J.D. and Richards, R.L., 1980a,
    Adjuvanticity of lipid A and lipid A fractions in liposomes,
    in: "Liposomes and immunobiology," B.H. Tom and H.R. Six, eds.,

Elsevier, New York.
Alving, C.R., Banerji, B., Shiba, T., Kotani, S., Clements, J.D. and
    Richards, R.L., 1980b, Liposomes as vehicles for vaccines,
    Progr. Clin. Biol. Res., 47: 339.
Alving, C.R. Iglewski, B.H., Urban, K.A., Moss, J., Richards, R.L.
    and Sadoff, J.C., 1980c, Binding of diphtheria toxin to phos-
    pholipids in liposomes, Proc. Nat., Acad. Sci. U.S.A., 77:
    1986.
Banerji, B. and Alving, C.R., 1981, Anti-liposome antibodies induced
    by lipid A.I. Influence of ceramide, glycosphingolipids and
    phosphocholine on complement damage, J. Immunol., 126: 1080.
Basten, A., Miller, J.F.A.P., Warmer, N.L. and Pye, J., 1971, Speci-
    fic inactivation of thymus-derived (T) and non-thymus-derived
    (b) lymphocytes by ^{125}-labelled antigen, Nature New Biol.,
    231: 104.
Blumenthal, R., Weinstein, J.N., Sharrow, S.O. and Henkart, P.,
    1977, Liposome-lymphocyte interaction: Saturable sites for
    transfer and intracellular release of liposome contents,
    Proc. Natl. Acad. Sci. U.S.A., 74: 5603.
Bomford, R., 1980, The comparative selectivity of adjuvants for
    humoral and cell-mediated immunity, Clin. Exp. Immunol., 39:
    426.
Boquet, P., 1979, Interaction of diphtheria toxin fragments A, B
    and protein crm 45 with liposomes, Eur. J. Biochem., 100: 483.
Bucher, D.J., Kharitonenkov, I.G., Zakomirdin, J.A., Grigoriev, V.B.,
    Klimenko, S.M. and Davis, J.F., 1980, Incorporation of influenza
    virus M-protein into liposomes, J. Virology, 36: 586.
Campbell, P.I., 1980, Liposome inhibition of 3H-thymidine incorpora-
    tion into DNA of L1210 cells in culture, IRCS Medic. Sci., 8:
    814.
Dancey, G.F., Yasuda, T. and Kinsky, S.C., 1977, Enhancement of
    liposomal model membrane immunogenicity by incorporation of
    lipid A, J. Immunol., 119: 1868.
Davies, M., Stewart-Tull, D.E.S. and Jackson, D.M., 1978, The binding
    of lipopolysaccharide from Escherichia coli to mammalian cell
    membranes and its effect on liposomes, Bioch. Bioph. Acta, 508:
    260.
Dresdner, G., Ehrenberg, A., Hammarstrom, L. and Smith, E., 1979,
    Interaction between lymphocytes and lecithin-cholesterol vesi-
    cles, Acta Chem. Scand. B., 33: 599.
Dresser, D.W., 1961, Effectiveness of lipid and lipidophilic substan-
    ces as adjuvants, Nature, 191: 1169.
Dresser, D.W. and Phillips, J.M., 1973, The cellular targets for
    the action of adjuvants: T-adjuvants and B-adjuvants, in:
    "Immunopotentiation," G.E.W. Wolstenholme and J. Knight, eds.,
    Elsevier, Amsterdam.
Edelman, R., 1980, Vaccine adjuvants, Rev. Infect. Dis., 2: 370.
Ferber, E. and Resch, K., 1977, Structure and physiologic role of
    lipids in the lymphocyte membrane, in: "The lymphocyte,"
    part II, J.J. Marchalonis, ed., Marcel Dekker, New York.

Fishman, Y. and Citri, N., 1975, L-Asparaginase entrapped in liposo-
    mes: Preparation and properties, FEBS Letters, 60: 17.
Gerlier, D., Sakai, F. and Dore, J.F., 1980, Induction of antibody
    response to liposome-associated Gross-virus cell-surface antigen
    (GCSAa) Br. J. Cancer, 41: 236.
Gregoriadis, G., 1980a, Tailoring liposome structure, Nature, 283:
    815.
Gregoriadis, G., 1980b, The liposome drug-carrier concept: its
    development and future, in: "Liposomes in biological systems,"
    G. Gregoriadis and A.C. Allison, eds., John Wiley and Sons,
    Chichester.
Gregoriadis, G., 1980c, Recent progress in liposome research, in:
    "Liposomes in biological systems," G. Gregoriadis and A.C.
    Allison, eds., John Wiley and Sons, Chichester.
Gregoriadis, G., 1980d, Targeting of drugs: Possibilities in viral
    chemotherapy and prophylaxis, Pharmacol. Therap., 10: 103.
Gregoriadis, G. and Allison, A.C., 1974, Entrapment of proteins in
    liposomes prevents allergic reactions in pre-immunised mice.
    FEBS Letters, 45: 71.
Gregoriadis, G. and Manesis, E.K., 1980, Liposomes as immunological
    adjuvants for hepatitis B surface antigens, in: "Liposomes
    and immunobiology," B.H. Tom and H.R. Six, eds., Elsevier,
    New York.
Gregoriadis, G. and Neerunjun, E.D., 1975, Homing of liposomes to
    target cells, Biochem. Biophys. Res. Com., 65: 537.
Gregoriadis, G., Siliprandi, N. and Turchetto, E., 1977, Possible
    implications in the use of exogenous phospholipids, Life Sci.,
    20: 1773.
Heath, T.D., Edwards, D.C. and Ryman, B.E., 1976, The adjuvant
    properties of liposomes, Biochem. Soc. Trans., 4: 129.
Heath, T.D., Macher, B.A. and Papahadjopoulos, D., 1981, Covalent
    attachment of immunoglobulins to liposomes via glycosphingo-
    lipids, Biochim. Biophys. Acta, 640: 66.
Heath, T.D., Robertson, D., Birbeck, M.S.C. and Davies, A.J.S.,
    1980, Covalent attachment of horseradish peroxidase to the
    outer surface of liposomes, Biochim. Biophys. Acta, 599: 42.
Hoekstra, D. and Scherphof, G., 1979, Effect of fetal calf serum
    and serum protein fractions on the uptake of liposomal phospha-
    tidylcholine by rat hepatocytes in primary monolayer culture,
    Biochim. Biophys. Acta, 551: 109.
Huang, A., Huang, L. and Kennel, S.J., 1980, Monoclonal antibody
    covalently coupled with fatty acid; a reagent for in vitro
    liposome targeting, J. Biol. Chem., 255: 8015.
Huang, L., and Kennel, S.J., 1979, Binding of immunoglobulin G to
    phospholipid vesicles by sonication, Biochemistry, 18: 1702.
Hudson, L.D.S., Fiddler, M.B. and Desnick, R.J., 1979, Enzyme therapy
    X. Immune response induced by enzyme- and buffer-loaded liposomes
    in C3H/HeJ Gus mice, J. Pharm. Exp. Ther. 208: 507.
Johnson, S.M., 1975, The inability of macrophages to digest liposomes
    containing a high proportion of cholesterol, Biochem. Soc.

Trans., 3: 160.

Katz, D.H. and Benacerraf, B., 1972, The regulatory influence of
    activated T cells on B cell responses to antigen, Adv. Immunol.,
    15: 1.

Kimelberg, H.K., Tracy, T.F., Biddlecome, S.M. and Bourke, R.S.,
    1976, The effect of entrapment in liposomes on the in vivo
    distribution of ^{3}H-methotrexate in a primate, Cancer Res., 36:
    2949.

Kinsky, S.C., 1980, Factors affecting liposomal model membrane
    immunogenicity, in: "Liposomes and immunobiology," B.H. Tom and
    H.R. Six, eds., Elsevier, New York.

Kramers, M.T.C., Patrick, J., Bottomley, J.M., Quinn, P.J. and
    Chapman, D., 1980, Studies of liposome interactions with rat
    thymocytes, Eur. J. Biochem., 110: 579.

Lawman, M.J.P., Naylor, P.T., Huang, L., Courtney, R.J. and Rouse,
    B.T., 1981, Cell-mediated immunity to Herpes simplex virus:
    induction of cytotoxic T lymphocyte responses by viral antigens
    incorporated into liposomes, J. Immunol., 126: 304.

Leserman, L.D., Barbet, J. and Kourilsky, F., 1980, Targeting to
    cells of fluorescent liposomes covalently coupled with mono-
    clonal antibody or protein A, Nature, 288: 602.

Morein, B., Helenius, A., Simons, K., Pettersson, R., Kaariainen, L.
    and Schirrmacher, V., 1978, Effective subunit vaccines against
    an enveloped animal virus, Nature, 276: 715.

Ng, M.H., Ng, W.S., Ho, W.K.K., Fung, K.P. and Lamelin, J.P., 1978,
    Modulation of phytohemagglutinin-mediated lymphocyte stimulation
    by egg lecithin, Exp. Cell Res., 116: 387.

Olsson, L., Kaplan, H.S., 1980, Human-human hybridomas producing
    monoclonal antibodies of predefined antigenic specificity,
    Proc. Natl. Acad. Sci. U.S.A., 77: 5429.

Onji, T. and Lium M.S., 1979, Changes in surface charge density on
    liposomes induced by Escherichia coli endotoxin, Biochim.
    Biophys. Acta, 558: 320.

Ostro, M.J., Bessinger, B., Summers, J.F. and Dray, S., 1980, Lipo-
    some modulations of surface immunoglobulins on rabbit spleen
    cells, J. Immunol., 124: 2956.

Ozato, K., Huang, L. and Pagano, R.E., 1978, Interactions of phospho-
    lipid vesicles with murine lymphocytes II. Correlation between
    altered surface properties and enhanced proliferative response,
    Membrane Chem., 1: 27.

Pagano, R.E. and Weinstein, J.N., 1978, Interactions of liposomes
    with mammalian cells, Ann. Rev. Biophys. Bioeng., 7: 435.

Paraskevas, F., Lee, S.T., Orr, K.B. and Israels, L.G., 1972, A
    receptor for Fc fragments on mouse B-lymphocytes, J. Immunol.,
    108: 1319.

Plesser, Y.M., Doljansky, F. and Polliack, A., 1979, Alteration in
    lymphocyte surface morphology and membrane fluidity induced by
    cholesterol depletion, Cell Molec. Biol., 25: 203.

Rivnay, B., Globerson, A. and Shinitzky, M., 1978, Perturbation of
    lymphocyte response to concanavalin A by exogenous cholesterol

and lecithin, Eur. J. Immunol., 8: 185.

Rottem, S., 1978, The effect of lipid A on the fluidity and permeability properties of phospholipid dispersions, FEBS letters,
95: 121.

Ryman, B.E. and Tyrrell, D.A., 1979, Liposomes - methodology and
applications, in: "Lysosomes in biology and pathology," vol. 6,
J.T. Dingle, P.J. Jacques and I.H. Shaw, eds., Elsevier,
Amsterdam.

Ryman, B.E. and Tyrrell, D.A., 1980, Liposomes - bags of potential,
Essays Biochem., 18: 49.

Sakai, F., Gerlier, D., Dore, J.F., 1980, Association of Gross
virus-associated cell-surface antigen with liposomes, Br. J.
Cancer, 41: 227.

Sanchez, Y., Ionescu-Matiu, I., Dreesman, G.R., Kramp, W., Six, H.R.,
Hollinger, F.B. and Melnick, J.L., 1980, Humoral and cellular
immunity to Hepatitis B virus-derived antigens: Comparative
activity of Freund complete adjuvant, alum and liposomes,
Infect. Immun., 30: 728.

Schieren, H., Weissmann, G., Seligman, M. and Coleman, P., 1978,
Interactions of immunoglobulins with liposomes: An ESR and dif-
fusion study demonstrating protection by hydrocortisone, Biochem.
Biophys. Res. Commun., 82: 1160.

Schuster, B.G., Neidig, M., Alving, B.M. and Alving, C.R., 1979,
Production of antibodies against phosphocholine, phosphatidylcholine, sphingomyelin, and lipid A by injection of liposomes
containing lipid A, J. Immunol., 122: 900.

Shi-Hua Chen, S. and Keenan, R.M., 1977, Effect of phosphatidylcholine liposomes on the mitogen-stimulated lymphocyte activation, Biochim. Biophys. Res. Commun., 79: 852.

Siddiqui, W.A., Taylor, D.W., Kan, S.C., Kramer, K., Richmond-Crum,
S.M., Kotani, S., Shiba, T., Kusumoto, S., 1978, Vaccination
of experimental monkeys against Plasmodium falciparum: A
possible safe adjuvant, Science, 201: 1237.

Six, H.R., Kramp, W.J.. Kasel, J.A., 1980, Effects of liposomes on
serological responses following immunization with adenovirus
purified type 5 subunit vaccines, in: "Liposomes and immunobiology," B.H. Tom and H.R. Six, eds., Elsevier, Amsterdam.

Strejan, G.H., Smith, P.M., Grant, C.W. and Surlan, D., 1979,
Naturally occurring antibodies to liposomes I. Rabbit antibodies
to sphingomyelin-containing liposomes before and after immunization with unrelated antigens, J. Immunol., 123: 370.

Sunamoto, J., Iwamoto, K., Kondo, H. and Shinkai, S., 1980,
Liposomal membranes VI. Polysaccharide-induced aggregation of
multilamellar liposomes of egg lecithin, J. Biochem., 88: 1219.

Szoka, F. and Papahadjopoulos, D., 1980, Comparative properties
and methods of preparation of lipid vesicles (liposomes), Ann.
Rev. Biophys. Bioeng., 9: 567.

Takeuchi, Y. and Nikaido, H., 1981, Persistence of segregated
phospholipid domains in phospholipid-lipopolysaccharide mixed
bilayers: Studies with spin-labelled phospholipids, Biochemistry,

20: 523.

Tom, B.H., 1980, An overview: liposomes and immunobiology - macrophages, liposomes and tailored immunity, in: "Liposomes and
immunobiology," B.H. Tom and H.R. Six, eds., Elsevier, Amsterdam.

Torchilin, V.P., Khaw, B.A., Smirnov, V.N. and Haber, E., 1979,
Preservation of antimyosin antibody activity after covalent
coupling to liposomes; Biochim. Biophys. Res. Commun., 89: 1114.

Torchilin, V.P., Berdichevsky, V.R., Barsukiv, A.A. and Smirnov, V.N.,
1980, Coating liposomes with protein decreases their capture
by macrophages, FEBS Letters, 111: 184.

Unanue, E.R., 1978, The regulation of lymphocyte functions by the
macrophage, Immun. Rev., 40: 227.

Van Houte, A.J., Snippe, H. and Willers, J.M.N., 1979, Characterization of immunogenic properties of haptenated liposomal model
membranes in mice. I. Thymus independence of the antigen,
Immunology, 37: 505.

Van Rooijen, N. and Streefkerk, J.G., 1976, Autoradiography and
immunohistoperoxidase techniques applied to the same tissue
section, J. Immunol. Meth., 10: 379.

Van Rooijen, N. and Van Nieuwmegen, R., 1977, Liposomes in immunology: The immune response against antigen-containing liposomes,
Immunol. Commun., 6: 489.

Van Rooijen, N. and Van Nieuwmegen, R., 1978a, Liposomes in immunology: Further evidence for the adjuvant activity of liposomes,
Immunol. Commun., 7: 635.

Van Rooijen, N. and Van Nieuwmegen, R., 1978b, Fluorochrome staining
of multilamellar liposomes, Stain Technol., 53: 307.

Van Rooijen, N. and Van Nieuwmegen, R., 1979a, Liposomes in immunology: Impairment of the adjuvant effect of liposomes by incorporation of the adjuvant lysolecithin and the role of macrophages, Immunol. Commun., 8: 381.

Van Rooijen, N. and Van Nieuwmegen, R., 1979b, Attempts to study the
localization of liposomes and liposome entrapped antigen in the
spleen, Acta Histochem., 65: 41.

Van Rooijen, N. and Van Nieuwmegen, R., 1980a, Liposomes in immunology: Evidence that their adjuvant effect results from surface
exposition of the antigens, Cell. Immunol., 49: 402.

Van Rooijen, N. and Van Nieuwmegen, R., 1980b, Liposomes in immunology: Multilamellar phosphatidylcholine liposomes as a simple,
biodegradable and harmless adjuvant without any immunogenic
activity of its own, Immunol. Commun., 9: 243.

Van Rooijen, N. and Van Nieuwmegen, R., 1980c, Endotoxin enhanced
adjuvant effect of liposomes, particularly when antigen and
endotoxin are incorporated within the same liposome, Immunol.
Commun., 9: 747.

Van Rooijen, N., Van Nieuwmegen, R. and Kors, N., 1981, The secondary
immune response against liposome associated antigens, Immunol.
Commun: in press.

Weissmann, G., Brand, A. and Franklin, E.C., 1974, Interaction of
immunoglobulins with liposomes, J. Clin. Invest., 53: 536.

Yasuda, T., Dancey, G.F. and Kinsky, S.C., 1977, Immunogenic proper-
    ties of liposomal model membranes in mice, J. Immunol.,
    119: 1863.
Zborowski, J., Roerdink, F. and Scherphof, G., 1977, Leakage of
    sucrose from phosphatidylcholine liposomes induced by inter-
    action with serum albumin, Biochim. Biophys. Acta., 497: 183.

ADJUVANT EFFECT OF LIPOSOME PRESENTATION OF

SOLUBLE TUMOUR ASSOCIATED ANTIGEN

D. Gerlier* and J.F. Doré

INSERM U218 Centre Léon Bérard
28 rue Laënnec
69373 Lyon Cedex 2, France

Lack of immunogenicity of cell surface antigen when dissociated from cell membranes has centred on the use of liposomes since they can mimic cell surface presentation (Curman et al., 1978, Enghelhard et al., 1978). Moreover, liposomes have been shown to act as an adjuvant (Kinsky and Nicolotti, 1977) and strong enhancement of the antibody response has been described for protein antigens such as diphtheria toxin (Allison and Gregoriadis, 1974), hepatitis B surface antigen (Gregoriadis and Manesis, 1980), and serum albumins or gamma-globulins (Heath et al., 1976, Van Rooijen and Van Nieuwmegen, 1977-1979). Therefore incorporation of tumour cell surface antigen into liposomes could prove to be of utmost interest. We have developed the association with liposomes of Gross Cell Surface Antigen (GCSAa) (Gerlier et al., 1978), a major cell surface antigen of protein nature, (Ledbetter and Nowinski, 1977, Snyder et al., 1977), associated with Gross virus induced lymphomas in mouse (Old et al., 1965) and rat (Geering et al., 1966). Immunogenicity of GCSAa sensitized liposomes has been studied in syngeneic animals (Gerlier et al., 1980a, b). GCSAa appears to play an important role in host tumour relationship and can induce high antibody response in syngeneic rats (Gerlier et al., 1977). Immunochemical characteristics of the association with liposome of GCSAa have been described previously (Sakai et al., 1980) and liposome presentation of this antigen has been shown to succeed in inducing cytotoxic antibodies to GCSAa reaching in some instances the level obtained following immunization with viable syngeneic tumour cells. Our present purpose is to further study the requirements for obtaining an adjuvant effect of liposome presentation in this tumour model.

---

* Attaché de Recherche at CNRS

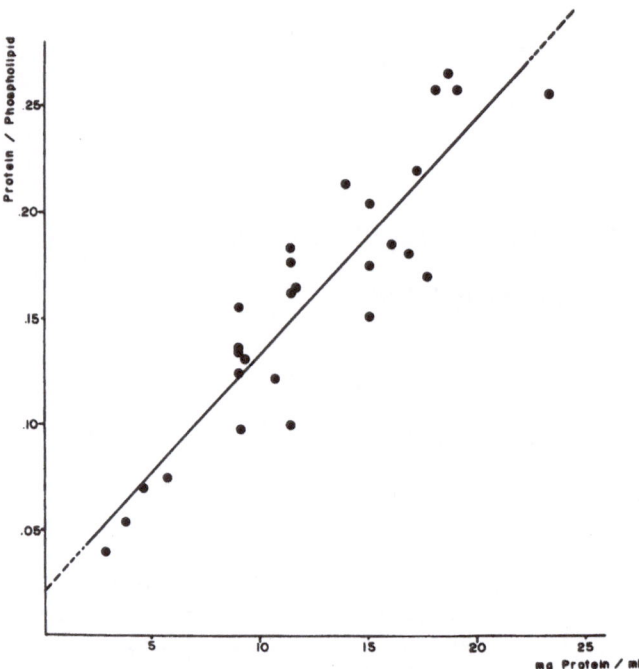

Fig. 1.   Association of proteins with liposomes as a function of
           protein concentration of the sensitizing cellular extracts.

ASSOCIATION OF GROSS VIRUS ASSOCIATED CELL SURFACE ANTIGEN WITH
LIPOSOMES.

     Gross Cell Surface Antigen (GCSAa) was extracted by solubiliza-
tion of (C58NT)D lymphoma cells or purified membranes with NP40
detergent and partially purified after 60% ammonium sulfate precipitation and Sephadex G200 filtration (Gerlier et al., 1978). Negatively charged multilamellar liposomes were prepared as described by
Gregoriadis et al., (1971); details of liposome sensitization with
GCSAa have been reported in previous work (Sakai et al., 1980).
Briefly, a film of dipalmitoyl phosphatidylcholine, cholesterol and
dicetylphosphate in 7:2:1 molar ratio, was dispersed in antigenic
extract. The amount of protein associated with liposomes was found
to be proportional to the protein concentration of the sensitizing
cellular extract (Fig. 1) and to the amount of phospholipids used and,
under defined conditions, 22-25% proteins of the cellular extract
could be associated with liposomes. Analysis of disrupted sensitized
liposomes showed that the GCSAa specific activity of the liposome
associated proteins was quite similar to that of the proteins of the
sensitizing cellular extract. Ultracentrifugation of disrupted liposomes showed that about 75% of the liposome associated GCSAa activity
was firmly associated with lipids and that little GCSAa was entrapped
within aqueous compartments between lipidic lamellae. 1.8-8.0% of

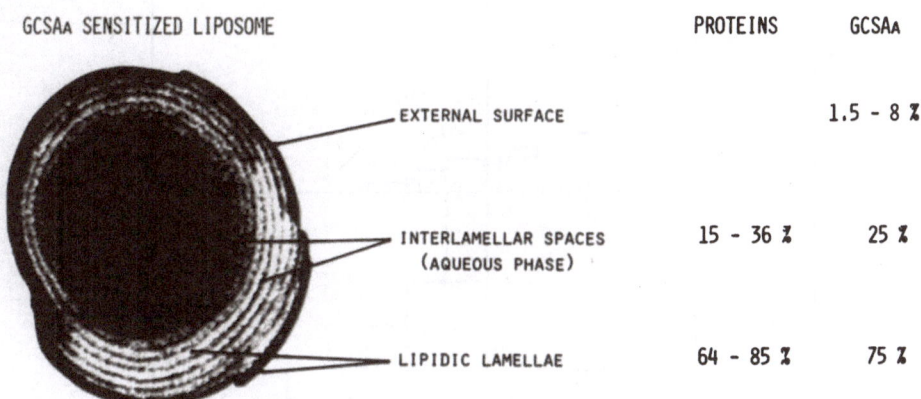

Fig. 2.   Distribution of protein and GCSAa activity within
          sensitized liposomes.

the liposome associated GCSAa was expressed at the liposome surface
(Fig. 2). Storage experiments at +4°C showed that GCSAa sensitized
liposomes were fairly stable.

IMMUNOGENICITY OF SOLUBILIZED OR LIPOSOME ASSOCIATED GCSAa

Influence of the Source of Antigen

     Groups of W/Fu rats were immunized by two subcutaneous injections
given at five week intervals with GCSAa preparations containing 0.5
to 2mg of proteins. Solubilized GCSAa was used as immunogen and
presented either as soluble antigen or as GCSAa sensitized liposomes
mixed in Complete Freund Adjuvant (CFA). Sera from animals under
immunization were tested for antibody to GCSAa using a complement
dependent cytotoxicity test as previously described (Gerlier et al.,
1977). Controls of the specificity of GCSAa detection in this cytotoxicity test were performed by absorbing sera on mouse normal
lymphoid cells, EδG2 lymphoma cells, or GCSAa negative lymphoma cells
as previously described (Gerlier et al., 1981).

     Injection of liposome containing GCSAa prepared from whole cells
and emulsified in CFA induced antibody titer (AT) of 32 or above 13/25
rats whereas most of the rats (24/26) receiving soluble antigen mixed
with CFA failed to develop a significant antibody response (Fig. 3a).

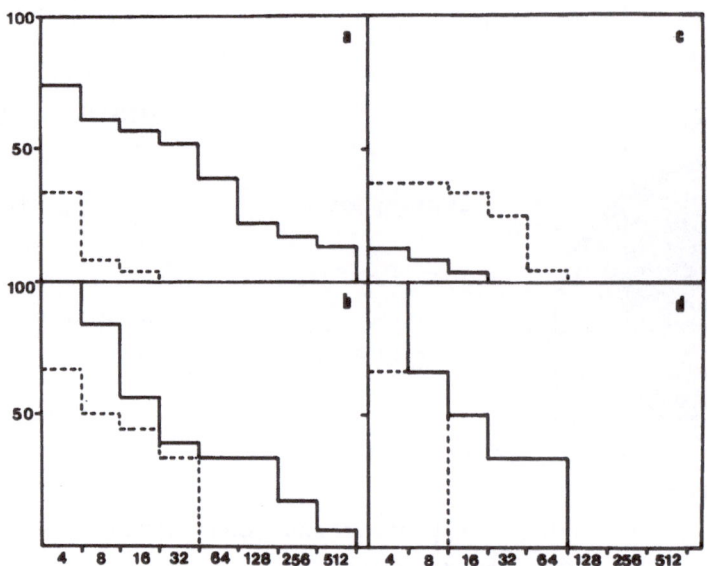

Fig. 3.   Cumulative percentage of antibody response (antibody titer)
           of rats immunized with GCSAa sensitized liposomes (————)
           or soluble antigen (------) extracted from (a) whole tumour
           cells, (b) cytosol, (c) purified cell membranes, (d) mixture
           of cytosol and purified cell membranes. All preparations
           were emulsified in CFA before injection.

Moreover, this strong adjuvant effect of liposomes was confirmed by
kinetic studies which showed that antibody response could mimic that
elicited by viable tumour cells (Gerlier et al., 1980a, b). In order
to determine the localisation of immunogenic GCSAa soluble antigenic
extracts were also prepared from the soluble part of cells (cytosol)
or from purified cell membranes. GCSAa solubilized by NP40 from cell
membranes, although containing a similar amount of serologically
detectable antigen (Gerlier et al. in preparation) were unable to
induce a significant antibody response even after association with
liposomes (Fig. 3c) whereas GCSAa prepared from cytosol showed a good
adjuvant effect of liposome presentation (AT $\geqslant$ 128 in 6/18 rats),
the soluble antigen eliciting poor antibody response (AT $\leqslant$ 8 in 11/18
rats, AT $>$ 32 in 0/18 rats) (Fig. 3b). To exclude an adverse effect
of antigen prepared from cell membranes on the immune response to
GCSAa, a control experiment was done where liposomes were sensitized
with a mixture of soluble antigen prepared from cell membranes and
cytosol (Fig. 3d) : this source of antigen was as immunogenic as
GCSAa prepared from whole cells when included in liposomes.

Requirement for a Macrophage Stimulating Agent

From these results it can be questioned as to the role of admixture of CFA on the expression of the adjuvant effect of liposome presentation. GCSAa prepared from whole cells or cytosol were injected into rats using the above procedure either as soluble antigen or as GCSAa sensitized liposomes mixed with saline, CFA, Incomplete Freund's adjuvant (IFA) or live BCG microorganisms. As previously described, a strong adjuvant effect of liposome presentation was observed when antigen preparations were injected mixed in CFA (Fig.4d) (AT$\geqslant$16 in 8/15 rats for sensitized liposomes, AT$\geqslant$16 in 2/16 rats for soluble antigen). Similar adjuvant effect of liposome presentation was observed when IFA was used instead of CFA (AT$\geqslant$8 in 6/6 for sensitized liposomes, AT$>$4 in 2/6 rats for soluble antigen, Fig. 4b). On the contrary no adjuvant effect of liposomes was obtained when antigen preparations were injected alone or mixed with live BCG microorganisms (2mg/rat) (Fig. 3a, 3c). Thus in this model, results suggest that expression of liposome adjuvant effect required the presence of a non antigenic macrophage stimulating agent.

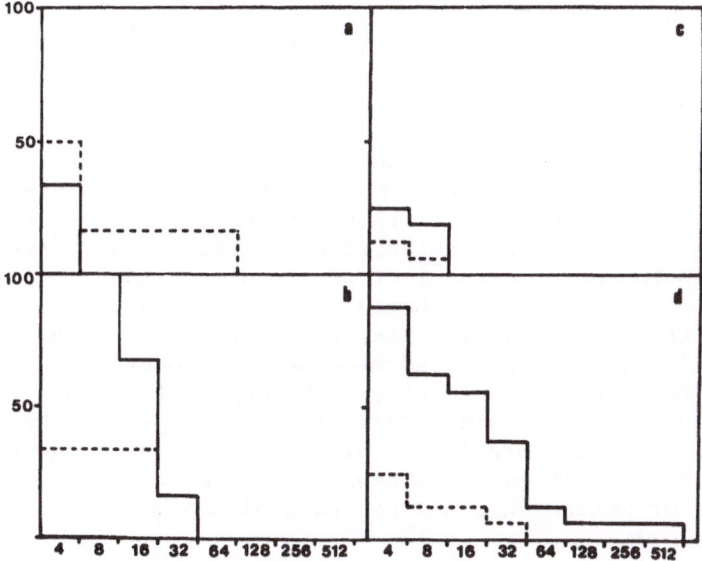

Fig. 4.   Cumulative percentage of antibody response of rats immunized with GCSAa sensitized liposomes (————) or soluble antigen (------) mixed with (a) saline, (b) Incomplete Freund's Adjuvant, (c) 2mg live BCG (d) Complete Freund's adjuvant.

Requirement for Constitutive Association with Lipids

To elucidate whether liposomes are a true secondary adjuvant by themselves or act as membrane presentation of antigen, the following experiment was carried out : rats were immunized twice with soluble antigen, soluble antigen mixed with empty liposomes or GCSAa sensitized liposomes, these preparations being emulsified in CFA, and secondary antibody responses were recorded. As shown in Fig. 5, injection of GCSAa sensitized liposomes elicited very good antibody response (AT $\geqslant$ 64 in 4/10 rats) whereas no significant antibody response was induced after immunization with either soluble antigen (AT = 8 in 1/10 rats) or soluble antigen and empty liposomes (AT $>$ 4 in 0/6 rats). Thus constitutive association with lipids is a prerequisite for the adjuvant effect of liposome presentation of solubilized tumour associated antigen.

Role of Phospholipid Composition

Liposomes made of four different phospholipids, dipalmitoyl phosphatidylcholine (DPPC), dimyristoyl phosphatidylcholine (DMPC), sphingomyelin (SM), and egg lecithin (EL) were tested in their ability to show an adjuvant effect. Antibody response evoked in rats receiving these sensitized liposomes mixed with CFA was compared with that of animals receiving soluble antigen emulsified in CFA. Results are shown in Fig. 6. A good adjuvant effect of liposome presentation was observed when DPPC, SM or EL were used (Fig. 6a, 6b, 6d). However liposomes made of DMPC showed no adjuvant effect (Fig. 6c).

DISCUSSION AND CONCLUDING REMARKS

Association of a protein tumour associated antigen with liposomes have clearly shown that liposomes may exert a strong adjuvant effect on the immunogenic properties of this antigen (Gerlier et al. 1980a,b). GCSAa, a cell surface tumour associated antigen can be extracted either from whole cells, cytosol or purified membranes, but only cytosol (and whole cells) extract showed good immunogenic properties when associated with liposomes. The lack of immunogenic properties of antigen solubilized from purified membranes was unexpected and it is not unlikely that the presence of a high amount of residual detergent in the membrane extract could interfere with the physicochemical structure of liposomes and might be toxic for macrophages. However in another tumour model it has also been described that cytosol was a better source of immunogenic antigen than plasma membranes (Dubois et al. 1980).

Our preliminary studies (Gerlier et al. 1980a,b) have raised the question of the mechanisms of liposome adjuvant effect and prerequisite of complete Freund's adjuvant was first established. From our recent results, the expression of liposome adjuvant effect appears to depend on two requirements : constitutive association with lipids

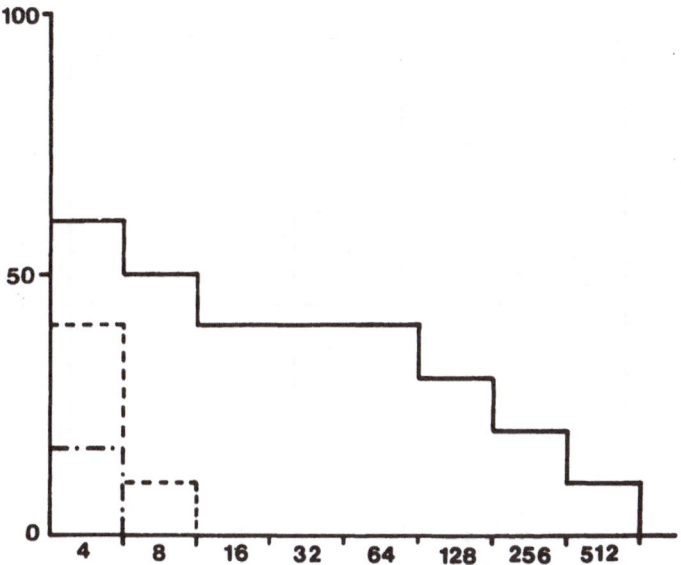

Fig. 5.   Cumulative percentage of antibody response of rats
immunized with GCSAa sensitized liposomes (————) soluble
antigen (-----) or soluble antigen and empty liposomes
(—·—·—·). All preparations were emulsified in CFA
before injection.

and presence of macrophage stimulating agent.   Constitutive
association with lipids can fulfil two roles : 1) a depot effect
i.e. a slow release system, or 2) a "membrane presentation effect".
Depot effect of liposomes have been previously suggested (Van Rooijen
and Van Nieuwmegen, 1977, Allison and Gregoriadis, 1974, Heath et al.
1976) and a progressive digestion of antigen sensitized plurilamellar
liposomes by macrophages is likely to occur (Tyrrell et al., 1976).
Membrane presentation effect is suggested by the findings of Curman
et al. (1978) and Enghelhard et al. (1978) who have shown that major
histocompatibility antigens must be exposed on membranes to stimulate
presensitized lymphocytes in vitro. In our system a depot effect per
se is unlikely to be sufficient to explain liposome adjuvant effect
on GCSAa since a similar slow release system represented by soluble
antigen emulsified in CFA was not able to induce a significant antibody response. This suggests that a membrane presentation effect of
liposomes may be at least one of the mechanisms of adjuvant effect.
Need of Freund's adjuvant has been also described to reveal adjuvant
properties of liposomes when used as hapten carriers (Nicolotti et al.
1976) and a macrophage activation by liposomes has been postulated
(Van Rooijen and Van Nieuwmegen, 1979). Results observed with GCSAa
indicated that a factor with activity towards macrophages should be

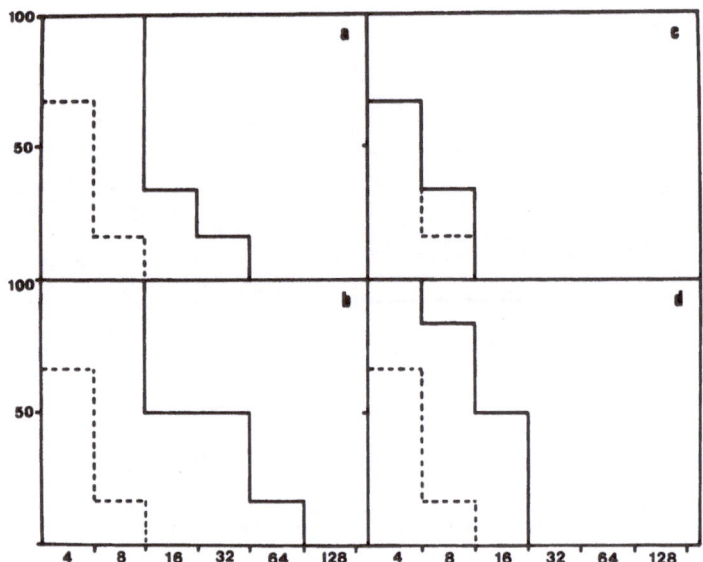

Fig. 6. Cumulative percentage of antibody response of rats immunized
with soluble antigen (-----) or GCSAa sensitized liposomes
(———) made of (a) dipalmitoyl phosphatidylcholine,
(b) sphingomyelin, (c) dimyristoyl phosphatidylcholine,
(d) egg lecithin. All preparations were emulsified in CFA
before injection.

present. The inability of live BCG to play this role may be related
to its strong antigenicity which could interfere with the anti-GCSAa
immune response. However preliminary results obtained in our laboratory have indicated that a powerful chemotactic product included in
the GCSAa sensitized liposomes can replace Freund's adjuvant. Then
it can be concluded that liposome presentation of tumour associated
antigen exerts an adjuvant effect by presenting the antigen on membranes and by acting as a slow release system, provided that a macrophage active product is present. The exact role of this macrophage
active product (chemotaxism, macrophage activation) is currently
under investigation.

     Conflicting reports have been made concerning the role of phos-
pholipid composition on adjuvant properties of liposomes. Transition
temperature of phospholipids has been described to be critical;
and for Heath et al. (1976) high transition temperature phospholipids
were less immunogenic but direct correlation between liposomal immunogenicity and transition temperature of the phospholipids was found by
Yasuda et al. (1977). No such correlations could be drawn from our

results with GCSAa.   Incorporation of two phospholipids with high
(DPPC 41.5°C, SM 42°C) and one low (EL) transition temperature was
successful in showing an adjuvant effect.   In this model it is more
likely that the physicochemical relations between antigen and phospholipids may be of importance as shown by the lack of adjuvant effect
of DMPC liposomes, the level of protein and antigen incorporation in
these liposomes being lower than observed with other phospholipids
(data not shown).

In conclusion, the adjuvant effect of liposomes exerted on tumour
associated cell surface antigen represents a good model to explore the
mechanisms of cell surface antigen immunogenicity and as a consequence,
a new approach for active immunotherapy of cancer.

ACKNOWLEDGEMENTS

The skilful technical assistance of Mrs. T. Avice and J. Geneve
is gratefully acknowledged.   This work was supported by a grant from
INSERM (CRL 78-4-186-2) and partly by a grant from DGRST (75-7-1369).

REFERENCES

Allison, A.C., and Gregoriadis, G., 1974, Liposomes as immunological
      adjuvants, Nature, 252: 252.
Curman, B., Ostberg, L., and Peterson, P.A., 1978, Incorporation of
      murine MHC antigens into liposomes and their effect in secondary
      mixed lymphocyte reaction, Nature, 272: 545.
Dubois, G.C., Appella, E., Law, L.W., Peleo, A.B. and Old, L.J.,
      1980, Immunogenic properties of soluble cytosol fractions of
      MethA sarcoma cells, Cancer Res., 40: 4204.
Engelhard, V.H., Strominger, J.L., Mescher, M., and Burakoff, S.,
      1978, Induction of secondary cytotoxic T lymphocytes by purified
      HL-A and HLA-B antigens reconstituted into phospholipid vesicles,
      Proc. Nat. Acad. Sci. USA., 75: 5688.
Geering, G., Old, L.J., and Boyse, E.A., 1966, Antigens of leukemias
      induced by naturally occurring murine leukemia virus : their
      relation to the antigen of Gross virus and other murine leukemia
      viruses, J. Exp. Med., 124: 753.
Gerlier, D., Gisselbrecht, S., Guillemain, B., and Doré, J.F., 1981,
      Measurement of Gross Cell Surface Antigen and p30 level in
      murine retrovirus-infected cell lines, Brit. J. Cancer, 43:
      in press.
Gerlier, D., Guibout, C., and Doré, J.F., 1977, Highly cytotoxic
      antisera obtained in W/Fu rats against a syngeneic Gross virus
      induced lymphoma, Europ. J. Cancer, 13: 855.
Gerlier, D., Sakai, F. and Doré, J.F., 1978, Inclusion d'un antigene
      de surface cellulaire associe au virus de Gross dans des
      liposomes, C.R. Acad. Sci., serie D 286: 439.
Gerlier, D., Sakai, F., and Doré, J.F., 1980a, Induction of antibody
      response to liposome associated Gross virus cell surface antigen

GCSAa, Brit. J. Cancer, 41: 236.

Gerlier, D., Sakai, F. and Doré, J.F., 1980b, Antibody response evoked in syngeneic animals by a cell surface tumour antigen induced into liposomes, in: "Biology of the Cancer Cell," K., Letnansky, ed., Kugler Publications, Amsterdam.

Gregoriadis, G., Leathwood, P.D., and Ryman, B.E., 1971, Enzyme entrapment in liposomes, FEBS Lett., 14: 95.

Gregoriadis, G., and Manesis, E.K., 1980, Liposomes as immunological adjuvants for hepatitis B surface antigens, in: "Liposomes and Immunobiology," B.H. Tom and H.R. Six, eds., Elsevier/North-Holland, New York.

Heath, T.D., Edwards, D.C. and Ryman, B.E., 1976, The adjuvant properties of liposomes, Biochem. Soc. Trans., 4: 129.

Kinsky, S.C. and Nicolotti, R.A., 1977, Immunological properties of model membranes, Ann. Rev. Biochem., 46: 49.

Ledbetter, J. and Nowinsky, R.C., 1977, Identification of the Gross Cell Surface Antigen associated with murine leukemia virus infected cells, J. Virol., 23: 315.

Nicolotti, R.A., Kochibe, N. and Kinsky, S.C., 1976, Comparative immunogeneic properties of N-substituted phosphatidylethanolamine derivatives and liposomal model membranes, J. Immunol., 117: 1898.

Old, L.J., Boyse, E.A. and Stockert, E., 1965, The G(Gross) leukemia antigen, Cancer Res., 25: 813.

Sakai, F., Gerlier, D. and Doré, J.F., 1980, Association of Gross virus associated cell surface antigen (GCSAa) with liposomes, Brit. J. Cancer, 41: 227.

Snyder, H.W., Stockert, E. and Fleissner, E., 1977, Characterization of molecular species carrying Gross cell surface antigen, J. Virol., 23: 302.

Tyrrell, D.A., Heath, T.D., Colley, C.M. and Ryman, B.E., 1976, New aspects of liposomes, Biochim. Biophys. Acta, 457: 259.

Van Rooijen, N., and Van Nieuwmegen, R., 1977, Liposomes in immunology: the immune response against antigen-containing liposomes, Immunol. Comm., 6: 489.

Van Rooijen, N., and Van Nieuwmegen, R., 1978, Liposomes immunology: Further evidence for the adjuvant activity of liposomes, Immunol. Comm., 7: 635.

Van Rooijen, N. and Van Nieuwmegen, R., 1979, Liposomes immunology: Impairment of the adjuvant effect of liposomes by incorporation of the adjuvant lysolecithin and the role of macrophages, Immunol. Comm., 8: 381.

Yasuda, T., Dancey, G.F. and Kinsky, S.C., 1977, Immunogenicity of liposomal model membranes in mice: dependence on phospholipid composition, Proc. Nat. Acad. Sci. USA., 74: 1234.

THERAPEUTIC POTENTIAL OF LIPOSOMES AS CARRIERS IN

LEISHMANIASIS, MALARIA, AND VACCINES

Carl R. Alving

Department of Membrane Biochemistry
Walter Reed Army Institute of Research
Washington, DC 20012, USA

INTRODUCTION

Since the first suggestion, approximately ten years ago, that lipid vesicles might have practical uses in medicine, liposomes have been a treatment in search of a disease. The approach of my laboratory since 1976 has been to search for clinical applications among infectious diseases. Because parenterally injected liposomes natually travel in great amounts to the liver and spleen I felt, at least at the beginning of our research, that attempts to tailor liposomes to particular diseases by artificially targeting the vesicles to areas other than the liver and spleen, might be difficult. Therefore, my colleagues and I have concentrated only on diseases in which the liver and spleen play an important, or even a crucial, role.

As it happens, parasites that cause two important diseases, namely visceral leishmaniasis (kala azar) and malaria, during some parts of their life cycles reside either exclusively or predominately in liver or spleen cells. Each of these diseases is among the six diseases targeted for particular attention by the World Health Organization.[1]

It was not purely a coincidence that we happened to select these parasitic diseases as research foci. Our efforts and thoughts were greatly aided by the traditional interest in tropical medicine, and large ongoing programs of research in leishmaniasis and malaria, at the Walter Reed Army Institute of Research (WRAIR). In particular, Drs. Edgar Steck, Larry Hendricks and Imogene Schneider, and Mr. Glenn Swartz at WRAIR, and Drs. William Hanson and Willie Chapman, and Miss Virginia Waits, under a drug testing contract from WRAIR to

the University of Georgia School of Veterinary Medicine in Athens,
Georgia, have been major contributors to various aspects of this
program. Publications from this research relating to leishmaniasis
are in refs. 2-4 (reviewed in 5), and on malaria in ref. 6.

Prior to our large scale commitment to tropical disease research, my laboratory had (and still has) a considerable interest in
basic aspects of the immunology of lipids and liposomes.[7] We have
now also performed numerous experiments directed to the use of liposomes as carriers of antigens and as adjuvants, that is, as vehicles
for vaccines. We have devised a useful model employing lipid A as
as an adjuvant, and cholera toxin as a model protein antigen.[8-10]
In the course of these immunological studies, we found that liposomes sometimes were immunosuppressive in animals, and both of
these effects, immunopotentiation and immunosuppression, will be
discussed.

This paper describes some of the strategy used and some of the
data obtained in each of the areas mentioned above, namely leishmaniasis, malaria, and immunological aspects of liposomes as carriers.

LEISHMANIASIS

The causative organism in leishmaniasis is a protozoan parasite
that lives almost exclusively in fixed macrophages of the reticuloendothelial system. The clinical disease is determined by the site
of infection, and the site is usually determined by the species of
leishmanial organism. Three general types of clinical leishmaniasis
occur: cutaneous, mucocutaneous, and visceral (kala azar). The
visceral form mainly infects macrophages in liver, spleen and bone
marrow, and in its untreated state is nearly 100% fatal. Treatment
of leishmaniasis, particularly in the less life-threatening cutaneous forms, often is difficult. This is partly because the drugs
employed can be quite toxic, and since doses are usually limited
treatment failures are common. In addition, a recurrent problem
is the emergence of leishmanial strains resistant to the standard
antimonial drug treatment. Depending on the patient population
examined, antimony-resistant visceral leishmanial infections can
constitute anywhere from 5% to 46% of the cases encountered.[11]

We, and others, have demonstrated that when standard antimonial
drugs, such as meglumine antimoniate (Glucantime®) or sodium stibogluconate (Pentostam®) are employed, the liposome-encapsulated drugs
are hundreds of times more effective than unencapsulated drugs in
treating experimental visceral leishmaniasis of rodents.[2-4,12,13]
Actually, the quantitative assessment of the relative effectiveness
of the drugs can be readily inflated, or deflated, depending on numerous variables in the rodent model. One such variable is the length
of time that elapses between infection and initiation of treatment.

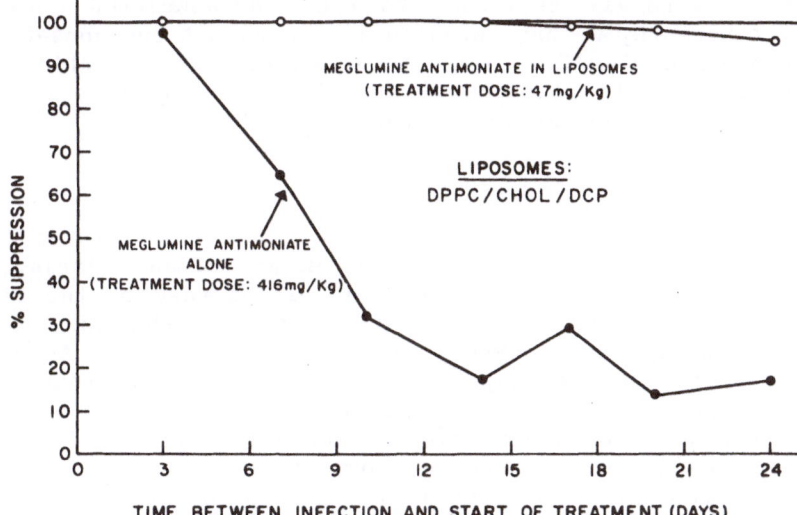

TIME BETWEEN INFECTION AND START OF TREATMENT (DAYS)

Fig. 1.   Effects of length of leishmanial infection on the efficacies of liposome-encapsulated and unencapsulated drugs.
Each point is the mean of 10-14 hamsters. The animals
were infected, treated with a single intracardial injection, and suppression of hepatic parasites was measured,
as described elsewhere.[2,3]

As shown in Fig. 1, in treating hamsters the relative efficacy
of therapy falls off as the infection becomes more chronic, regardless of whether encapsulated or unencapsulated drug is employed.
However, under the conditions shown, even at almost a tenfold greater dose, the unencapsulated drug loses effectiveness much more
rapidly than the liposome-encapsulated drug. In fact, it is easily
possible to select an infection that is sufficiently chronic that
the encapsulated drug is thousands of times better than the unencapsulated drug. That is to say, liposome-encapsulated drugs can be
highly effective when the infection is so far advanced that unencapsulated drugs are essentially useless. The effectiveness of liposomes in advanced leishmanial infections may be fortuitous since
chronic infections are the most likely types to be encountered in
the field, and are most likely to present severe clinical problems.

Will the liposomes be as effective in clinical practice in humans as they are in the experimental animal models? Only time will
tell, of course, but there are many additional optimistic signs.
For example, as mentioned above, one notable problem frequently
encountered in chemotherapy of leishmaniasis is the appearance of
antimony-resistant organisms. In recent preliminary unpublished
testing we found outstanding efficacy of a liposome-encapsulated
antimonial drug against an infection that had been carefully deve-

loped to be strongly resistant to the unencapsulated antimonial
drug. Furthermore, we have previously shown that one nonantimonial
drug, an 8-aminoquinoline called WR 6026, has marked antileishmanial effectiveness in liposomes,[4] and this effectiveness also will
probably extend to antimony-resistant infections.

MALARIA

In the life cycle of all forms of mammalian malaria, after
sporozoite forms are injected into the bloodstream by the bite of
an anopheline mosquito, the parasite must pass through the liver
prior to entering erythrocytes. In rodents, the parasite resides
in the liver for several days, and in humans for more than a week.
During this prolonged period in the liver the organism multiplies
and is transformed morphologically, biochemically and biologically
from a sporozoite to a hepatic form (hepatic schizont). After
leaving the liver the parasite enters the blood where it is then
free to enter erythrocytes to become an erythrocyte schizont. The
erythrocyte schizonts are easily visualized and quantified on a

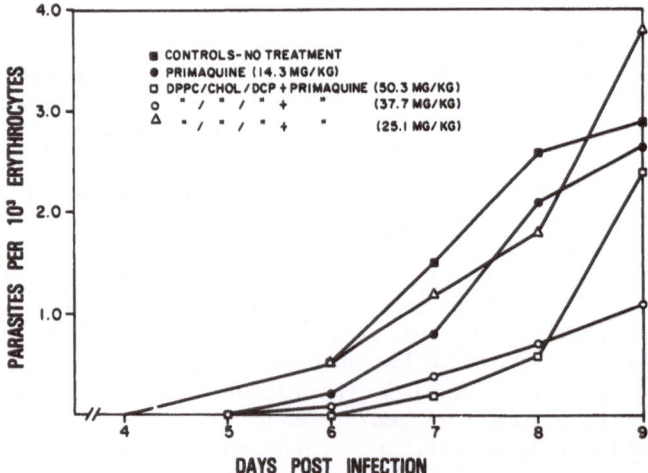

Fig. 2.   Anti-malarial effects of liposome-encapsulated primaquine
           diphosphate. The liposomes were prepared, drug was encap-
           sulated, and extraction of liposomes for drug analysis was
           done, as described before.[2,3] The drug was quantified by
           phosphate analysis. The mice (3-7 animals for each point)
           were injected i.v. with sporozoites (Plasmodium berghei);
           the indicated drugs were injected i.v. 1 day later; and
           parasitemia was checked each day.[6]

blood smear, and an animal that has these forms is said to have a "patent" infection.

Chemotherapy of malaria typically is keyed to a single stage of the life cycle.[14] For example, chloroquine affects only erythrocytic forms, whereas primaquine affects only hepatic schizonts. Our initial approach was to utilize liposome-encapsulated primaquine to treat sporozoite-induced malaria. All of the work on malaria was performed in collaboration with Dr. Imogene Schneider, Director of the Mosquito Colony and Sporozoite Laboratory at WRAIR.

Sporozoites (Plasmodium berghei) obtained from salivary glands of mosquitos were injected into mice. One day later a therapeutic formulation, such as primaquine or a liposome preparation, was injected i.v., and therapeutic efficacy was assessed by quantifying the number of erythrocytic forms that appeared over a period of weeks. As shown in Fig. 2, the parasitemia that appeared was not substantially changed by liposome-encapsulated primaquine compared to unencapsulated primaquine. This conclusion has also been reported by Pirson et al.[15] We also found a substantial drop in the lethal toxicity (LD$_{50}$) of liposome-encapsulated primaquine (not shown), and this again confirms results of Pirson et al.[15]

Undaunted by the above failure (Fig. 2) to obtain increased efficacy of primaquine by liposomes, we decided to try "intrahepatic targeting" of liposomes. Our reasoning was as follows. The hepatic schizont stage is known to reside in hepatocytes. The liposome-encapsulated drug might have been taken up by Kupffer cells (and other macrophages) and degraded or diluted in body fluids at a distance from hepatocytes. We felt that if the liposomes contained a glycoconjugate, such as a glycolipid, then they might have an increased affinity for hepatocytes because of the carbohydrate-binding lectin on hepatocyte plasma membranes earlier described by Ashwell and colleagues.[16] Previous reports indeed have shown increased hepatic uptake of liposomes containing glycolipids.[17,18]

We found, to our amazement, that control liposomes that contained glycolipid in the lipid bilayer, but which lacked primaquine, had strong antimalarial properties (Fig. 3).[6] Although not shown, even glycolipids alone, without liposomes, were equally effective as antimalarial agents.

Why did the striking antimalarial effects of liposomal glycolipids occur? Originally, we thought that all of the parasites had entered into hepatocytes prior to onset of treatment with liposomes. We suggested[6] that the hepatocyte lectin, much of which reportedly is in cytoplasmic structures,[19,20] was recognized by the parasite, and that the lectin served some vital role in the intrahepatic development of the organism. The liposomal glycolipids may have blocked parasite development at a crucial stage by binding to the lectin.[6]

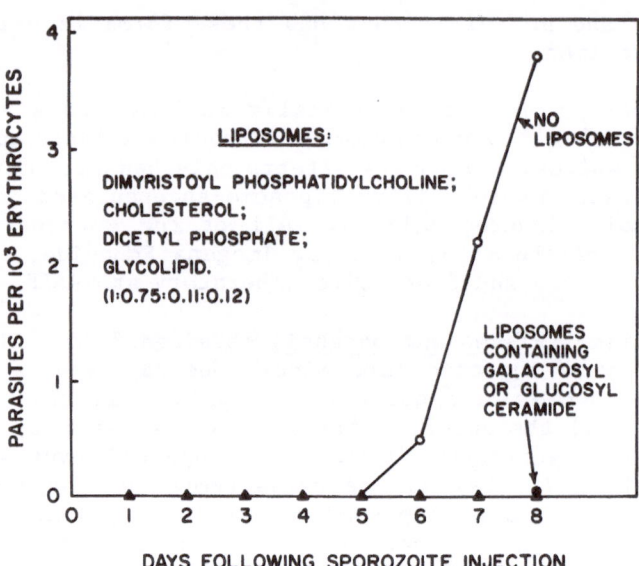

Fig. 3.   Antimalarial effects of liposomes containing glycolipids
           but lacking primaquine.   See legend to Fig. 2 for experi-
           mental details.   From Alving et al.[6]

An alternative hypothesis to the one given above is that the
hepatocyte lectin serves as a plasma membrane receptor for entry of
the parasite, and that glycolipids block the receptor. This hypothesis is based on the suggestion by Danforth et al.[21] that the
parasite enters the Kūpffer cell prior to transferring through the
space of Disse to the hepatocyte.   In collaboration with Dr.
Masamichi Aikawa at Case-Western Reserve University, we have found
electron microscopic evidence supporting this hypothesis. We observed parasites in Kūpffer cells at 24 hours after injection, and
in the interhepatocyte space at 44 hours after injection of parasites into mice. If the Danforth mechanism of intrahepatic parasite
movement were true, then one might expect that the liposomal glycolipids would only be effective during a relatively short interval
starting at approximately 24 hrs after injection of parasites, and
this was observed. The glycolipids only cured the infection when
they were used 24 hrs after injection of parasites, and they were
not effective when injected 1 day before, at the same time as, or
3 days after, injection of parasites.[6,22]

After obtaining the above results, the question arose whether
liposomal glycolipids would enhance the therapeutic efficacy of
liposome-encapsulated primaquine? The answer is that they cause an
enormous enhancement.   Figure 4 shows that liposomal glycolipids
still cause 50% suppression (SD_{50}) when diluted by 1:46,000. The

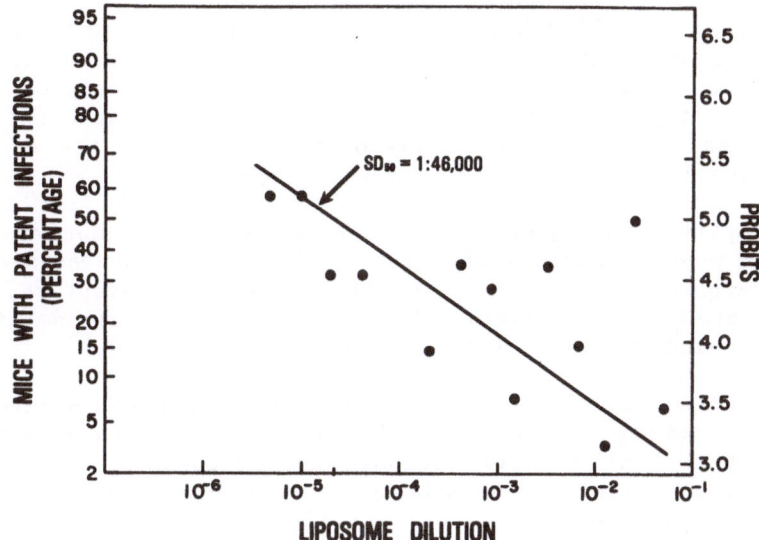

Fig. 4.   Antimalarial effects of diluted liposomes containing galactosyl ceramide. See Figs. 2 and 3 for liposome composition and experimental details. Each point is the mean of
7-27 mice. SD_{50} is dose that reduces the number of animals having blood forms (patency) by 50% compared with
control animals treated only with isotonic saline.

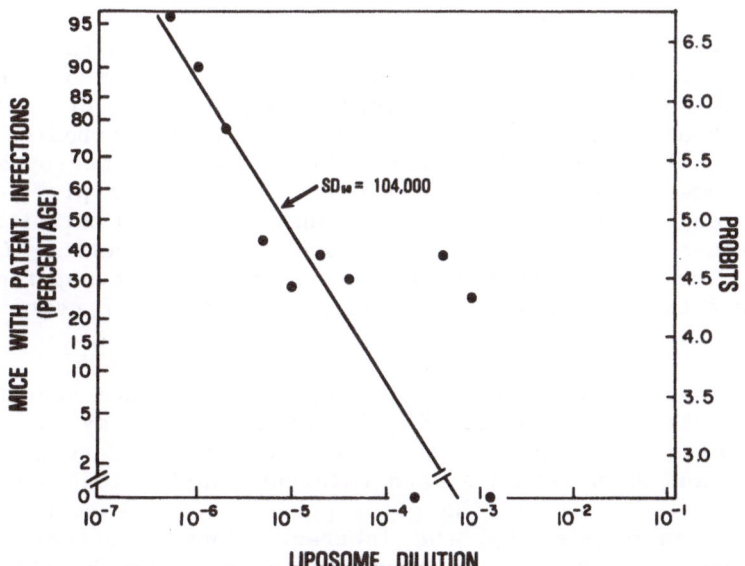

Fig. 5.   Effects of liposomes containing both galactosyl ceramide
and encapsulated primaquine. See Figs. 2-4 for experimental details. Each point is a mean of 8-24 mice.

same liposomes, containing primaquine, caused 50% suppression at a dilution of 1:104,000 (Fig. 5). Thus, it can be said that primaquine increased the efficacy of liposomal glycolipids by approximately two-fold. Based on the lack of increased efficacy of liposomal primaquine in the absence of glycolipids (Fig. 2), apparently it can also be said that liposomal glycolipids increased the efficacy of primaquine by approximately more than 46,000 fold!

Despite these interesting observations, it has not yet been determined whether glycolipids alone, or liposome-encapsulated primaquine targeted by liposomal glycolipids, are equivalent to, superior to, or inferior to standard clinical methods for oral administration of primaquine in treating hepatic stages of malaria.

Although primaquine acts exclusively on hepatic schizonts, and causes a radical cure of established infection, the mechanism, and indeed, the exact site of action, of primaquine is still unknown. Liposomal glycolipids also apparently cure 24 hr sporozoite-induced infections in mice. It is evident that liposomes might be useful in helping to elucidate not only the mechanism of action of primaquine, or other drugs,[23] but also may help to clarify certain biological aspects of the malaria infection itself. If the glycolipids only block entry of the parasite into the hepatocyte, then it is unlikely that they would have any clinical application.

IMMUNOLOGY

Another area in which macrophages play an important role is in the field of immunology.[24] As shown in Fig. 6, enormous quantities of liposomes can be ingested by macrophages. Uptake of liposomes is strikingly enhanced by coating the vesicles with antibodies and complement.[25] Because of the great attraction that macrophages have for liposomes, and the central role that macrophages play in immunology, three important immunological questions stand out with respect to liposomes as carriers. Can liposomes be antigenic? Can liposomes be immunosuppressive? Can liposomes be immunopotentiators? The answer to each question is: yes, at least under certain conditions.

Numerous laboratories, including mine, have demonstrated adjuvant properties of liposomes.[26] A partial list of my collaborators in this area are Drs. Brian Schuster, Benoy Banerji, Roberta Richards, and John Clements, and relevant publications are in refs. 8-10 and 27. In summarizing our experience, we have noted, but we have not been dazzled by, the inherent adjuvant effects of liposomes. However, we have been _extremely_ impressed by the adjuvant effects of liposomes containing certain known immunopotentiators, particularly lipid A.

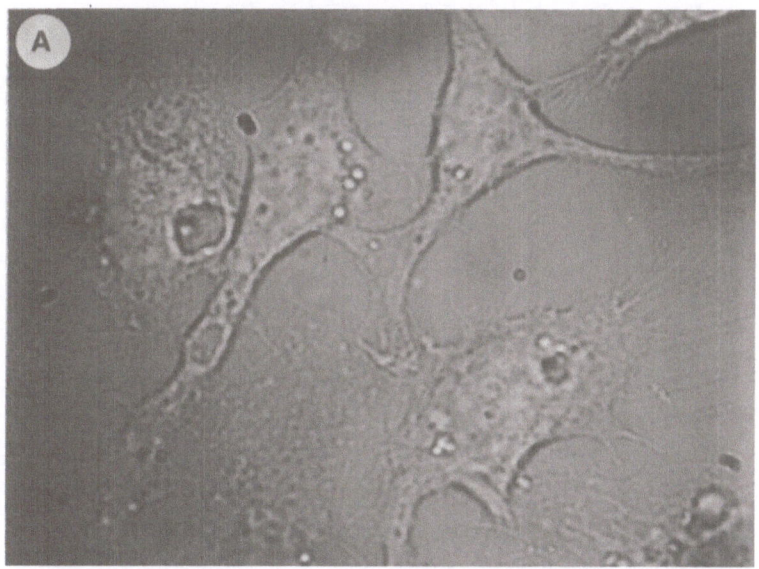

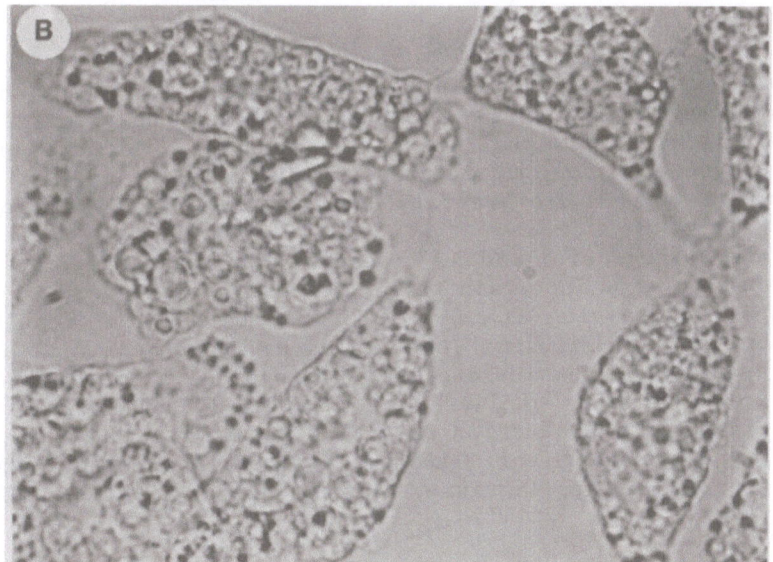

Fig. 6.   Antibody and complement-dependent phagocytosis of lipo-
           somes. Liposomes containing Forssman antigen (320 nmols
           sheep erythrocyte phospholipid) were incubated with 10^6
           mouse peritoneal macrophages in the presence of anti-
           Forssman serum (0.9 ml) and guinea pig complement (2 ml)
           as described earlier.[25]   Light microscopy prior to adding
           liposomes (A), and 24 hrs. after adding liposomes (B).

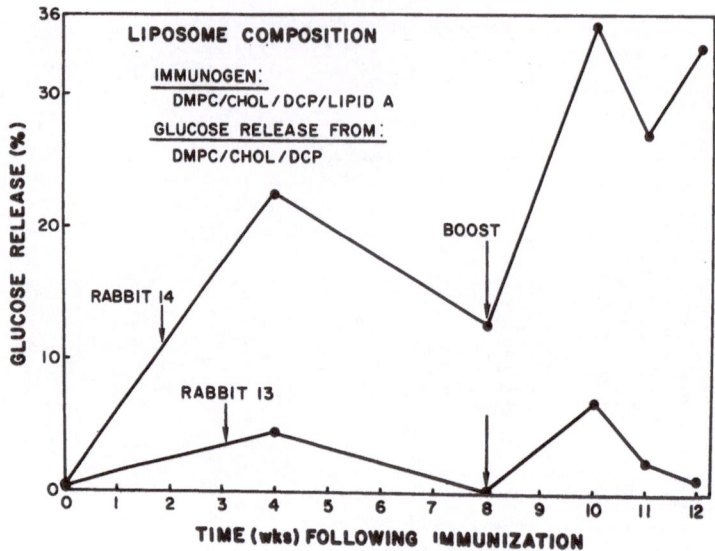

Fig. 7.   Complement-mediated immune damage to liposomes lacking
lipid A after injection of rabbits with liposomes containing lipid A.   From Schuster et al.[8]

Lipid A is the lipid portion of a very potent adjuvant, bacterial lipopolysaccharide (LPS).   Virtually all of the powerful adjuvant activity of LPS is provided by lipid A.[28,29] Lipid A consists
of a heterogeneous group of glycophospholipid molecules, and all of
the molecular types are readily incorporated into liposomes.[30]

In the absence of lipid A, liposomes are apparently nonimmuno-
genic upon injection into rabbits[8] or rodents[31].   However, injection
of liposomes containing lipid A into rabbits or mice resulted in
production of "anti-liposome" antibodies having specificity against
phosphocholine, phosphatidylcholine, sphingomyelin[8], and even to a
slight extent against cholesterol, and dicetyl phosphate[10].   An
illustration of the production of anti-liposome antibodies is shown
in Fig. 7.   A hybridoma anti-liposome antibody having anti-phospha-
tidylinositol phosphate activity was produced with the help of
lipid A.[32,33]

Obviously, the appearance of anti-liposome antibodies could be
considered undesirable for certain applications of liposomes.   We
have never observed adverse effects of such antibodies in rabbits,
even over the course of a year, and naturally-occurring antibodies
against sphingomyelin[34] or phosphatidylcholine,[35,36] have been observed frequently in rabbits and humans.   The possible occurrence,
and possible effects, of such antibodies must be considered during
any clinical applications of liposomes.

To illustrate the efficacies of liposomes as adjuvants for protein antigens, a model immunogenic particle was constructed that
utilized cholera toxin (CT) as an antigen.[9,10] Liposomes containing
the receptor for CT, ganglioside G_{M1}, were coated with CT in such a
concentration that all of the CT was bound to the outer surface of
the liposomes, and all of the G_{M1} molecules had CT attached to them.
These vesicles were then injected i.v. or s.c. into rabbits, and
serum antibody levels against CT were measured by a solid-phase
radioimmunoassay.[10] Some of the potential advantages of using this
system are shown in Table 1.

Table 1.   Some Characteristics and Advantages of a Model
            That Uses Liposomes Containing CT Bound to G_{M1}

1. Amount of CT bound can be controlled by altering G_{M1}.

2. Toxicity of CT can be blocked by liposomal G_{M1}.[37]

3. Antigenicity of G_{M1} can be suppressed by CT.[9]

4. No problem with "leaky" liposomes causing premature re-
    lease of antigen.

5. Surface exposure of protein antigens may be superior to
    encapsulation for inducing antibodies.[26,38]

6. Adjuvant effects of immunopotentiators, such as lipid A,
    or lipid-conjugated MDP derivatives,[9] can be studied.

Some of the results that we obtained are shown in Table 2
(which is partially derived from ref. 10). When lipid A was included as an adjuvant in the liposomal lipid bilayer, a very strong
anti-CT response was obtained, and the response was approximately
equivalent to that found when the same amount of CT was emulsified
with complete Freund's adjuvant. When lipid A was omitted, the
anti-CT response of the liposome-bound CT was greater (by 18-fold)
than CT alone, but it was not strikingly impressive when compared
with complete Freund's adjuvant as a standard.

The results in Table 2 show that the immune response against a
liposomal antigen can be approximately the same as that induced by
complete Freund's, provided that the liposomes contain lipid A.

Table 2. Enhancement of the Antigenicity
of CT Bound to Liposomes

Composition of immunogen[a]	3 week bleeding after 1° immunization	
	Antibody bound to CT (RIA units x 10^{-3})[b]	Fold increase compared to CT alone
CT alone	9	–
L(G_{M1}) + CT	162	18
L(G_{M1} + lipid A) + CT	5,850	629
Complete Freund's + CT	9,130	1,026

[a]Abbreviations used: L, liposomes (DPPC/CHOL/DCP); L(G_{M1}) + CT, liposomes containing G_{M1} to which CT is attached; L(G_{M1} + lipid A) + CT, the same liposomes also containing lipid A in the lipid bilayer.

[b]The RIA units are defined as CPM x 1/antiserum dilution in a linear region of the dose-response curve.[10] Each value shown is an average from two rabbits.

Table 3. Immunosuppression by Liposomes

Composition of immunogen[a]	3 week bleeding after 2° immunization
	Antibody bound to CT (RIA units x 10^{-3})
1) CT alone	3,320
2) L(G_{M1}) + CT	2,118
3) L(G_{M1} + lipid A) + CT	>10,000
4) L + CT	292
5) L(lipid A) + CT	283

[a]See Table 2 for abbreviations. Two rabbits were injected with each immunogen.

At this point I should like to inject a note of caution. All of us in the field of liposomal vaccines are quite alert to immuno-enhancement effects induced by liposomes. Because of this it is possible that the reverse effect, immunosuppression, or even lack of enhancement, could be overlooked. We have seen several instances of immunosuppression, and one such example is illustrated in Table 3. This experiment was part of a larger experiment in which 8 rabbits were injected with liposomes containing various formulations of lipids, including G_{M1}, and coated with CT. As controls, 8 additional rabbits were injected simultaneously with identical formulations, except G_{M1} was not present in the liposomes, and therefore CT was not bound. Each of the 8 rabbits injected with liposomes lacking G_{M1} was strongly immunosuppressed. That is, the anti-CT response was much less than that observed with CT alone (4 of the 8 rabbits are illustrated in Table 3, groups 4 and 5). When this experiment was repeated later, immunosuppression was not observed in any of the rabbits. We do not know the reason for the immuno-suppression, nor why it could not be reproduced. The rabbits in the two groups of experiments differed in that the nonsuppressed rabbits were much older than the suppressed ones, and the possibility that age played a role is being investigated.

The data for Table 3 were obtained after the rabbits had been given a boosting injection. After the boost, the immune response against CT alone was markedly increased, compared to Table 2, and the increased antigenicity of CT bound to liposomes was no longer apparent. The lack of antigenic difference (Table 3, groups 1 and 2) was not due to a ceiling in the ability to produce antibodies, or in the ability to assay the immune response, because a marked increased antigenicity of CT was still observed when the liposomes contained lipid A (Table 3, group 3). This observation suggests that the adjuvant effect of liposomes may be much greater, and more important as a phenomenon, when lipid A is present (as in Table 2).

Finally, what is the potential clinical practicality of utilizing lipid A, which is the active ingredient of bacterial endotoxin, as an adjuvant in liposomes? Does lipid A retain in vivo endotoxic activity in liposomes?

One of the most severe, and even life-threatening, aspects of endotoxic shock is the appearance of the generalized Schwartzman reaction, and one of the prominent features of the Schwartzman reaction is a marked reduction in the leukocyte count (neutropenia).[39] As shown in Fig. 7, which is taken from ref. 40, neutropenia can be induced in rabbits by injection of lipid A, but the neutropenia does not occur after injection of lipid A incorporated in liposomes. Therefore, by the criterion of elimination of neutropenia, we have shown that liposomes can block at least one endotoxic effect, that is, one aspect of the Schwartzman reaction induced by lipid A in vivo.

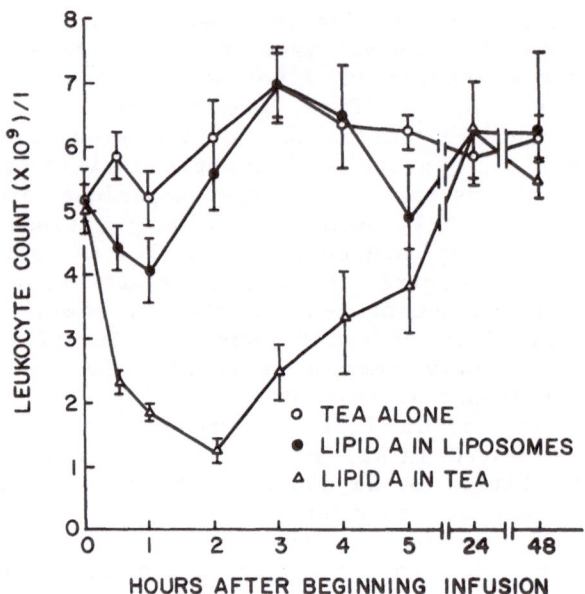

Fig. 8.   Effect of infusion of lipid A (0.01 mg/kg) on leukocyte
counts (mean ± SEM) in rabbits. Lipid A that was in 0.5%
triethylamine (TEA), or in liposomes, was infused during
1 hr into 4 rabbits.   Six controls received 0.5% TEA.
From Ramsey et al.[40]

It is unlikely that any potential toxic effects of liposomes
will approach the highly toxic potential of certain vaccines already
in general use. For example, if liposomes containing lipid A are
pyrogenic, I do not believe that the reaction could be as bad as the
sore arm and fever reaction that many of us have experienced following injection of vaccines containing massive amounts of endotoxin.
If lipid A (or other liposomal lipids) are good adjuvants, the
potential advantages of application in certain viral or parasitic
diseases probably would outweigh minor pyrogenic reactions. Although the immunology of liposomes is very complex, in my opinion
liposomes could have a role in certain vaccines.

REFERENCES

1. H.   C. Goodman, Immunology and tropical diseases: Challenges and
        opportunities, Ann. Immunol. (Inst. Pasteur) 129C:267 (1978)
2. C.   R. Alving, E. A. Steck, W. L. Chapman, Jr., V. B. Waits, L.
        D. Hendricks, G. M. Swartz, Jr., and W. L. Hanson, Therapy
        of leishmaniasis: Superior efficacies of liposome-encapsu-
        lated drugs, Proc. Natl. Acad. Sci. U.S.A. 75:2959 (1978).

3. C. R. Alving, E. A. Steck, W. L. Hanson, P. S. Loizeaux, W. L. Chapman, Jr., and V. B. Waits, Improved therapy of experimental leishmaniasis by use of a liposome-encapsulated antimonial drug, Life Sci. 22:1021 (1978).

4. C. R. Alving, E. A. Steck, W. L. Chapman, Jr., V. B. Waits, L. D. Hendricks, G. M. Swartz, Jr., and W. L. Hanson, Liposomes in leishmaniasis: Therapeutic effects of antimonial drugs, 8-aminoquinolines, and tetracycline, Life Sci. 26:2231 (1980).

5. C. R. Alving and E. A. Steck, The use of liposome-encapsulated drugs in leishmaniasis, Trends Biochem. Sci. 4(8):N175 (1979).

6. C. R. Alving, I. Schneider, G. M. Swartz, Jr., and E. A. Steck, Sporozoite-induced malaria: Therapeutic effects of glycolipids in liposomes, Science 205:1142 (1979).

7. C. R. Alving, Immune reactions of lipids and lipid model membranes, in:"The Antigens, vol. 4", M. Sela, ed., Academic Press, NY, p.1 (1977).

8. B. G. Schuster, M. Neidig, B. M. Alving, and C. R. Alving, Production of antibodies against phosphocholine, phosphatidylcholine, sphingomyelin, and lipid A by injection of liposomes containing lipid A, J. Immunol. 122:900 (1979).

9. C. R. Alving, Liposomes as vehicles for vaccines, in:"New Developments With Human and Veterinary Vaccines", A. Mizrahi, M. A. Klingberg, I. Hertman, and A. Kohn, eds., Alan R. Liss, Inc., NY, (1980).

10. C. R. Alving, B. Banerji, J. Clements, and R. L. Richards, Adjuvanticity of lipid A and lipid A fractions in liposomes, in:"Liposomes and Immunobiology", B. H. Tom and H. R. Six, eds., Elsevier/North-Holland, NY, (1980).

11. R. K. Sanyal and R. R. Arora, Assessment of drug therapy of kala-azar in current epidemic in Bihar, J. Com. Dis. 11:198 (1979).

12. C. D. V. Black, G. J. Watson, and R. J. Ward, The use of Pentostam liposomes in the chemotherapy of experimental leishmaniasis, Trans. R. Soc. Trop. Med. Hyg. 71:550 (1977).

13. R. R. C. New, M. L. Chance, S. C. Thomas, and W. Peters, Antileishmanial activity of antimonials entrapped in liposomes, Nature 272:55 (1978).

14. W. H. Wernsdorfer, Long-term aims of malaria research, Trends Biochem. Res. 4(3):N49 (1979)

15. P. Pirson, R. F. Steiger, A. Trouet, J. Gillet, and F. Herman, Primaquine liposomes in the chemotherapy of experimental murine malaria, Ann. Trop. Med. Parasit. 74:383 (1980).

16. G. Ashwell and A. G. Morell, The role of surface carbohydrates in the hepatic recognition and transport of circulating glycoproteins, Adv. Enzymol. 41:99 (1974).

17. A. Surolia and B. K. Bachhawat, Monosialoganglioside liposome-entrapped enzyme uptake by hepatic cells. Biochim. Biophys. Acta 497:760 (1977).

18. M. M. Jonah, E. A. Cerny, and Y. E. Rahman, Tissue distribution of EDTA encapsulated within liposomes containing glycolipids or brain phospholipids, Biochim. Biophys. Acta 541:321 (1978).

19. J. R. Riordan, L. Mitchell, and M. Slavik, The binding of asialo-glycoprotein to isolated Golgi apparatus, Biochem. Biophys. Res. Comm. 59:1373 (1974).

20. W. E. Pricer, Jr. and G. Ashwell, Subcellular distribution of a mammalian hepatic binding protein specific for asialoglyco-proteins, J. Biol. Chem. 251:7539 (1976).

21. H. D. Danforth, M. Aikawa, A. H. Cochrane, and R. S. Nussenzweig, Sporozoites of mammalian malaria: Attachment to, interiorization and fate within macrophages, J. Proto-zool. 27:193 (1980).

22. I. Schneider, and C.R. Alving, unpublished data.

23. R. F. Steiger, D. G. Layton, P. Pirson, J. Gillet, and F. Herman, Therapeutic activity of DAPI on experimental murine malaria, J. Parasitol. 66:352 (1980).

24. B. H. Tom, An overview: Liposomes and immunobiology--macro-phages, liposomes and tailored immunity, in:"Liposomes and Immunobiology", B. H. Tom and H. R. Six, eds., Elsevier, North-Holland, NY, (1980).

25. C. R. Alving, J. J. Mooney, and G. E. Olson, Use of liposomes as a model for studying immune phagocytosis, Fed. Proc. 30:693 (1971).

26. N. van Rooijen and R. van Nieuwmegen, Immunoadjuvant properties of liposomes, this volume.

27. B. Banerji and C. R. Alving, Anti-liposome antibodies induced by lipid A. I. Influence of ceramide, glycosphingolipids, and phosphocholine on complement damage, J. Immunol. 126: 1080 (1981).

28. J. M. Chiller, B. J. Skidmore, D. C. Morrison, and W. O. Weigle, Relationship of the structure of bacterial lipopoly-saccharides to its function in mitogenesis and adjuvanti-city, Proc. Natl. Acad. Sci. U.S.A. 70:2129 (1973).

29. Y. Cho, K. Tanamoto, Y. Oh, and J. Y. Homma, Differences of chemical structures of Pseudomonas aeruginosa lipopolysac-charide essential for adjuvanticity and antitumor and inter-feron-inducing activities, FEBS Lett. 105:120 (1979).

30. B. Banerji and C. R. Alving, Lipid A from endotoxin: Antigenic activities of purified fractions in liposomes, J. Immunol. 123:2558 (1979)

31. K. Uemura, R. A. Nicolotti, H. R. Six, and S. C. Kinsky, Anti-body formation in response to liposomal model membranes sen-sitized with N-substituted phosphatidylethanolamine deriva-tives, Biochemistry 13:1572 (1974).

32. F. Roerdink, B. J. Berson, R. L. Richards, G. M. Swartz, Jr., J. A. Lyon, and C. R. Alving, Specificity of a hybridoma monoclonal antibody against liposomes containing phosphati-dylinositol monophosphate, Fed. Proc. 40:996 (1981).

33. R. L. Friedman, F. Roerdink, B. H. Iglewski, and C. R. Alving, Suppression of cytotoxicity of diphtheria toxin by mono-clonal antibodies against phosphatidylinositol phosphate, Biophys. J., in press.

34. G. H. Strejan, P. M. Smith, C. W. Grant, and D. Surlan, Natur-ally occurring antibodies to liposomes. I. Rabbit antibo-dies to sphingomyelin-containing liposomes before and after immunization with unrelated antigens, J. Immunol. 123:370 (1979).

35. R. L. Richards and C. R. Alving, Immune reactivities of anti-bodies against glycolipids. Natural Antibodies, in:"Cell Surface Glycolipids", ACS Symposium Series No. 128, C. C. Sweeley, ed., American Chemical Society, Washington, (1980).

36. R. L. Richards and C. R. Alving, unpublished data.

37. C. R. Alving, J. Moss, R. L. Richards, and L. I. Alving, Lipo-somes as vehicles for vaccines. Increased antigenicity and lack of toxicity of a toxin bound to liposomes, Clin. Res. 29(2):531A (1981).

38. N. van Rooijen and R. van Nieuwmegen, Liposomes in immunology: evidence that their adjuvant effect results from surface exposition of the antigens, Cell. Immunol. 49:402 (1980).

39. D. C. Morrison, R. J. Ulevitch, The effects of bacterial endo-toxins on host mediation systems, Am. J. Pathol. 93:525 (1978).

40. R. B. Ramsey, M. B. Hamner, B. M. Alving, J. S. Finlayson, C. R. Alving, Effects of lipid A and liposomes containing lipid A on platelet and fibrinogen production in rabbits, Blood 56:307 (1980).

INTERACTION OF LIPOSOMES WITH CELLS: MODEL STUDIES

Catherine Vakirtzi-Lemonias and Kalliope Sekeris-Pataryas

Biology Division, Nuclear Research Center Demokritos
Aghia Paraskevi Attikis, Athens, Greece

GENERAL CONSIDERATIONS

It is well documented to date that the mode of interaction of a given cell type with liposomes is affected by the chemical composition of the latter. Thus, it has been shown that "fluidity", charge and size of the vesicles are important parameters in determining the mechanism by which liposomes interact with their target cells.[1]

During the life cycle of a cell however important changes may occur in the chemical composition and properties of its membrane. These must also influence and alter the mode of cell-liposome interaction and therefore the potential use of liposomes as drug carriers.

A starting point in the analysis of the mode of cell-liposome interaction from this point of view may be provided by studies with cells which undergo natural changes in their membrane composition and properties, as a function of their developmental stages.[2-4] Another starting point may be provided by studying cell lines differing in membrane properties and composition as exemplified by drug resistant cell lines.[5] A third possibility is provided by cells in which artificial changes in their membrane composition may be induced by introducing different substances into their membranes.[6-8]

EXPERIMENTAL APPROACHES

The question of the relation of changes in membrane composition and properties during the life cycle of a cell and the mode of cell-liposome interaction was investigated with three different types of cells:

a)   The slime mold <u>Dictyostelium discoideum</u>

b)   The insect trypanosomatid <u>Crithidia fasciculata</u>

c)   Two cell variants of <u>Pseudomonas aeruginosa</u>

STUDIES WITH <u>DICTYOSTELIUM DISCOIDEUM</u>

The life of <u>D. discoideum</u> is known in considerable detail.[9,10]
The organism, in its vegetative form, is a unicellular amoeba
dividing about every three hours, (9 hours in axenic cultures), and
this part of the life cycle is called the non social phase. Upon
food deprivation the amoebae differentiate into an aggregation competent state in the course of about 9-12 hours.

Cell differentiation between vegetative and aggregation competent
cells is expressed in changes of the properties of the cells which
include:

1)   Ability for aggregation and fusion[10,11]

  - vegetative cells do not aggregate. They are able to
    fuse when they reach the stationary phase and are kept
    in the nutrient medium.

  - aggregation competent cells appear after 9-12 hours of
    starvation. They have adhesive but not fusing ability.

2)   Surface chemical composition and structure expressed by altera-
     tions during differentiation in:

   a) plasma membrane proteins and glycoproteins[12-16]

   - quantitative and qualitative changes in the protein
     composition.

   - increased activity of various enzymes, e.g. C-AMP,
     phosphodiesterase, glycosyl transferases.

   b) Cell surface charge[17]

   - decrease in the density of negatively charged groups,
     (COO$^-$), accompanied by an increase in that of the
     amino groups.

   c) plasma membrane lipids[18-20]

   - slight increase in lysophosphatidylethanolamine,
     phosphatidylinositol and phosphatidylglycerol with
     slight decrease in phosphatidylethanolamine and its
     plasmalogen form.

   - slight increase in diunsaturated fatty acids with a
     corresponding decrease in the monounsaturated ones.

- no appreciable change in total phospholipid and
  sterol content of cells but changes in percentage
  distribution. Increase in total cellular neutral
  lipid.

d) plasma membrane fluidity[18]

- there seems to be no appreciable change in membrane
  fluidity.

3) Membrane ultrastructure[4,21]

- the flexible, with phagocytic caps membrane of the
  vegetative cells becomes very wrinkled and filled
  with many filopods.

4) Ability for phagocytosis[21]

- vegetative cells are typically phagocytic. After
  a 2 hour starvation period they inject twice as
  many yeast cells as during growth. Afterwards
  phagocytic activity decreases and their digestive
  apparatus is transformed into an autophagic one.

To study cell-liposome interaction with vegetative and aggregation competent cells of D. discoideum appropriate cell samples (see
legends of Figures and Table) were incubated in the presence of multilamellar negative liposomes prepared by entrapment of tracer amounts
of ^{125}I-albumin (sp.act. 1.25 x 10^7 cpm) into a mixture of PC:Chol:PA,
7:2:1 molar ratio and sonication (MSE sonicator 4 min, 0°C, titanium
probe 2 cm). Liposomes were collected by centrigugation at 198000xg
for 45 min. washed and resuspended in PBS to the desired volume. A
biodegradable compound was chosen as a liposome marker in order to
allow the cells to perform normally their metabolic functions. It
must be added that starved cells, although they have the competence
for it, do not aggregate but remain as single cells when kept under
continuous shaking (150 rotations/min)[10].

The kinetics of uptake of liposome-associated radioactivity,
(the sum of cell-associated plus that catabolized and excreted in the
incubation media), are shown in Fig. 1A and 1B. It is clear that:

a) Both types of cells take up liposome-associated radioactivity
   at a rigorous rate (35% and 42% of added radioactivity at the
   end of a five hour incubation period for the vegetative and
   aggregation competent cells respectively).

b) When incubations are performed in the presence of inhibitors of
   metabolism, vegetative cells do not show any inhibition in total
   uptake, (Fig. 1A). On the contrary, uptake by aggregation competent cells is circa 30% inhibited (Fig. 1B). The same results

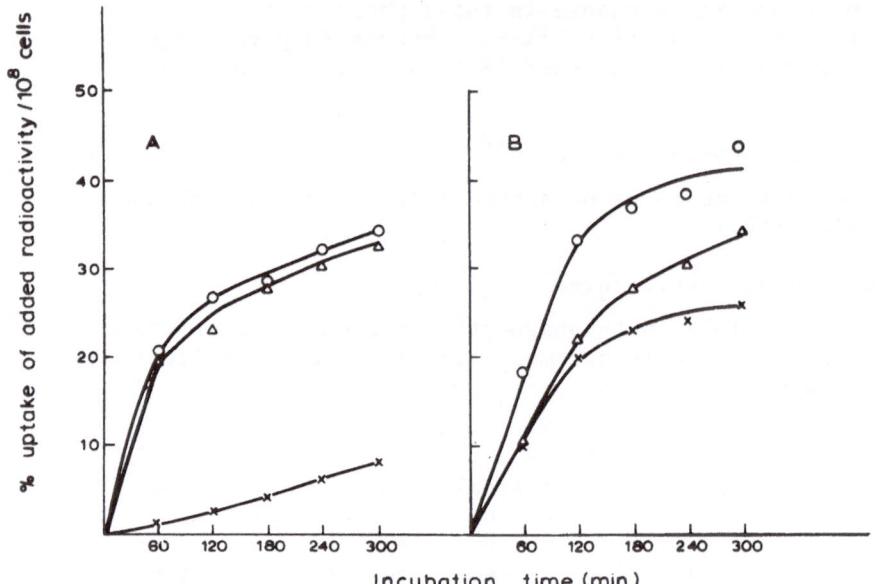

Fig. 1.   Total uptake of liposome entrapped ^{125}I-albumin by vegetative (A) and aggregation competent (B) cells of <u>Dictyostelium
discoideum</u>.(o-o) cells incubated at 25°C, (Δ-Δ) cells incubated at 25°C in the presence of inhibitors, (x-x) cells
incubated at 0°C. Incubation mixtures contained per ml 5-8
x 10^8 vegetative or aggregation competent cells suspended in
medium or buffer respectively and the appropriate liposome
dispersion (0.3 mg liposomal lipids, 1000 cpm). The concentration of inhibitors, when present, was 0.03M NaF and 0.01M
NaN$_3$. Aliquots of 2 ml were taken at the appropriate times,
centrifuged at 1500xg for 5 min and the cell pellets washed
three times with 1% saline. The first washing was added to
the cell supernatant and proteins were precipitated by TCA.
Total uptake was estimated as the sum of cell-associated and
TCA soluble radioactivity recovered in the supernatant.

were obtained at a 10-fold higher concentrations of inhibitors.

c)   When incubations are performed at 0°C vegetative cells appear to
have a low linear rate of association with liposomes amounting to
about 25% of total uptake at the end of the incubation period
(Fig. 1A). On the contrary, more than half of the radioactivity
taken up by aggregation competent cells is due to adsorption on
the cell surface. Kinetics of uptake also differ in comparison
with vegetative cells. An explanation of this mode of reaction
may be found in the known adhesive properties of the aggregation
competent cells and in their highly wrinkled surface.

d)   Free albumin is not taken up by either type of cells under our
      experimental conditions.

      Assay conditions had no effect on the cells as could be judged
by phase microscopy examination and by the ability of the cells to
aggregate.

      Fig. 2 shows the radioactivity – from liposomal ^{125}I-albumin –
which is associated with the two types of cells at various times,
under the experimental conditions given in Fig. 1.   As indicated,
(Fig. 2B), aggregation competent cell-associated radioactivity increases continuously during a five hour incubation period and reaches
over 30% of the added radioactivity for 10^8 cells at the end of the
incubation period.   Incubation at 0°C shows that most of the radioactivity is due to adsorption on the cell surface (23% of added at 5
hours) and only a small amount (5-7%) is taken up by the cells by
other mechanisms (endocytosis and/or fusion).

      Incubation of these cells in the presence of metabolic inhibitors
shows no change in cell-associated radioactivity.   Comparison of
Fig. 1B with Fig. 2B shows that total and cell-associated radioacti-

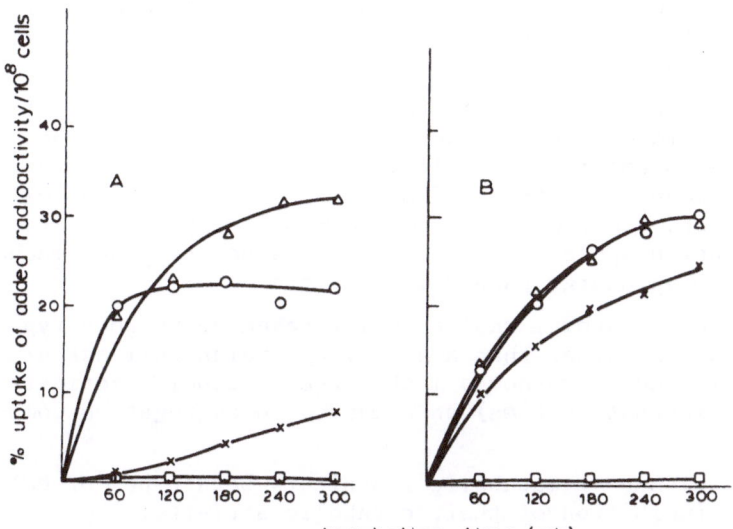

Fig. 2.   Cell-associated radioactivity from liposome-entrapped
          ^{125}I-albumin by vegetative (A) and aggregation competent(B)
          cells of <u>Dictyostelium discoideum</u> at 25°C (o-o), at 25°C
          in the presence of metabolic inhibitors (Δ-Δ) and at 0°C
          (X-X). Uptake of free albumin (□-□). Experimental condi-
          tions as given in Fig. 1.

vity coincide under conditions in which respiration and glycolysis
are presumably inhibited. It appears therefore that, under our
experimental conditions, metabolic inhibitors repress also catabolism
of the material taken up.

Contrary to the aggregation competent cells, vegetative cells
show a higher initial rate of association with liposomes, but then
cell-associated radioactivity reaches a plateau, after the first hour
of incubation, as shown in Fig. 2A. The same figure shows furthermore that vegetative cells accumulate far more liposomal radioactivity
when incubated in the presence of metabolic inhibitors. A comparison
of Fig. 1A and 2A reveals that the role of inhibitors is to repress
catabolism rather than uptake, and the question remains if liposomes
are taken up by other than a phagocytic process by vegetative cells.

An evaluation of the different modes by which liposomal radioactivity is associated with the two types of cells with time is
summarized in Table 1. Adsorption, phagocytosis and/or fusion as
well as catabolized radioactivity are expressed as percentaged of
total radioactivity taken up by the cells at each incubation time.

It can be seen that:

1)   Vegetative cells take up a high percentage of liposomal radioactivity by mechanisms other than adsorption over the whole incubation
period. Adsorption is of relatively minor importance as a mechanism
of uptake of liposomes.

2)   Aggregation competent cells take up a high percentage of liposomes by adsorption especially during the first hours of incubation.
With time other mechanisms of cell-liposome interaction come into
play. They account for about 40% of total uptake, half of which is
energy dependent. In the presence of metabolic inhibitors the percentage of adsorption appears to be higher because the other mechanisms
are inhibited when energy supply is affected.

3)   Most of the liposomal radioactivity taken up by both types of
cells by mechanisms other than adsorption remains cell-associated.
Vegetative cells however show a much higher catabolic activity (x3
at five hours incubation time) as compared to aggregation competent
cells.

4)   In the presence of metabolic inhibitors both types of cells
show complete inhibition of their catabolic activity.

CONCLUSION

Vegetative cells of D. discoideum interact with negatively
charged liposomes by mechanisms involving mainly endocytosis and/or
fusion while aggregation competent cells interact mainly by adsorption.

TABLE 1. Percentage distribution of liposomal radioactivity taken
          up by vegetative and aggregation competent cells of
          <u>Dictyostelium discoideum</u> in relation to its mode of uptake.

% radioactivity taken up by

	Phagocytosis and/or Fusion		Adsorption	
	Vegetative cells			
Time (hours)	−Inhibitors	+Inhibitors	−Inhibitors	+Inhibitors
1	95.1 (4.2)*	94.9 (0.0)*	4.9	5.1
2	91.4 (13.0)	92.6 (0.1)	8.6	7.4
3	74.0 (16.5)	81.5 (0.4)	6.0	18.5
4	78.0 (29.6)	80.0 (0.2)	22.0	20.0
5	76.0 (32.0)	75.4 (0.3)	24.0	24.6
	Aggregation competent cells			
1	24.0 (3.1)	11.3 (0.3)	76.0	88.7
2	28.3 (5.9)	18.9 (0.2)	71.7	81.1
3	34.5 (7.5)	21.0 (0.4)	65.5	78.9
4	40.5 (11.0)	24.0 (0.4)	63.2	75.9
5	41.6 (10.9)	19.5 (0.1)	58.4	80.5

*Percentage taken up by the cells and catabolized.

Energy-dependent phagocytosis as a mechanism of liposomal uptake by
vegetative cells cannot be supported under our experimental conditions,
using as criterion the inhibition of phagocytosis in the presence of
inhibitors of metabolism.

STUDIES WITH <u>CRITHIDIA FASCICULATA</u>

Experiments analogous to those reported with <u>D. dictyostelium</u>
were undertaken with the insect trypanosomatid <u>Crithidia fasciculata</u>,
having in mind the, ultimately, pharmacological utilization of liposomes as carriers of trypanocidal drugs.

The importance of trypanosomes in causing parasitic diseases and
difficulties in treating them are well known,[22-24] the main reason
being the continuously changing properties of the cells, mainly their
antigenic variation.[25,26] This variation does not permit successful
immunological approaches and the development of the vaccines[27] and
thus chemotherapy is the only way practiced to-date with its many
side effects.[22,28] Recently successful uses of liposomes as drug
carriers have been reported for leishmaniasis.[29-31]

During their life cycle the parasites of the trypanosomatidae family pass through several stages of development characterized by changes in morphology and composition,[32,33] many of which are not well characterized. The genus Crithidia was, up to recently, one of the very few genera capable for growth and multiplication in mono-phasic media for studies in culture and during its life cycle the organism passes through two distinct stages of development, the choanomastigote stage during active multiplication(exponential growth) and the amastigote or spheromastigote stage of stationary phase cells.[33]

We chose therefore to study Crithidia using the species Crithidia fasciculata, an organism easy to grow in defined media[34,35], and rather extensively studied for chemical composition,[36,39] morphology[40,41] and metabolism.[42-46] We have also isolated and characterized the surface membrane of the choanomastigote (L-form) and the spheromastigote (S-form) cells and some of the main differences in their lipid chemical composition are listed in Table 2. These differences in phospholipid class, sterol and fatty acid content suggested the possibility of different modes of interaction of the two developmental stages of the cells with various liposomal preparations. Most of the work to be reported on the interaction of liposomes with G. fasciculata was done in collaboration with Dr. G. Gregoriadis.[47]

First linearity of uptake of liposomes by cells was established for up to 10^9 cells/ml regardless of the developmental stage and the charge of liposomes. Next negatively charged multilamelar liposomes, (PC:Chol:PA 7:2:1 molar ratio), and liposomes made up from lipids extracted from C. fasciculata, both labeled with trace amounts of ^{131}I-albumin, were incubated with L- and S- form cells and Figure 3 shows total liposomal uptake after a 12 hour incubation period. Results may be summarized as follows:

a)   S-form cells incubated with negatively charged liposomes take up 4-fold more radioactivity as compared to L-form cells. The contrary holds true for liposomes made up from Crithidia lipids where L-form cells take up more, (2-fold) radioactivity compared to S-form cells.

b)   S-form cells take up about 5-fold more radioactivity from negatively charged liposomes as compared to Crithidia lipid liposomes. On the contrary L-form cells take up less radioactivity from negatively charged liposomes as compared with those made up from Crithidia lipids.

c)   The presence of metabolic inhibitors has relatively small effect on the uptake of negative liposomes by L-form cells compared with the inhibition in uptake of Crithidia lipid liposomes which is decreased by about 7-fold. Uptake by S-form cells is also energy-dependent for both types of liposomes. Differences however are not so pronounced, as in the case of L-cells and

TABLE 2.   Chemical composition of plasma membranes isolated from
L- and S-form cells of Crithidia fasciculata

Compound	Plasma Membrane Content of	
	L-form cells	S-form cells
Phosphatidylcholine[1]	139	201
Phosphatidylinositol[1]	82	130
Sphingomyelin[1]	55	93
Ergosterol[1]	13.3	6.3
Erg/PL[2]	0.71	0.36
Diunsaturated fatty acids[3]	10.0	7.0
Polyunsaturated fatty acids[3]	7.9	5.0
9,10 methylene-octadecanoic acid[3]	3.1	2.1

Crithidia fasciculata were grown under standardized conditions[39]
to the respective developmental stages. Surface membranes were
isolated, purified and characterized chemically and enzymatically
(N. Frantzis and C. Vakirtzi-Lemonias, unpublished results). Some
of the main differences in their chemical composition are listed in
the table. 1. μg/mg membrane protein; 2. Molar ratio; 3. Percent
distribution of surface membrane fatty acids.

Crithidia lipids liposomes

The findings imply endocytotic activity which is the main mode
of interaction of L-form cells with Crithidia lipid liposomes.
Considering now the metabolism of the liposomal uptake (TCA soluble
products) we may observe that negatively charged liposomes are degraded by the cells to a great extent (70-90%). This finding implies
also that adsorption is not the main mechanism for liposome association with the cells. Catabolism is still extensive even in the
presence of metabolic inhibitors, implying degradation of liposomal
albumin in the digestive apparatus of the organism. Separate control
experiments (incubation of C. fasciculata cells with liposomes for 12
hours and column fractionation of the incubation media had shown that
liposomes and their contents were not degraded in the incubation media
by phospholipases and proteases excreted by the cells in the media.

Catabolism of Crithidia lipid liposomal albumin is considerably
lower (20-35%) compared to catabolism of negative liposome albumin
and metabolic inhibitors suppress completely catabolic activity. It
is clear therefore that intracellular metabolism is different for the

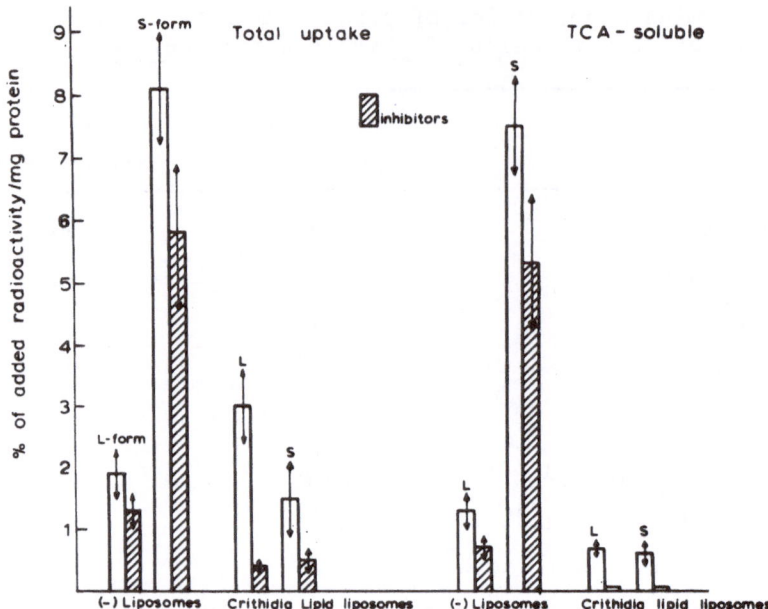

Fig. 3.   Incubation mixtures, 2.8 ml contained 4-5 x 10^8 cells of
L-form, (0.98 mg protein/10^8 cells), or S-form (0.71 mg
protein/10^8 cells), negative liposomes (PC:Chol:PA, 7:2:1
molar ratio, 0.5-0.6 mg total lipid) or Crithidia total
lipid extract liposomes (0.5 mg lipid) labeled with a trace
amount of ^{131}I-albumin (8-75 x 10^7 cpm, 9.4 μCi/mg sp. act.)
and 0.03M NaF and 0.015M NaN$_3$ when inhibitors were present.
Total uptake and TCA soluble radioactivity as in Fig. 1 and
(47). Results recalculated from (47) per mg cell protein.

two types of liposomes.

The above differences prompted comparison of the mode of interaction with Crithidia of other types of liposomes made up from
commercial lipids. Thus neutral, (PC:Chol 7:2 molar ratio), and
positive (PC:Chol:St, 7:2:1 molar ratio), liposomes were prepared,
and their interaction with L- and S-form cells was investigated.

Figure 4 shows that, in general, liposomes made from commercial
lipids interact with L-and S-form C. fasciculata cells in the same
general manner as negative liposomes.

Thus, S-form cells take up 8-fold (neutral) and 5-fold (positive)
more liposome-associated radioactivity compared to the L-form cells.
Catabolism of uptaken material is again very extensive, over 90% for
neutral and a little lower for positive liposomes. The effect of
metabolic inhibitors show that energy-dependent endocytosis is a
major mode of association of neutral liposomes (L-form and S-form

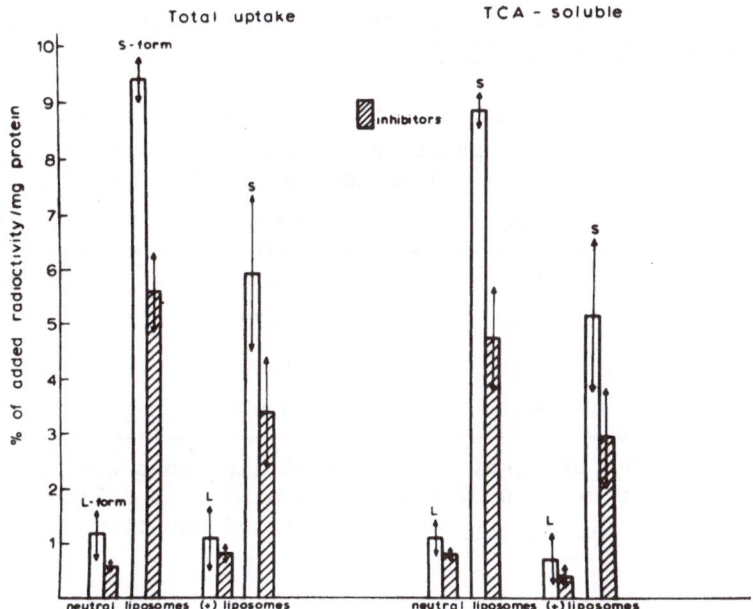

Fig. 4.   Neutral and positive liposomes were incubated with L- and
          S-form cells of C. fasciculata. Experimental details as in
          Fig. 3.

cells) and positive liposomes (S-form) cells.

The interaction of positively charged liposomes with L-form cells
appears to be different because it is not energy-dependent. Almost
complete catabolism of uptaken liposomes implies that their association with the cells must involve mainly a fusion mechanism. Fusion
has also been proposed as a mechanism for the interaction of positive
fluid liposomes with Trypanosoma brucei plasma membranes.[48]

The effect of size of liposomes on their uptake by C. fasciculata
was studied having in mind efficacy of drug entrapment and fate of
liposomes in vivo. Table 3 shows total uptake of negatively charged
liposomes by L-form cells with time and similar results were obtained
with the other liposomal preparations and the S-form cells.

Table 3 shows first that large liposomes are taken up at higher
quantities compared to small ones and second that larger liposomes
are taken up faster than smaller ones.

Efficacy of liposomes to introduce larger amounts of entrapped
drug as compared to the free compound is shown in Table 4. It is
clearly shown that uptake of entrapped radioactivity was 15-fold
greater than uptake of the free drug. It may be noted also that
when respiratory and glycolytic inhibitors are used separately they
are without effect in inhibiting liposomal uptake[1].

TABLE 3.   Effect of size of liposomes on their uptake with time by Crithidia fasciculata

Incubation time, hours	Total uptake (% of added radioactivity) of liposomes sonicated for		
	20 sec.	2 min	15 min
3	5.50	3.70	0.35
7	10.25	4.70	2.75
12	8.85	11.00	6.45
15	7.90	8.00	5.20

Three different sizes of negatively charged liposomes were prepared by sonication for 20 seconds, 2 min and 15 min[47]. The liposomes were incubated with C. fasciculata as described and total liposomal uptake was assayed.

CONCLUSION

    S-form cells take up much more PC-liposomal albumin than L-form cells. The opposite was observed with liposomes make up from a total lipid extract of the organism. Changes in the net charge of the carrier did not have any significant effect on the uptake of either

TABLE 4.   Uptake of free and liposome entrapped tritiated Colchicine by Crithidia fasciculata

Preparation	Total uptake % of added radioactivity ± S.D.
Free colchicine	0.18 ± 0.040
Entrapped in negative liposomes	2.85 ± 0.165 p < 0.001
Negative liposome + NaF_3	2.49 ± 0.410
Negative liposomes + NaN	2.49 ± 0.410

L-form cells, (4×10^8, 2.2 mg protein), were incubated for 2 hours at 37°C in media containing either free, (6×10^5 dpm), or entrapped, ($9-2 \times 10^5$ dpm), in liposomes, (PC:Chol:PA, 7:2:1 molar ratio, 24 mg lipid/ml), colchicine (ring G-methoxyl-^{3}H, sp.act. 5.9 Ci/mmol). Total uptake was measured as described in Fig. 3.

of the two forms of cells.

At least for some of the liposomal preparations endocytosis is a major mode of their association with the trypanosomatids. Other mechanisms of liposome-cell interaction may co-exist.

The ability of C. fasciculata to incorporate much more drug when the latter is presented in the entrapped form could render chemo-therapy of trypanosomasis via liposomes a more effective treatment under the presupposition that the interaction of Crithidia fasciculata with liposomes observed in this study is also exhibited by pathogenic trypanosomes.

STUDIES WITH PSEUDOMONAS AERUGINOSA

In the third section of this report we wish to discuss some preliminary work done with two strains of the gram negative bacterium Pseudomonas aeruginosa. The work has been done in collaboration with Drs. N. Legakis and Th. Pataryas. Our interest in P.aeruginosa was aroused because of the increased frequency of infections caused by this bacterium in hospitals and because of recent reports which des-cribe strains of P. aeruginosa resistant to gentamicin and carbeni-cillin, the choice antibiotics for the organism.[49,50]

Resistance of bacteria to antibiotics may be due to an alteration of some cellular component in such a way that the antibiotic either does not reach or does not interact with its target site within the cell. Another mechanism of resistance is due to an acquired ability of the bacterium for modification and subsequent inactivation of the antibiotic[51]. In the case of gram negative bacteria there is evidence suggesting that the external membrane acts as barrier in many antibiotics which thus cannot reach their target.[52,53]

A membrane barrier to the entrance of antibiotics rather than drug modification appears to be the resistance mechanism in the strain $P_{28-600Cb}$ of P. aeruginosa derived by habituation from the parent strain P_{28-0}, a clinical isolate sensitive to carbenicillin and gen-tamicin. Experiments on the adherence to various spithelial cells provided evidence for alterations in the surface structure of the trained strain to carbenicillin[54] while changes in composition of the proteins of the external membranes of the $P_{28-600Cb}$ cells as well as absence of hydrolysis of carbenicillin by B-lactamases suggested that resistence of the trained strain $P_{28-600Cb}$ is due to a permeability defect (Th. Pataryas, N. Legakis and K. Sekeri-Pataryas, unpublished results).

These findings regarding differences in the surface structure of the two strains together with the increasing frequency of emergence of resistance to aminoglycosides of clinical isolates of P. aeruginosa

made it very attractive to study the mode of interaction of the bacteria with liposomes and to consider the possiblity of introducing
the antibiotics into the cells by the use of liposomes as carriers.

The methodology used for cell cultures, incubations and cell
fractionation was as follows:

TABLE 5.   Uptake of free and liposome-entrapped ^{125}I-albumin by
viable cells of Pseudomonas aeruginosa, P_{28-0}.

Time	% uptake of ^{125}I-labelled liposomes		
(minutes)	Pseudomonas lipids	Synthetic lipids	Free albumin
0	0.8	1.2	0.0
10	6.2	4.6	0.1
40	7.1	7.1	0.2
60	15.2	20.6	1.1
120	18.4	45.6	2.5

Incubation mixtures contained per ml 0.9-1.3 mg bacterial protein
and about 0.8 mg liposomal lipid (4-5 x 10^4 cpm). Negatively charged
liposomes (PC:Chol:PA, 7:5:1) in which tracer amount of ^{125}I-albumin
(spec. act. 1.25 x 10^7 cpm/mg) was entrapped were prepared by sonication for 15 min. Incubations were done at 37°C. Aliquots of 2 ml
taken at the appropriate times were centrifuged at 1500xg for 10 min
and the cell pellets washed three times. Other conditions as in
Fig. 1.   Liposomal ^{125}I-albumin was not degraded by P. aeruginosa
since all radioactivity of incubation media was TCA precipitable.
Therefore cell-associated and total radioactivity uptake coincide.

The clinical isolate P_{28-0} sensitive to carbenicillin, minimal
inhibitory concentration (MIC) 6.25 μg/ml, was trained by serial
passage to grow in carbenicillin (MIC 600 μg/ml) in Muller-Hinton
broth containing gradually increasing concentrations of the drug.[54]
The strain may be reverted to the parent type when allowed to grow in
antibiotic free media for, at least, three serial passages. Assay
cultures of the two strains were grown statically in Muller-Hinton
broth in the absence of the antibiotics for 24 hrs at 37°C.

Preliminary experiments showed that P. aeruginosa takes up
liposomes entrapped albumin very fast while uptake of free albumin
is negligible (Table 5). Furthermore, synthetic lipid liposomes are
taken up as efficiently as liposomes prepared from a P. aeruginosa
total lipid extract. Zero time uptake is quite high although pre-

cautions had been taken to stop liposome-cell interaction (x3 dilution of sample with saline, 0°C immediate centrifugation). Zero time values are reported therefore instead of correcting figures for zero time uptake. Our results are in agreement with the findings that incubation of Salmonella typhimurium with bilayer phospholipid vesicles results in significant transfer of vesicle lipids to the cells.[55,56]

In an attempt to follow the fate of radioactivity uptake we undertook a crude fractionation of the cells after a 30 min incubation with liposomes. The results showed, Table 6, that about 90% of the label was found in the cytosol. Further fractionation of the cytosol at a higher speed showed a 50/50% distribution of the label between supernatant and sediment. The second sediment must contain small envelope fractions.[57] It may also contain liposomes separated from the surface of the cells during their sonication. These liposomes must be sedimented at the speed of 160.000xg for 120 min. It is improbable that smaller liposomes formed during the disruption of the cells may account for the 50% of the radioactivity found in the supernatant after the second centrifugation. A series of experiments are under way now to clarify this point.

TABLE 6. Distribution of radioactivity in subcellular fractions of Pseudomonas aeruginosa, P_{28}, after incubation of the cells with ^{125}I-albumin labelled liposomes.

Preparation	P_{28-0}		$P_{28-600Cb}$
	0 min	30 min	30 min
Cytosol (33000xg, 30 min)	88.6	85.0	86.0
1st sediment	11.3	15.0	14.0
Cytosol (160.000xg, 120 min)	ND	52.0	42.5
2nd sediment	ND	48.0	57.5

Cells were incubated for 30 min. with liposomes. They were then collected by centrifugation, washed three times and resuspended in Tris/HCl, pH 8.2. They were disrupted by sonication (MSE, Sonicator, Titanium probe, 2 cm d., 20 kg/s, 4 min), and fractionated as indicated. ND, not done.

In Table 7 a comparison of the uptake of liposomes by the parent strain P_{28-0} and the variant strain $P_{28-600Cb}$ is made. It can be seen that the carbenicillin resistant strain shows a higher rate of uptake of liposome-associated radioactivity as compared with the parent strain. Furthermore, carbenicillin resistant cells are associated with at least 2-fold higher quantities of liposomal albumin in comparison with the parent cells. A redistribution of membrane components in such a manner so that more phospholipids are exposed to the surface of the cell[58] may account for the higher association of liposomes by these cells. The high uptake of liposomal radioactivity by the resistant cells at zero time must be emphasized and shows again the higher affinity of the liposomes for these cells. As in the case of the parent strain, free albumin is not associated with the carbenicillin resistant strain.

TABLE 7.   Uptake of free and liposome entrapped ^{125}I-albumin by viable cells of <u>Pseudomonas aeruginosa</u>, strains P_{28-0} and $P_{28-600Cb}$.

Time (mins)	% cpm/mg bacterial protein			
	Liposomal albumin		Free albumin	
	P_{28-0}	$P_{28-600Cb}$	P_{28-0}	$P_{28-600Cb}$
0	3.1	14.5	0.03	0.02
10	15.0	43.9	0.05	0.04
20	20.5	50.7	0.07	0.05
30	24.5	56.0	0.10	0.08
60	26.1	53.4	0.50	0.60

Conditions are given in Table 5.

CONCLUSION

Liposome-entrapped albumin is associated with <u>Pseudomonas aeruginosa</u> cells while free albumin is not. Liposomal albumin is associated with habituated, carbenicillin-resistant strain of <u>P. aeruginosa</u> with a higher rate and at higher quantities when compared with the parent strain. Liposomes may be used therefore, to facilitate association of larger quantities of entrapped compounds with cultured cells than cell envelope barriers permit.

GENERAL SUMMARY

The results presented above make it clear that the same cell in the course of its life cycle may change composition and properties including its mode of interaction and processing of liposomes. The stage of the development of the cell therefore is an important factor to be considered when liposomes are to be used as drug carriers.

REFERENCES

1. G. Poste, The interaction of lipid vesicles (liposomes) with
    cultured cells and their use as carriers for drugs and
    macromolecules in: "Liposomes in Biological Systems", G.
    Gregoriadis and A.C. Allison, eds., John Wiley, Chichester,
    New York (1980).
2. H. Kutchai, Y. Barenholz, T.F. Ross and D.E. Wermer, Develop-
    mental changes in plasma membrane fluidity in check embryo
    heart, Biochim. Biophys. Acta, 436: 101 (1976).
3. Y. Kawasaki, N. Wakayama, T. Koike, M. Kawai and T. Amano, A
    change in membrane microviscosity of mouse neuroblastoma
    cells in association with morphological differentiation,
    Biochim. Biophys. Acta, 509: 40 (1978).
4. A. Ryter and P. Brachet, Cell surface changes during early
    development stages of Dictyostelium discoideum: A scanning
    electron microscopic study, Biol. Cellul., 31:265 (1978)
5. H.B. Bosmann, Mechanism of cellular drug resistance, Nature, 233:
    566 (1971).
6. D.V. Mohan Das and G. Weeks, Effects of polyunsaturated fatty
    acids on the growth and differentiation of the cellular
    slime mould, Dictyostelium discoideum, Exp. Cell. Res.
    118: 237 (1979).
7. A. Kennedy and C. Rice-Evans, A spectrofluorimetric study of
    the interaction of glycerol mono-oleate with human erythro-
    cyte ghosts, FEBS Letters, 69: 45 (1976).
8. B.E. Schaeffer and A.S.G. Curtis, Effects on cell adhesion and
    membrane fluidity of changes in plasmalemmal lipids in
    mouse L929 cells, J. Cell. Sc. 26: 47 (1977).
9. W.F. Loomis, "Dictyostellium discoideum. A developmental system",
    Academic Press, New York (1975).
10. G. Gerisch, Cell aggregation and differentiation in Dictyostel-
    ium, Curr. Top. Develop. Biol., 3: 157 (1968).
11. J. Fukui and J. Takeuchi, Drug resistant mutants and appearance
    of heterozygotes in the cellular slime mould Dictyostelium
    discoideum., J. Gen. Microb. 67: 307 (1971).
12. K. Muller and G. Gerisch, A specific glycoprotein as the target
    site of adhesion blocking Fab in aggregating Dictyostelium
    cells, Nature, 274: 445 (1978).
13. R.W. Parish and S. Schmidlin, Synthesis of plasma membrane pro-
    eins during development of Dictyostelium discoideum. FEBS
    Letters, 98: 257 (1979).
14. N.R. Gilkes, K. Laroy and G. Weeks, An analysis of the protein,
    glycoprotein and monosaccharide composition of Dictyostelium
    discoideium plasma membranes during development, Biochim.
    Biophys. Acta, 551: 349 (1979).
15. E.J. Henderson, the cyclic adenosine 3'5'-monophosphate receptor
    of Dictoystelium discoideum, J. Biol. Chem., 250: 4730 (1975).
16. S. Sierers, H.J. Risse and K. Sekeri-Pataryas, Mol. Cell. Biochem.
    20: 103 (1978).

17. K.L. Lee, Cell electrophoresis of the cellular slime mould
Dictyostelium discoideum, J. Cell. Sc. 10: 229 (1972).

18. G. Weeks and F.G. Herring, The lipid composition and membrane
fluidity of Dictyostelium discoideum plasma membranes at
various stages during differentiation. J. Lip. Res. 21:
681 (1980).

19. H.B. Long and E.L. Coe, Changes in neutral lipid constituents
during differentiation of the cellular slime mould
Dictyostelium discoideum, J. Biol. Chem. 249 521 (1974).

20. J.S. Ellingson, Changes in the phospholipid composition in the
differentiating cellular slime mould Dictyostelium discoideum, Biochim. Biophys. Acta, 337: 60 (1974).

21. C. de Chastellier and A. Ryter, Changes of the cell surface and
of the digestive apparatus of Dictyostelium discoideum
during the starvation period triggering aggregation. J.
Cell Biol. 75: 218 (1977).

22. A. Newton, The chemotherapy of trypanosomiasis and leishmaniasis, CIBA Found. Symp. (new series), 20: 285 (1974).

23. A.M. Fairlamb, F.R. Opperdoes and O. Borst, New approach to
screening drugs for activity against African Trypanosomiasis,
Nature, 265: 270 (1977).

24. C.J. Bacchi, H.C. Nathan, S.H. Hutner, P.P. McCann and A.
Sjoerdsma, Polyamine metabolism; A potential therapeutic
target in Trypanosomes, Science, 210:332 (1980).

25. G.A.M.Cross, Antigenic variation in trypanosomes, Proc. R. Soc.
London B. 202: 55 (1978).

26. J.D. Barry and K. Vickerman, Trypanosoma brucei: Loss of variable antigens during transformation from bloodstream to
procyclic forms in vitro, Exp. Parasitol., 48: 313 (1979).

27. K. Vikerman, Antigenic variation in trypanosomes, Nature, 273:
613 (1978).

28. H. Van de Bossche, Chemotherapy of parasitic infections, Nature,
273: 626 (1978).

29. C.D.V. Black, G.J. Watson and R.J. Ward, The use of pentostam
liposomes in the chemotherapy of experimental leishmaniasis, Trans. Roy. Soc. Trop. Med. Hyg. 71: 550 (1977).

30. R.R.C. New, M.L. Chance, S.C. Thomas and W. Peters, Antileishmanial activity of antimonials entrapped in liposomes,
Nature, 272: 55 (1978).

31. C.R. Alving, E.A. Steck, W.L. Chapman Jr., V.B. Waits, L.D.
Hendricks, G.M. Swartz Jr., and W.L. Hanson, Therapy of
leishmaniasis: Superior effecacies of liposome-encapsulated drugs, Proc. Nat. Acad. Sci. USA, 75: 2959 (1978).

32. K. Vickerman, The ultrastructure of pathogenic flagellates,
CIBA Found. Symp. (new series), 20: 171 (1974).

33. R.B. McGhee and W.B. Cosgrove, Biology and Physiology of the
lower Trypanosomatidae, Microbiol. Rev. 44: 140 (1980).

34. G.W. Kidder and B.N. Dutta, The growth and nutrition of
Crithidia fasciculata, J. Gen. Microbiol., 18: 621 (1958).

35. K.M. Tamburro and S.H. Hunter, Carbohydrate-free media for

Crithidia, J. Protozool, 18: 667 (1971).

36. N.S. Constantsas, G.M. Levis and C. Vakirtzi-Lemonias,
     Crithidia fasciculata tyrosine transaminase, 1. Develop-
     ment, characterization and differentiation from alanine
     transaminase, Biochim. Biophys. Acta., 230: 137 (1971).

37. F.B. St. C. Palmer, Lipids of Crithidia fasciculata, The
     occurrence and turnover of phosphoinosides, Biochim.
     Biophys. Acta., 316: 396 (1973).

38. P.A.J. Gorin, J.O. Previato, L. Mendosa-Previato and L.R.
     Travassos, Structure of the D-mannan and D-arabino- -
     galactan in Crithidia fasciculata, Changes in composition
     with age of culture, J. Protozool, 26: 473 (1979).

39. N. Frantzis and C. Vakirtzi-Lemonias, Concanavalin A receptors
     of the surface membrane of Crithidia fasciculata. Biochem.
     Soc. Trans., 9: 135 (1981).

40. K.B. Easterbrook, The ultrastructure of Crithidia fasciculata,
     A freeze-etching study, Canad. J. Microbiol. 17: 277 (1971).

41. B.E. Brooker, The cell coat of Crithidia fasciculata, Parasit-
     ology 72: 259 (1976).

42. C. Vakirtzi-Lemonias, C.C. Karahalios and G.M. Levis, Fatty
     acid oxidation by Crithidia fasciculata, Can. J. Biochem.,
     50: 501 (1972).

43. C.J. Bacchi, C. Lambros, B. Goldberg, S.G. Hutner and G.D.F.
     de Carvalho, Susceptibility of an insect Leptomonas and
     Crithidia fasciculata to several established antitrypano-
     somatid agents, Antimicrob. Ag. Chemother. 6: 785 (1974).

44. M. Midgley, The transport of -aminobutyrate into Crithidia
     fasciculata, Biochem. J. 174: 191 (1978).

45. V.C. Dewey, G.W. Kidder and L.L. Nolan, Mechanism of inhibition
     of Crithidia fasciculata by adenosine and adenosine ana-
     logs, Biochem. Pharmacol.,27: 1479 (1978).

46. M. Midgley and M.C. Stephenson, Measurement of membrane poten-
     tial component of the transmembrane proton electrochemical
     gradient in Crithidia fasciculata, Biochem. Soc. Trans.,

47. C. Vakirtzi-Lemonias and G. Gregoriadis, Uptake of liposome
     entrapped agents by the trypanosome Crithidia fasciculata,
     Biochem. Soc. Trans., 6: 1241 (1978).

48. J. Gruenberg, D. Coral, A.L. Knupfer and J. Deshusses, Inter-
     actions of liposomes with Trypanosoma brucei plasma mem-
     branes, Biochem. Biophys. Res. Commun., 88: 1173 (1979).

49. P. Chadwick, Resistance of Pseudomonas aeruginosa to gentamicin,
     Can. Med. Ass. Journal, 109: 585 (1973).

50. N.J. Legakis, J. Tselentis, K.J. Courtis, J. Papavassiliou,
     Cross resistance of clinical isolates of Pseudomonas aerug-
     inosa to five aminoglycosides, J. Antimicrob. Chem. 5:
     487 (1979).

51. R. Benviste and J. Davies, Mechanisms of antibiotic resistance
     in bacteria, Ann. Rev. Biochem. 42: 471 (1973)

52. T.R. Korfhagen, J.C. Lopez and J.A. Ferrel, Pseudomonas aerug-
     inosa R factors determining gentamicin plus carbenicillin

resistance from patients with urinary tract colonization.
Antimicr. Agents Chemoth., 7: 64 (1975).

53. J.W. Payne and C. Gilvarg, Size restriction on peptide util-
     ization in E. coli, J. Biol. Chem. 243: 6291 (1968).

54. P.E. Lianous, H.P. Bassaris, G.K. Kaikos, T.A. Katsorchis
     and N.J. Legakis, Increased adherence to human epithelial
     cells of resistant Pseudomonas aeruginosa strains, J.
     Infect. 2: 354 (1980).

55. N.C. Jones and M.J. Osborn, Interaction of Salmonella typhimur-
     ium with phospholipid vesicles, J. Biol. Chem.252: 7398
     (1977).

56. N.C. Jones and M.J. Osborn, Translocation of phospholipids
     between the outer and inner membranes of Salmonella
     typhimurium, J. Biol. Chem. 252: 7405 (1977).

57. H. Nikaido and T. Nakae, The outer membrane of gram negative
     bacteria, Adv. Microb. Physiol., 20: 164 (1979).

58. T.I. Nicas and R.E.W. Hancock, Outer membrane protein H_1 of
     Pseudomonas aeruginosa: involvement in adaptive and muta-
     tional resistance to ethylenediaminetetracetate, Polymyxin
     B, and gentamicin, J. Bacter., 143: 872 (1980).

DEVELOPMENT OF LIPOSOMES AS AN EFFICIENT CARRIER SYSTEM:
NEW METHODOLOGY FOR CELL TARGETING
AND INTRACELLULAR DELIVERY OF DRUGS AND DNA

D. Papahadjopoulos[+], T. Heath, F. Martin,
R. Fraley*, and R. Straubinger
Cancer Research Institute, and [+]Department of
Pharmacology, University of California, San Francisco,
CA 94143 and *Monsanto Company, St. Louis, Missouri 63166

Liposomes are a valuable carrier system for enhancing the pharmacological activity of drugs and the functional incorporation of macromolecules into cells. During the last few years, we have concentrated on developing new liposome methodology designed to optimize their properties as a carrier system. We will describe some of these procedures related to the following specific topics: (1) efficiency of encapsulation: the reverse phase evaporation method produces large unilamellar vesicles (0.2-0.4 μdiameter) encapsulating approximately 50% of the initial aqueous phase. This procedure is particularly valuable for the encapsulation of large macromolecules such as RNA and DNA which can be entrapped with very high efficiency and no appreciable degradation. (2) control of vesicle size: extrusion of liposomes through nucleopore membranes produces vesicles which conform to the membrane pore diameter without loss of material. This allows the preparation of reasonably homogeneous populations of unilamellar vesicles in the range of 0.1-0.2 μ in diameter. (3) control of liposome permeability: minimizing permeability by increasing the cholesterol content increases dramatically in vivo anti-tumour effects. This has been tested with Ara-C containing vesicles against L1210 leukemia in mice. (4) intracellular delivery of macromolecules: the infectivity of liposome-encapsulated SV40 DNA is enhanced up to 1000-fold over free DNA and is dependent on the vesicle lipid compositions and the incubation conditions. The highest infectivity is achieved with vesicles composed of phosphatidylserine and cholesterol (1:1 mole ratio) in the presence of chloroquine, and in conjunction with a short post-incubation treatment with high concentrations of glycerol. Under these conditions, the infectivity of SV40 DNA (3 x 10^5 pfu/ g DNA) is comparable or greater than can be obtained using the $Ca_3(PO_4)_2$techniques for DNA delivery. (5) targeting to specific cells: the covalent attachment of cell specific $F(ab')_2$ and Fab'

fragments of IgG to the liposome surface induces nearly quantitative
uptake of liposomes by target cells. These new procedures increase
by 100-fold the uptake of liposomes and their contents by the target
cells. Current studies involve monoclonal antibodies against a
variety of human and murine antigenic determinants.

INTRODUCTION

        Liposomes were developed originally as a model membrane system,
not as a drug carrier. It should not be surprising therefore that
the original preparative methodology has not been optimal in relation
to use of liposomes as a carrier system. The most commonly used
methods for preparation of liposomes are the multilamellar vesicles
(MLV) originally described by Bangham et al.(1965) and the small
sonicated unilamellar vesicles initially described by Papahadjopoulos
and Miller (1967) and later characterized in more detail by Huang
(1969). The main drawbacks of these "classical" liposome preparations
are the wide heterogeneity in size distribution and number of lamellae
(Olson et al., 1979), the relatively low trapping efficiency of
aqueous space (Szoka and Papahadjopoulos, 1978), and/or their inability to encapsulate large macromolecules due to their small internal
volume (Adrian and Huang, 1979). Several new methods have been published recently describing the preparation of large unilamellar vesicles
(LUV) which exhibit a relatively high ratio of internal aqueous space
per unit lipid (Papahadjopoulos et al., 1975; Deamer and Bangham,
1976; Szoka and Papahadjopoulos, 1978; Enoch and Strittmater, 1979;
Szoka et al., 1980). These methods produce liposomes which can be
considered to have inherent advantages as carrier systems, and will
be valuable for future uses of liposomes in cellular systems. In this
paper, we will discuss recent methodology developed in our laboratory
in relation to two parameters: efficiency of encapsulation and control of particle size.

        Perhaps the two most important aspects of liposomes as a carrier
system are the efficiency by which they deliver their contents (drugs
or other macromolecules) into cells, and the ability to recognize
specific cell types. Although numerous studies have shown already
that liposome encapsulation can increase cellular delivery,
(Gregoriadis, 1976; Poste et al., 1976; Tyrrell et al., 1976) no
systematic effort has been undertaken so far to optimize these
effects. We will discuss here our own work on the delivery of functionally intact viral DNA into cells using liposomes, with special
emphasis on the use of this system for optimizing conditions for
liposome delivery. Finally, we will describe new methods for covalent
binding of antibody molecules (IgG) on liposome surface with promising
new evidence for increased cellular specificity.

Efficiency of Encapsulation

        The reverse phase evaporation method (REV) was developed in an attempt to maximize the efficiency of encapsulation of the available aqueous space (Szoka and Papahadjopoulos, 1978). Table I summarises the percentage of aqueous space encapsulated by various methods of liposome preparation at identical lipid concentrations. It is obvious that the REV procedure yields a much higher efficiency (in the range of 40-60% depending on the ionic conditions and lipid composition). The resulting vesicles are in the range of 0.2-0.8 μ in diameter and have a very high ratio of internal aqueous volume per lipid (14 ml/g). Calculations of the expected internal aqueous space for vesicles of this diameter give very similar values if it is assumed that each vesicle is composed of one bilayer (Szoka and Papahadjopoulos, 1978). More recent experimental evidence based on chemical reactivity (Szoka et al., 1980) and proton NMR spectrum broadening (unpublished observations) indicate that 50% of the phospholipid head groups are exposed to the exterior of the vesicles, a finding consistent with a predominantly unilamellar configuration.

Table 1. Comparison of Various Liposome Preparations

	MLV	SUV	LUV*	REV
Diameter[+] (microns)	0.2-10	0.02-0.05	0.2-1.0	0.2-0.8
Encapsulation[++] Efficiency (%)	5-15	0.5-1.0	5-15	35-65
Captured[++] Volume (μl/mg)	4	0.5	9	14

Vesicle preparations were composed of PG/PC/Chol (1/4/5 mole ratios) prepared at 66 μmoles/ml in phosphate buffered saline.

* Prepared from PS/Chol (1/1) by fusion of SUV with Ca^{2+}, followed by EDTA.
+ Diameter range was based on EM observation by negative stain and freeze fracture.
++ Encapsulation efficiency and captured volume were obtained with radioactive sucrose as marker.
MLV: Multilamellar vesicles; SUV: Small unilamellar vesicles;
LUV: Large unilamellar vesicles; REV: Vesicles prepared by Reverse Phase Evaporation.

The REV procedure is relatively simple, quick, and can be applied to a variety of lipid compositions. The resultant vesicles are quite stable and predictably impermeable to molecules such as sucrose or araC (Mayhew et al., 1979). Special care should be taken, however,

to use freshly re-distilled ether (to avoid peroxides) and to dialyze
or gel-filtrate the vesicles soon after their preparation (to remove
any traces of ether not eliminated by evaporation). A unique
advantage of the method is that high trapping efficiency is obtained
both for compounds of small molecular weight, as well as large macromolecules such as ferritin (0.5×10^6 daltons) or SV40 DNA (3.5×10^6
daltons). The procedure does not appear to denature the DNA (see
below) or some encapsulated enzymes, and has been used recently for
the reconstitution of purified rhodopsin (Darszon, et al., 1979).
In summary, the REV method has a number of desirable characteristics
and considerable advantages over other methods for the production of
well-defined unilamellar liposomes capable of efficiently encapsulating large macromolecules. Its use will be described in the sections
below.

Homogeneity and Control of Particle Size

     Of all the commonly used liposome preparations, only the small
unilamellar vesicles (SUV) exhibit any appreciable homogeneity in
particle size distribution. In an attempt to produce a narrower size
distribution from preparations of liposomes with diameters in the
micron range, we have developed a method involving extrusion through
polycarbonate membranes (Olsen et al., 1979). During extrusion of
liposomes through straight pore (nucleopore) membranes under pressure,
the larger vesicles give rise to smaller ones. Sequential extrusion
through membranes of decreasing pore diameter produces liposomes which
conform closely to the diameter of the pore through which they have
been extruded. The lipid recovery is nearly quantitative, and if the
extrusion is done in the presence of the material to be encapsulated
there is no loss in efficiency of trapping. The method can be applied
to both MLV and LUV (Szoka and Papahadjopoulos, 1978; Szoka et al.,
1980) and produces populations of liposomes within a well-controlled
size range from 1.0 to 0.1 microns in diameter. The extrusion is
easy to perform, highly reproducible, involves no losses or degradation and can be used to sterilize the liposome preparations.

Liposome-mediated Delivery of DNA to Cells

     Previous studies from this laboratory have demonstrated that
large unilamellar PS vesicles are capable of encapsulating poliovirus
RNA and delivering it efficiently to both primate and nonprimate cells
(Wilson et al., 1979; Papahadjopoulos et al., 1980). The biological
activity of the liposome-encapsulated polio RNA was high ($1-2 \times 10^4$
pfu/ng RNA) and the data suggested that infection could be initiated
by a single RNA molecule. Liposome-mediated DNA delivery may be useful in increasing the efficiency of transfection in existing cell
genetic systems as well as extending genetic studies to those cells
which are not transformable using current techniques for gene delivery.
For our initial studies we have examined SV40 DNA in liposomes for the
following reasons: 1) The existence of sensitive plaque and fluore-

scent assays makes possible the quantitation of DNA delivery; 2) its relatively small size (3.5 x 10^6 daltons) facilitates encapsulation in lipid vesicles and 3) the availability of a variety of recombinant SV40 DNA molecules and its potential use as a gene vector make it an important molecule to study. Liposomes containing SV40 DNA were prepared by the reverse evaporation procedure described above and were separated from free DNA by flotation on discontinuous Ficoll gradients. These gradients provided a rapid and quantitative separation of vesicles from DNA (and other large macromolecules) that is not easily achievable by molecular sieve chromatography or velocity centrifugation (Fraley et al., 1980). The biological activity of the liposome-encapsulated SV40 DNA was determined by plaque assays on CV-1P African Green Monkey Kidney cells (Mertz and Berg, 1974) and was compared to control SV40 DNA. The infectivity of control and liposome-extracted SV40 DNA using the DEAE/Dextran procedure, was identical (approx. 5 x 10^6 pfu/μg). The incubation of 10 ng of liposome-encapsulated SV40 DNA with AGMK cells resulted in a low frequency of infection (1.5 x 10^3 pfu/μg), while naked SV40 DNA (100 ng) was not infective (10 pfu/μg) when incubated with cells under the same conditions. Buffer-loaded vesicles did not increase the infectivity of naked SV40 DNA (100 ng). The infectivity of the liposome-encapsulated SV40 DNA was not affected by DNAse whereas the infectivity of a DEAE-Dextran DNA complex was very sensitive to DNAse digestion.

The infectivity of the liposome encapsulated SV40 DNA was 100-1000 fold less efficient that was found for encapsulated polio RNA under similar conditions, which may partly reflect the requirement for delivery of SV40 DNA to the nucleus for its replication. Since a number of different vesicle lipid compositions have been reported to promote liposome-mediated delivery of molecules to cells (Pagano and Weinstein, 1978), we examined whether vesicles formed from other phospholipids or lipid mixtures would be more efficient in delivering SV40 DNA to cells than pure PS vesicles. The results of a number of experiments using different vesicle lipid compositions are summarized in Table 2. Vesicles made from egg PC, a neutral phospholipid, were at least 10 fold less efficient that PS vesicles in promoting DNA delivery, and the inclusion of 10 mol% stearylamine in the egg PC vesicles to make them positively-charged, lowered infectivity even further (not shown). The infectivity of SV40 DNA encapsulated in a variety of other negatively-charged lipid vesicles (see Table 2) was much lower (10-100 fold) than observed for PS vesicles. The efficiency of encapsulation of SV40 DNA in these various preparations was similar and the large differences observed in infectivity must therefore reflect differences in the extent of cell binding, or differences in the ability of liposomes to delivery their contents. A detailed analysis and comparison of the cell binding for the various liposome preparations has revealed that the relatively high efficiency of DNA delivery promoted by the PS vesicles is due to their high binding affinity and their resistance to cell-induced leakage of contents (Fraley et al., 1981). As a result, a greater amount of the liposome-

Table 2. Infectivity of SV40 DNA encapsulated in various
          liposomes*

Vesicle Lipid Composition	μg DNA per μmol LIPID[a]	pfu/μg DNA[b]	pfu/μg DNA[c]
Free DNA	---	1.0	2×10^2
Free DNA + PS	0.4	1.0	---
PC	0.31	1.1×10^2	4.9×10^2
PG	0.36	40	1.7×10^3
PS	0.44	1.5×10^3	2.3×10^4
PS:Chol (1:1)	0.35	1.8×10^3	3.4×10^4

*Incubation and plaque assays were performed as described by Mertz
and Berg (1974). Liposomes were prepared by the reverse phase evaporation technique and employed 10 μmol of phospholipid and 10 μg SV40
DNA in the preparation. The liposome preparations were sized and
sterilized by passage through 0.4 μm Unipore filters and were separated from unencapsulated DNA by flotation on Ficoll gradients.
[a]The amount of encapsulated DNA per μmole of phospholipid.
(1, 10 or 100 ng of DNA were added to each plate).
[b]The infectivity of liposome-encapsulated SV40 DNA in the
absence of glycerol.
[c]The infectivity of liposome-encapsulated SV40 DNA following
a 20% glycerol wash.

encapsulated SV40 DNA remains available for intracellular delivery.

Treatments which have been used to increase vesicle fusion or
promote the uptake of DNA into cells (Fraley et al., 1980) were tested
to determine if they enhanced the infectivity of liposome-encapsulated
SV40 DNA. Treatment of the cells with either DMSO (25% v/v), PEG
(45% w/v) or glycerol (20% v/v) after a 30 min incubation of vesicles
with cells increased SV40 infectivity an additional 10-20 fold and
the use of 40% w/v glycerol increased infectivity an additional 10-
fold to 3×10^5 pfu/μg (Fraley et al., 1981).

The enhancement of the infectivity of liposome-encapsulated SV40
DNA by glycerol is relatively specific for negatively-charged liposomes (Table 2). The infectivity of PS and PG liposomes containing
SV40 DNA is enhanced 100-200 fold by exposure of cells to glycerol,
whereas the infectivity of SV40 DNA encapsulated in PC or PC-SA

liposomes was only increased 2-5 fold following the glycerol treatment.

Glycerol also increases the infectivity of liposome-encapsulated polio RNA, which shows the same proportional enhancement by glycerol following incubation with either AGMK or HeLa cells. Glycerol stimulation of liposome delivery of DNA occurs via an energy-dependent pathway (inhibitable by Na-Azide plus 2-deoxyglucose), and is largely unaffected by agents which disrupt microtubule structure (Fraley, et al., 1981). Treatment of cells with chloroquine, which alters lysosomal activity, enhances infectivity of liposome-encapsulated SV40 DNA an additional 5-fold following glycerol treatment which suggests a lysosomal processing step following uptake in glycerol-treated cells and illustrates the possibilities for altering liposome-cell interactions to engineer more efficient delivery by liposomes.

The percentage of cells which can be infected by liposome-containing SV40 DNA is critically dependent on the number of DNA copies per vesicle (Fraley et al., 1980). Under optimal conditions, 30% of the cell population are infected when incubated with liposomes containing approx. 10 SV40 DNA molecules per vesicle, which is substantially higher than using either the DEAE dextran or calcium phosphate methods for transfection. Liposome-mediated DNA delivery will have practical application by increasing the efficiency of transformation in several other mammalian cell systems. The recent demonstration that liposomes efficiently deliver DNA (Dellaporta et al., 1982), and RNA (Fraley et al., 1982) to plant protoplasts is the first demonstration of the potential use of liposomes in plant genetics.

Targeting to Specific Cells

Several attempts have been made to increase the efficiency by which liposomes are taken up by cells. These include specific glycolipids (Bussian and Wriston, 1977), dinitrophenylated phospholipids and immunoglobulins (Weinstein et al., 1978), glycoproteins and lectins (Juliano and Stamp, 1976) heat-aggregated immunoglobulins (Weissmann et al., 1975) and immunoglobulins recognizing specific cell surface antigens (Gregoriadis, 1975; Magee, 1978). The latter approach seems to be the most promising, especially because of the recent development of monoclonal antibodies.

Previous attempts at conjugation of immunoglobulin to liposomes have relied mostly on non-covalent interactions during co-sonication of liposomes with immunoglobulins (Gregoriadis, 1975; Magee, 1978) which is not likely to yield an efficient interaction (Huang and Kennel, 1979), or on the use of bifunctional reagents (Dunnick et al., 1975; Torchilin et al., 1978; 1979) which produces homopolymers of vesicles and protein as a biproduct. We have recently developed new methods for covalent attachment of IgG molecules on liposomes,

which circumvent the above difficulties and yield liposomes with a
relatively high (100-200 μg protein per μmole lipid) protein to lipid
ratio (Heath et al., 1980; Martin et al., 1981; Martin and
Papahadjopoulos, 1981).

One of the new methods involves an initial periodate oxidation
of liposomes containing either phosphatidylglycerol or various glycolipids to produce reactive aldehyde residues. The protein is then
attached to the vesicles via free amino groups by Schiff-base formation and reduction (Heath et al., 1980a). We have shown that under
optimal conditions the conjugation occurs without leakage of the
liposome contents, and without appreciable degradation of any oxidi-
zable molecules within the interior of the vesicles. The unreacted
protein can be removed by flotation of the conjugated liposomes on
Dextran density gradients following centrifugation. The procedure
applies equally well to IgG and to F(ab')$_2$ fragments, and possibly
to other proteins (Heath et al., 1980a).

Another efficient method for covalently cross-linking 50K Fab
antibody fragments to the surface of liposomes was described more
recently (Martin et al., 1981). Coupling up to 600 μg Fab'/ mole
phospholipid (about 6000 Fab' molecules per 0.2 μ vesicle) is achieved
via a disulfide interchange reaction between the thiol group exposed
on each Fab' fragment and a pyridyl-dithiol derivative of phosphatidylethanolamine present in low concentration in the membranes of preformed large unilamellar vesicles. The coupling reaction is efficient,
proceeds rapidly under mild conditions and yields well-defined products. Each vesicle-linked Fab' fragment retains its original antigenic specificity and full capacity to bind antigen. We have used
Fab' fragments, coupled to vesicles by this method, to achieve
immunospecific targeting of liposomes to cells in vitro. Vesicles
bearing anti-human erythrocyte Fab' fragments bind quantitatively to
human erythrocytes (at multiples of up to 5000 vesicles per cell)
while essentially no binding is observed to sheep or ox red blood
cells. Vesicle-cell binding is stable over a pH range from 6 to 8
and is virtually unaffected by the presence of human serum (50%).
Cell-bound vesicles retain their aqueous contents and can be eluted
intact from cells by treatment with reducing agents (dithiothreitol
or mercaptoethanol) at alkaline pH (Martin et al., 1981). A very
recent report (Martin and Papahadjopoulos, 1981) describes another
conjugation method which has the advantage that the binding is
irreversible and stable even in the presence of reducing agents.

We have already described (Heath et al., 1980a) the binding of
anti-human erythrocyte F(ab')$_2$-conjugated vesicles to human erythrocytes. When 10^8 cells are incubated with up to 500 nmole lipid, 80%
of a lipid label (^{3}H-DPPC) and encapsulated marker (^{14}C-sucrose)
binds to the cells. Vesicle binding is extremely low (200 fold less)
if the vesicles are conjugated to normal rabbit F(ab')$_2$. This clearly
demonstrates that vesicles conjugated to antibody by this method bind

efficiently to the target cells. This system, however, can give little information about the number of antibodies per vesicle required for efficient binding, the cell antigen density, or the extent of inactivation of the antibody during vesicle conjugation.

To answer these questions we have conjugated antifluorescein antibody to vesicles and studied their binding to erythrocytes conjugated with fluorescein isothiocyanate. Antifluorescein may readily be immunopurified (Lopatin and Voss, 1971) to give preparations in which all the antibodies are specific for the antigen. Antifluorescein activity may be measured by the quenching of fluorescein. Using this technique, we have compared the activity of unmodified antifluorescein with vesicle-bound and residual unbound antifluorescein. Conjugation partially inactivates the antibody, and vesicle-bound antibody is inactivated more than the residual unbound antibody which has been exposed to vesicles and sodium cyanoborohydride. In a series of experiments we have observed that the vesicle-bound antibody retains 35-60% of its activity.

We have also examined vesicle-binding to cells with a series of preparations in which vesicles were conjugated to antifluorescein mixed with varying amounts of normal rabbit IgG. In such an experiment it is possible to control the number of active antifluorescein antibodies per vesicle, which can be measured directly by fluorescence quenching. Preparations containing 33 to 186 active antibodies per vesicle show 75% binding to 10^8 erythrocytes when up to 200 nmole lipid is added to the cells, while a preparation with 2 molecules per vesicle bound poorly to cells. Some differences are observed in the extent of binding of the various preparations when 10^7 or 10^6 cells are used. However, the most striking differences are observed in hapten inhibition studies. Carboxyfluorescein added before vesicle

Table 3. Inhibition of vesicle binding by carboxyfluorescein*

Number of Active Antibodies/Vesicle	Vesicle Binding to Cells (% of maximal)	
	10^8 Cells	10^7 Cells
186	73	66
67	68	23
33	54	9

* 50 nmole lipid was incubated with 10^7 or 10^8 cells in the presence of 10^{-6}M carboxyfluorescein. Binding is expressed as the % of that observed for 50 nmole lipid in the absence of carboxyfluorescein.

cell mixing at concentrations between 10^{-8} and 10^{-3} M reduces specific
binding from 100% in the absence of CF (observed at 10^{-9} M CF) to 0
(observed at 10^{-3} M CF). 10^{-6} M carboxyfluorescein will reduce
specific binding to a variable extent depending upon the number of
antibody molecules per liposome (Table 3). Differences are most
striking for incubations with 10^7 erythrocytes where the vesicle with
33 active molecules per vesicles are 91% inhibited whereas the vesicles with 186 molecules per vesicle are only 34% inhibited. This
demonstrates that high numbers of antibody molecules per liposome may
increase the affinity of vesicles for the cell surface and enable the
vesicles to bind in the presence of soluble antigen. This may be a
decisive factor in the use of antibody targeted vesicles against
tumors which shed soluble antigen, for example CEA or HCG.

Targeting and delivery of Methotrexate with monoclonal antibodies

The above experiments clearly demonstrate that antibody conjugation to liposomes can promote binding of the liposomes to a cellular
target, but do not address whether delivery may be achieved by such
binding. To perform such experiments we have investigated the interaction of liposomes conjugated to a monoclonal mouse antiH2K^k antibody
(Oi et al., 1978) with a variety of cells in culture. We have also
examined the toxicity of methotrexate (MTX) encapsulated in targeted
liposomes on L929 fibroblasts.

Table 4 shows the binding of 20 nmole targeting and non-targeted
liposomes to a variety of cells in the presence or absence of serum.
There is no evidence that conjugation to a nonspecific (anti-sheep
RBC) monoclonal increases liposome binding to cells. This is interesting since some of the cell types tested (spleen cells, S49.1) are
known to express Fc receptors. Evidently, conjugation of antibody to
liposomes does not provide any triggering of Fc interaction, which is
useful since it may avoid unwanted interaction of targeted liposomes
with the RE system.

Anti H2K^k targeted liposomes show increased interaction only
with cells of the relevant H2 haplotype (L929, R1.1, CBA splenocytes).
Amongst the control lines tested is a variant of R1.1 (R1E/T18 x 1)
which is a deletion mutant lacking the K-D region (Hyman and Stallings,
1976), and this confirms most closely the specificity of the interaction.

In previous studies with erythrocytes the difference between
specific and nonspecific binding was much greater than is observed
here. This is in part due to nonspecific liposome binding to cultured
cells which is higher than is observed for erythrocytes. However,
nonspecific binding may be reduced, without affecting targeted interaction by the addition of serum to the incubation medium. Binding of
targeted liposomes to L929 is only 6-fold greater than non-targeted
binding in the absence of serum, but 18-fold greater than non-targeted

Table 4. Binding of monoclonal antibody targeted liposomes to cells.

Cell Type	Serum[a]	nMole Lipid Bound[a]			
		Uncoated[d]	SRBC[e]	H2K^{k}[f]	Binding[g]
L929[b]	−	2.7	2.1	12.4	5.9
	+	1.2	0.6	10.6	17.6
R1.1[c]	−	0.3	0.5	2.8	5.6
	+	−	0.1	4.2	42
CBA Splenocytes[c]	+	0.1	0.1	3.4	34
Balb/c Splenocytes[c]	+		0.1	0.2	0.1
Balb/c 3T6[b]	+	0.4	0.5	0.4	0.8
R1E/T18 x .1[c]	+	0.2	0.3	0.1	0.3
Balb/c S49.1[c]	+	0.5	0.1	0.1	1

[a] Cells were incubated with 20 nMole lipid in 0.2 ml PBS $\pm$ 50% newborn calf serum.
[b] 5×10^{6} cells in monolayer.
[c] 2×10^{6} cells in suspension.
[d] 5:5:1 PC: cholesterol:ganglioside vesicles labelled with ^{3}H-DPPC (2000 cpm/nmole).
[e] vesicles conjugated to monoclonal antisheep erythrocyte IgG$_{2a}$.
[f] Vesicles conjugated to monoclonal antiH2K^{k} IgG$_{2a}$.
[g] Binding=nmole antiH2K^{k} coated liposomes bound divided by nmole antiSRBC coated liposomes bound.

binding in the presence of serum. Similarly for R1.1 addition of serum increased the difference between specific and nonspecific binding from 6-fold to 42-fold. Such levels of enhancement of binding are comparable to those seen with erythrocytes. Moreover, the effects of serum are clearly advantageous when considering liposome targeting in vivo.

There are numerous compounds which one might use for examining the delivery of contents of antibody targeted liposomes to cells, including SV40 DNA (Fraley et al., 1980). In our initial experiments, we chose to investigate the delivery of a drug of proven potency to see whether antibody targeting could promote its delivery sufficiently to achieve enhanced toxicity (Table 5). In all our experiments, soluble MTX has proved to be the most potent preparation, with an ID$_{50}$ of 1.8×10^{-8}M. When encapsulated at 0.2mM in non-targeted vesicles, the MTX had an ID$_{50}$ of 1.5×10^{-6}M, whilst drug encapsulated at 26mM had an ID$_{50}$ of 3.8×10^{-8}M. This difference is most likely a reflection of the rate at which the drug leaks from the liposomes since it is well known that the effects of encapsulated drug in non-targeted liposomes may largely be ascribed to leakage (Allen et al., 1981). When the vesicles are targeted there is a 25-fold increase in the toxicity of MTX when encapsulated at 0.2mM while a 2-fold increase is observed when MTX is encapsulated at 26mM. It is not yet clear to what extent the increase in toxicity is due to delivery or leakage. It seems most likely that both factors are involved and indeed any enhancement of leakage may be due to the internalization and lysosomal processing of the vesicles. It is clear that weakly acidic molecules such as MTX and carboxyfluorescein (Fraley et al., 1981) may rapidly escape the lysosomal compartment into the cytoplasm. Furthermore, MTX is known to be transported out of cells rapidly (Goldman et al., 1968) and may therefore leak from the cells after delivery to the cytoplasm. The effective delivery of such a drug may require a sustained uptake of vesicles and cytoplasmic delivery of their contents, which may only be achieved at an optimal drug-vesicle ratio. This may explain why the toxicity of drug encapsulated at 0.2 mM is increased more by antibody targeting than the drug encapsulated at 26mM.

Table 5. Toxicity of methotrexate in targeted liposomes

Encapsulated	Targeted	Encapsulation Concentration (mM)	ID_{50} (M)	Lipid Concentration at ID_{50} (nmole/ml)
---	---	---	1.8×10^{-8}	---
+	---	0.2	1.5×10^{-6}	1910
+	+	0.2	6×10^{-8}	76
+	---	26	3.8×10^{-8}	0.18
+	+	26	2.2×10^{-8}	0.11

Methotrexate was encapsulated in phosphatidylcholine: cholesterol: MPB-PE (10:10:1) liposomes at concentrations indicated. Targeted vesicles were conjugated to 60 μg/μmole monoclonal antiH2K[k]. Toxicity was determined on L929 fibroblasts seeded at 10^5 per well, left 24 hours before treatment, and treated 48 hours before resuspension and counting. ID_{50} = drug concentration required to inhibit growth by 50%.

CONCLUSION

We have described several interrelated approaches to the ultimate goal of increasing the efficiency of liposomes as a carrier
system for the intracellular delivery of drugs and macromolecules.
It is clear that each of the methods we discussed enhances the usefulness of liposomes for the specific cases we have studied so far. Some
of these procedures are generally applicable and should be valuable
for future experimentation in other systems. It will be particularly
interesting to establish whether liposome targeting can be applied
against specific cell types in vivo.

REFERENCES

Adrian, G., Huang, L., 1979, Entrapment of proteins in phosphatidyl-
    choline vesicles, Biophys. J. 25: A292.
Allen, T.M., McAllister, L., Mausolf, S. and Gyoffry, E., 1981,
    A study of the interactions of liposomes containing entrapped
    anti-cancer drugs with the EMT6, S49 and AE_1 (transport deficient)
    cell lines, Biochim. Biophys. Acta, 643: 346.
Bangham, A.D., Standish, M.M., Watkins, J.C., 1965, Diffusion of
    univalent ions across the lamellae of swollen phospholipids,
    J. Mol. Biol., 13: 238.
Bussian, R.W., and Wriston, J.C., 1977, Influence of incorporated
    cerebrosides on the interactions of liposomes with HeLa cells,
    Biochim. Biophys. Acta, 471: 336.
Deamer, D., Bangham, A.D., 1976, Large volume liposomes by an ether
    vaporization method, Biochim. Biophys. Acta, 443: 629.
Dellaporta, S., Giles, K., Fraley, R., Papahadjopoulos, D., Powell,A.,
    Thomashow, M., Nester, G. and Gordon, M., 1982 (Submitted for
    publication).
Darszon, A., Vandenberg, C.A., Ellisman, M.H. and Montal, M., 1979,
    Incorporation of membrane proteins into large single bilayer
    vesicles; application to rhodopsin, J. Cell. Biol., 81: 446.
DeGier, J. Blik, M.C., Van Dijck, P.W.M., Mombers, C., Verkley, A.,
    Van der NeutKok, E.C.M., Van Deenen, L.L.M., 1978, Relations
    between liposomes and biomembranes, Ann. N.Y. Acad. Sci.,
    308: 85.
Dunnick, J.K., McDougall, I.R., Aragon, S., Goris, M.L., and Kriss,
    J.P., 1975, Vesicle interactions with polyamino acids and anti-
    body: in vitro and in vivo studies, Nucl. Med., 16: 483.
Enoch, H.G., Strittmatter, P., 1979, Formation and properties of 1000
    A^o diameter single bilayer phospholipid vesicles, Proc. Natl.
    Acad. Sci. USA, 76: 145.
Finkelstein, M.C., Weissmann, G., 1978, The introduction of enzymes
    into cells by means of liposomes, J. Lipid Res. 19: 289.
Finkelstein, M.C., Weissmann, G., 1979, Enzyme replacement via lipo-
    somes. Variations in lipid composition determine liposomal
    integrity in biological fluids, Biochim. Biophys. Acta, 587: 202.
Fraley, R., Straubinger, R., Rule, G., Springer, L. and

Papahadjopoulos, D., 1981, Liposome-mediated delivery of DNA to cells: enhanced efficiency of delivery by changes in lipid composition and incubation conditions, Biochemistry, (in press).

Fraley, R., Delaporta, S., Gordon, M., Nester, E. and Papahadjopoulos, D., 1981, Liposome-mediated delivery of TMV RNA into tobacco protoplasts: a sensitive assay for monitoring liposome-protoplast interactions, Proc. Nat. Acad. Sci. USA, (in press).

Fraley, R., Subramani, S., Berg, P. and Papahadjopoulos, D., 1980, Introduction of liposomes-encapsulated SV40 DNA into cells: Effect of vesicle composition and incubation conditions, Biol. Chem., 255: 10431.

Goldman, I.D., Lichtenstein, N.S. and Oliveiro, V.T., 1968, Carrier mediated transport of the folic and analogue methotrexate in the L1210 leukemia cell, J. Biol. Chem., 243: 5007.

Gregoriadis, G., 1975, Homing of liposomes to target cells, Biochem. Soc. Trans., 3: 613.

Gregoriadis, G., 1976, The carrier potential of liposomes in biology and medicine, New Engl. J. Med., 295: 704.

Gregoriadis, G. and Davis, C., 1979, Stability of liposomes in vivo and in vitro is promoted by their cholesterol content and the presence of blood cells, Biochem. Biophys. Res. Commun., 89: 1287.

Heath, T.D., Fraley, R.T., and Papahadjopoulos, D., 1980, Antibody targeting of liposomes: Specific interaction of vesicles conjugated to anti-erythrocyte F(ab')$_2$, Science, 210: 539.

Heath, T.D., Macher, B.A. and Papahadjopoulos, D., 1981, Covalent attachment of proteins to liposomes via glycosphingolipids, Biochim. Biophys. Acta, 640: 66.

Heath, T.D., Robertson, D., Birbeck, M.S.C. and Davies, A.J.S., 1980, The covalent attachment of horseradish peroxidase to the outer surface of liposomes, Biochim. Biophys. Acta, 599: 42.

Huang, L., Kennel, S.T., 1979, Binding of immunoglobulin G to phospholipid vesicles by sonication, Biochemistry, 18: 1702.

Hunt, C.A., Rustum, Y.M., Mayhew, E. and Papahadjopoulos, D., 1979, Retention of cytosine arabinoside in mouse lung following intravenous administration in liposomes of different size, Drug. Metab. Dispos., 7: 124.

Hyman, R., and Stallings, V., 1976, Characterization of a TL variant of a homozygous TL$^+$ mouse lymphoma, Immunogenetics, 3: 75.

Juliano, R.L., and Stamp, D., 1976, Lectin-mediated attachment of glycoprotein-bearing liposomes to cells, Nature, 261: 235.

Kimelberg, H. Mayhew, E. and Papahadjopoulos, D., 1975, Distribution of liposome entrapped cations in tumor-bearing mice, Life Sciences, 17: 715.

Kimelberg, H. Papahadjopoulos, D., 1971, Phospholipid-protein interactions: Membrane permeability correlated with monolayer penetration, Biochim. Biophys. Acta, 233: 805.

Kosloski, M.J., Rosen, F., Milholland, D. and Papahadjopoulos, D., 1978, Liposome encapsulation of methotrexate enhances its chemotherapeutic efficacy in solid rodent tumors, Cancer Res.

38: 2848.

Lopatin, D. and Voss, E.W., Jr., 1971, Fluorescein hapten and antibody active site probe, Biochemistry, 10: 208.

Magee, W.E., 1978, Potentiation of interferon production and stimulation of lymphocytes by polyribonucleotides entrapped in liposomes, Ann. NY Acad. Sci., 308: 308.

Martin, F., Hubbell, W. and Papahadjopoulos, D., 1981, Immunospecific Targeting of Liposomes to Cells: A novel and efficient method for covalent attachment of Fab' fragments via disulfide bonds. Biochemistry, 20: 4229.

Martin, F. and Papahadjopoulos, D., 1981, Irreversible coupling of immunoglobulin fragments to preformed vesicles: An improved method for liposome targeting, J. Biol. Chem. (in press).

Mason, J.T., Huang, C., 1978, Hydrodynamic analysis of egg phosphatidylcholine vesicles, Ann. NY Acad. Sci., 308: 29.

Mayhew, E., Papahadjopoulos, D., Rustum, Y.M., and Dave, C., 1976, Inhibition of tumor cell growth in vitro and in vivo by cytosine arabinoside entrapped within phospholipid vesicles, Cancer Res., 36: 4406.

Mayhew, E.G., Szoka, F.C., Rustum, Y. and Papahadjopoulos, D., 1979, Role of cholesterol in enhancing the anti-tumor activity of 1-B-D-Arabinofuranosyl cytosine entrapped in liposomes, Cancer Treat. Rep., 63: 1923.

Mertz, J., and Berg, P., 1974, Defective simian virus 40 genomes: Isolation and growth of individual clones, Virology, 62: 112.

Oi, V.T., Jones, P.P., Goding, J.W. and Herzenberg, L.A., 1978, Properties of monoclonal antibodies to mouse Ig allotypes, H2 and Ia antigens, Curr. Topics Microbiol. Immun., 81: 115.

Olson, F., Hunt, C.A., Szoka, F.C., Vail, W.J. and Papahadjopoulos, D., 1979, Preparation of liposomes of defined size distribution by extrusion through polycarbonate membranes, Biochim. Biophys. Acta, 557: 9.

Pagano, R.E., Weinstein, J.N., 1978, Interactions of liposomes with mammalian cells, Ann. Rev. Biophys. Bioeng., 7: 435.

Papahadjopoulos, D., Cowden, M., Kimelberg, H.K., 1973, Effects on phospholipid-protein interactions, membrane permeability and enzymatic activity, Biochim. Biophys. Acta, 330: 8.

Papahadjopoulos, D., Jacobson, K., Nir, S. and Isac, T., 1973, Phase transitions in phospholipid vesicles: fluorescence polarization and permeability properties concerning the effect of temperature and cholesterol, Biochim. Biophys. Acta, 311: 330.

Papahadjopoulos, D., Mayhew, E., Poste, G., Smith, S. and Vail, W.J., 1974, Incorporation of lipid vesicles by mammalian cells provides a potential method for modifying cell behaviour, Nature, 252: 163.

Papahadjopoulos, D., Miller, N., 1967, Phospholipid Model Membranes. 1. Structural characteristics of hydrated liquid crystals. Biochim. Biophys. Acta, 135: 624.

Papahadjopoulos, D., Nir, S. and Ohki, S., 1972, Permeability properties of phospholipid membranes: Effect of cholesterol and temperature, Biochim. Biophys. Acta, 266: 561.

Papahadjopoulos, D., Vail, W.J., Jacobson, K. and Poste, G., 1975, Cochleate lipid cylinders: Formation by fusion of unilamellar lipid vesicles, Biochim. Biophys. Acta, 394: 483.

Papahadjopoulos, D., Watkins, J.C., 1967, Phospholipid model membranes. II. Permeability properties of hydrated liquid crystals, Biochim. Biophys. Acta, 135: 639.

Papahadjopoulos, D., Wilson, T., Taber, R., 1980, Liposomes as macromolecular carriers for the introduction of RNA and DNA into cells, in: "Transfer of Cell Constituents into Eukaryotic Cells," J.E. Cellis, ed., Plenum Press, New York.

Poste, G., 1980, Interaction of lipid vesicles (liposomes) with cultured cells and their use as carriers for drugs and macromolecules, in: "Liposomes in Biological Systems," G. Gregoriadis and A.C. Allison, eds., John Wiley, Chichester, New York.

Poste, G., Papahadjopoulos, D. and Vail, W.J., 1976, Lipid vesicles as carriers for introducing biologically active materials into cells, Methods Cell Biol., 14: 33.

Scherphof, G., Roerdink, F., Waite, M. and Parks, J., 1978, Transfer in vitro of lecithin from liposomes to high-density lipoproteins, Biochim. Biophys. Acta, 542: 296.

Szoka, F.C., Jacobson, K. and Papahadjopoulos, D., 1979, The use of aqueous space markers to determine the mechanism of interaction between phospholipid vesicles and cells, Biochim. Biophys. Acta, 551: 295.

Szoka, F., Olson, F., Heath, T.D., Vail, W.J., Mayhew, E. and Papahadjopoulos, D., 1980, Preparation of unilamellar liposomes of intermediate size ($0.1-0.2\mu$) by a combination of reverse phase evaporation and extrusion through polycarbonate membranes, Biochim. Biophys. Acta, 601: 559.

Szoka, F.C., and Papahadjopoulos, D., 1978, A new procedure for preparation of liposomes with large internal aqueous space and high capture, by Reverse Phase Evaporation (REV), Proc. Natl. Acad. Sci. USA, 75: 4194.

Szoka, F.C. and Papahadjopoulos, D., 1980, Comparative properties and methods of preparation of lipid vesicles (liposomes), Ann. Rev. Biophys. Bioengin., 9: 467.

Tall, A.R., Hogan, V., Askinazi, L. and Small, D.M., 1978, Interactions of plasma high density lipoproteins with dimyristoyl lecithin multilamellar liposomes, Biochemistry, 17: 322.

Torchilin, V.P., Khaw, B.A., Smirnov, V.N. and Haber, E., 1979, Preservation of antimyosin in antibody activity after covalent coupling to liposomes. Biochem. Biophys. Res. Commun., 89: 1114.

Tyrrell, D.A., Heath, T.D., Colley, C.M. and Ryman, B.E., 1976, New aspects of liposomes, Biochim. Biophys. Acta, 457: 259.

Weinstein, J.N., Blumenthal, R., Sharrow, S.O. and Henkart, P.A.,

1978, Antibody-mediated targeting of liposomes. Binding to lymphocytes does not insure incoroporation of vesicle contents into cells, Biochim. Biophys. Acta, 509: 272.

Weinstein, J.N ., Magin, R.L., Yatvin, M.B., and Zaharko, D.S., 1979, Liposomes and local hyperthermia: Selective delivery of methotrexate to heated tumors, Science, 204: 188

Weissmann, G., Bloomgarden, D., Kaplan, R., Cohen, C., Hoffstein, S., Collins, T., Gottlieb, A. and Nagle, D., 1975, A general method for the introduction of enzymes by means of immunoglobulin-coated liposomes into lysosomes of deficient cells, Proc. Natl. Acad. Sci. USA, 72: 88.

Wilson, T., Papahadjopoulos, D. and Taber, R., 1977, Biological properties of poliovirus encapsulated in lipid vesicles: Antibody resistance and infection in virus resistant cells, Proc. Natl. Acad. Sci. USA, 74: 3471.

Wilson, T., Papahadjopoulos, D. and Taber, R., 1979, The introduction of poliovirus RNA into cells via lipid vesicles (liposomes), Cell, 17: 77.

LIPOSOME-MEDIATED DNA TRANSFER IN EUKARYOTIC CELLS:

GENE UPTAKE AND EXPRESSION IN THE HOST CELL

Claude Nicolau and Claude Sené

Centre de Biophysique Moleculaire, C.N.R.S.
45045 Orléans Cedex, France and Max Planck Institut für
Strahlenchemie, 4330 Mülheim a.d. Ruhr, FRG

INTRODUCTION

Liposomes have been used to introduce drugs (Poste and Papa-hadjopoulos, 1976), enzymes (Gregoriadis and Buckland, 1973), mRNA (Dimitriadis, 1978), viruses (Lonberg-Holm et al., 1976; Wilson et al., 1977), and allosteric effectors (Nicolau and Gersonde, 1979; Gersonde and Nicolau, 1979) in a number of different cells. Recently, chromosomes have been entrapped in liposomes and transferred to cells (Mukherjee et al., 1978) and DNA has been introduced into bacterial cells (Fraley et al., 1979) and into plant cells (Lurquin, 1979). Also the expression of the tetracycline resistance gene (Tet^R) has been observed in E. coli after liposome-mediated transfer of the plasmid pBR322 to these cells (Fraley et al., 1979). Fraley et al. (1981) have used liposomes to encapsulate with high efficiency DNA isolated from SV40 virus. Infection of a permissive monkey cell line with these DNA-loaded liposomes resulted in the expression of the SV40 DNA encapsulated in liposomes with efficiencies comparable to the calcium phosphate method. Wong et al. (1980) isolated, from E. coli a restriction fragment, 875 bp, which encodes for a β-lacta-mase activity, and entrapped it in liposomes. Incubation of the DNA-loaded liposomes with avian, murine and human cells resulted in the uptake by the cells of the DNA and the expression of a β-lactamase activity as determined by spectroscopic and microbiological methods. Recently, Schaeffer-Ridder et al. (1981) transformed mouse LMTK⁻ cells with the liposome-encapsulated thymidine kinase gene and Nicolau and Rottem (1981) transformed M. capriolum with the pBR322 plasmid encapsulated in liposomes, conferring thus tetracycline resistance to this tetracycline sensitive organism. We will discuss here several aspects of the transformation of eukaryotic cells with liposome encapsulated genetic material.

UPTAKE OF THE BLA-GENE   OR OF THE pBR322 PLASMID BY EUKARYOTIC CELL

Preparation of DNA-loaded Liposomes

   10 μM phosphatidyl choline (Sigma) purified according to Singleton et al. (1965) and phosphatidyl serine (Ox brain, Sigma, high
purity) at the molar ratio of 9:1 were dissolved in 10 ml of chloroform (Merck, p.a.). The lipids were then evaporated to dryness under
a nitrogen stream at 36°C and redissolved in 10 ml of ether.

   2 μM of bla DNA (Wong et al., 1980) with traces of ^{32}P-labelled
DNA (0.44 x 10^6 cpm/10 μl) were dissolved in 5 ml of Tris-histidine-
NaCl buffer (25 mM Tris-HCl, 2 mM histine, 145 mM NaCl pH 7.4) and
heated at 60°C in a water-bath. 10 ml of the ether solution of the
PC-PS mixture were slowly injected (0.19 ml/min) into the warm DNA
solution: liposomes formed under these conditions, entrapping DNA
molecules (Deamer and Bangham, 1976). After injection, nitrogen was
bubbled until the ether was completely removed. The same procedure
 was repeated with 10 μg pBR322 plasmid. The bla-gene (875 bp) was
entrapped in liposomes also by cosonication with the lipids. Traces
of ^{32}P-labelled DNA (0.44 x 10^6 cpm/10 μl) were added to the sonication suspension. After sonication, an aliquot of the ^{32}P-DNA liposome suspension was taken and analyzed by electrophoresis through
1% horizontal agarose gels (Loening, 1967).

   10 μM egg phosphatidyl choline were used to prepare, by the same
procedure, liposomes which are taken up by the cells by endocytosis.
The PC-PS liposomes are taken up by the cells both by endocytosis
and by an energy-independent mechanism (fusion ?) which cannot be
inhibited by cytochalasin B.

   3.5 ml of the liposome suspension was run through a Sepharose
4B column, in order to check the incorporation of the gene within the
liposome. 1.5 ml of the same suspension was incubated for 30 min
with 50 μg/ml of DNase I (Sigma) in PBS supplemented with 10 mM of
MgCl$_2$. After incubation, this suspension was chromatographed on a
Sepharose 4B column and the ^{32}P radioactivity of DNA was counted.
The presence of liposomes was monitored by following the optical
density at 650 nm of the samples. The liposome-DNA suspension was
eluted from the column with a Hepes buffer (5 mM Hepes, 0.1 M NaCl/
KCl, pH 7.4). The fraction containing the liposomes and the associated DNA was used for the transformation experiments.

Cell-Liposome Interaction

   The DNA loaded liposomes were incubated with Hela and Detroit-6
cells. Before 4 ml of the liposome suspension were added to 10^7
cells, the cells were washed with 20 ml of DMEM without serum. After
incubation for 2 h at 37°C, the liposome suspension was decanted and
the cells were washed twice with 10 ml of PBS before they were fed

with serum free DMEM.

In order to remove non-entrapped DNA adsorbed on the cell surface, the cells were treated with DNase I. After washing away the liposome suspension, aliquots of cells were mixed with 4 ml of a DNase I solution (50 μg/ml in PBS supplemented with 10 mM of MgCl$_2$) and the mixture was incubated for 30 min. The cells were then washed twice with 10 ml Tris-histidine-NaCl buffer (pH 7.4) trypsinized and pelleted by centrifugation. After washing twice with 5 ml of Tris-histidine-NaCl buffer, the cell pellet was resuspended in 1 ml of PBS and counted for ^{14}C and ^{32}P. The controls in which DNA was used without liposomes entrapment were counted as well.

Extraction of Total Nucleic Acids

After incubation, cells were washed in PBS, trypsinized and pelleted by centrifugation.

The cells were suspended in buffer (10 mM NaCl, 10 mM Tris-HCl, pH 7.5, 1.5 mM MgCl$_2$) containing 1% Triton X-100 and lyzed by homogenizing with 20 strokes in a Dounce homogenizer or by brief sonication. Nuclei were pelleted at 1000 g for 5 min and washed twice with PBS buffer.

In order to avoid a possible redistribution between ^{32}P DNA released by the detergent from liposome and membrane, the lysis was performed after addition of an excess of unlabelled DNA (300 μg/ml). These conditions virtually eliminate non-specific binding of DNA to nuclei as indicated by Lurquin (1979).   Total nucleic acid extracts were obtained by treating the cells with 2 M sodium dodecyl sulfate in 0.1 M Tris-HCl, 0.2 M NaCl (pH 9.0) (followed by 1 h incubation at 37°C in the presence of 100 mg/ml proteinase I).

Deproteinization was performed twice with an equal volume of phenol (equilibrated in the buffer). Nucleic acids were then precipitated with 10% trichloroacetic acid (TCA) and the precipitates were collected on Whatman GF/C glass fiber filters and washed with 5% TCA and subsequently with 95% ethanol.

Synchronization of Cells

In order to obtain a mitotic population, the Hela cells were synchronized by a single thymidine block of 2.5 mM for about 20 h. Four hours after reversal of the thymidine block, the cells were incubated for about 10 h with colcemid (0.05 μg/ml). The mitotic cells and the part-G$_2$ cells were used for the incorporation experiments. After 5 h in regular culture conditions the Hela cells were in the G$_1$ phase.

Mitotic index were performed on the cells fixed in absolute methanol/glacial acetic acid, 3:1, v/v, and stained with GIEMSA 2%.

Assay of β-Lactamase

The β-Lactamase activity was followed spectrophotometrically.
After 14-24 h of incubation at 37°C, 10^7 cells were trypsinized and
pelleted by centrifugation. After resuspending in 1 ml of PBS (pH
7.0), the cells were sonicated briefly for disruption. After treating
the cell suspensions with 1% Triton X-100, the cell suspensions were
centrifuged (10000 rpm, 10 min, 4°C). Aliquots of the supernatant
were reacted with 10^{-4} M cephalosporin (O'Callaghan et al., 1972).
The reaction proceeded for 30 min. The optical absorption spectra of
the reaction mixture were recorded with a Hitachi 100-80 recording
spectrophotometer.

Microbiological tests were carried out as follows. The supernatant of the cell extracts was prepared as that for spectroscopic
measurement except that Triton X-100 was omitted. The supernatant,
1 ml, was incubated with ampicillin for 30 min at 37°C before it was
transferred to the 10 ml of LB medium which had been inoculated with
0.1 ml of an overnight culture of E. coli C600. The final concentration of ampicillin in the incubation mixture was adjusted to 30 g/ml.
The culture was incubated at 37°C for overnight in order to detect
for bacterial growth.

In order to check whether the sonication method is appropriate
for the entrapment of the DNA fragment bearing the bla gene, electrophoresis of the DNA before and after sonication was carried out.
Figures 1a, b and c show that the DNA is not fragmented by sonication.
This procedure of entrapping solutes in liposomes can be applied to
genes like bla because its molecular weight is rather low (around
0.57×10^6 daltons). Larger DNA pieces, with molecular weights above
0.6×10^6 daltons, cannot be entrapped in liposomes by cosonication
with the lipid suspensions, as they are broken down to fragments
during the sonication (H. Hauser, I. Wilke and C. Nicolau, unpublished observation). In these cases, other methods can be used (for
review, see Poste et al., 1976).

In order to show that after sonication the DNA molecules have
been entrapped into liposomes, the DNA-liposomes were chromatogra-
phied on a Sepharose 4B column before and after DNase I treatment.
Figure 2a shows that before DNase I treatment, the DNA peak overlaps
the liposomes peak (fraction 12-16), but much of it is present out-
side the liposome-containing fractions (fractions 16-29). Incubation
with DNase I changed completely this picture as shown in Fig. 2b.
Most of the DNA is degraded and has completely shifted to fractions
21 to 30. However, part of the DNA contained in the liposome fractions still elutes at the same position. Thus, the DNA must be
protected against DNase I, i.e. entrapped into liposomes.

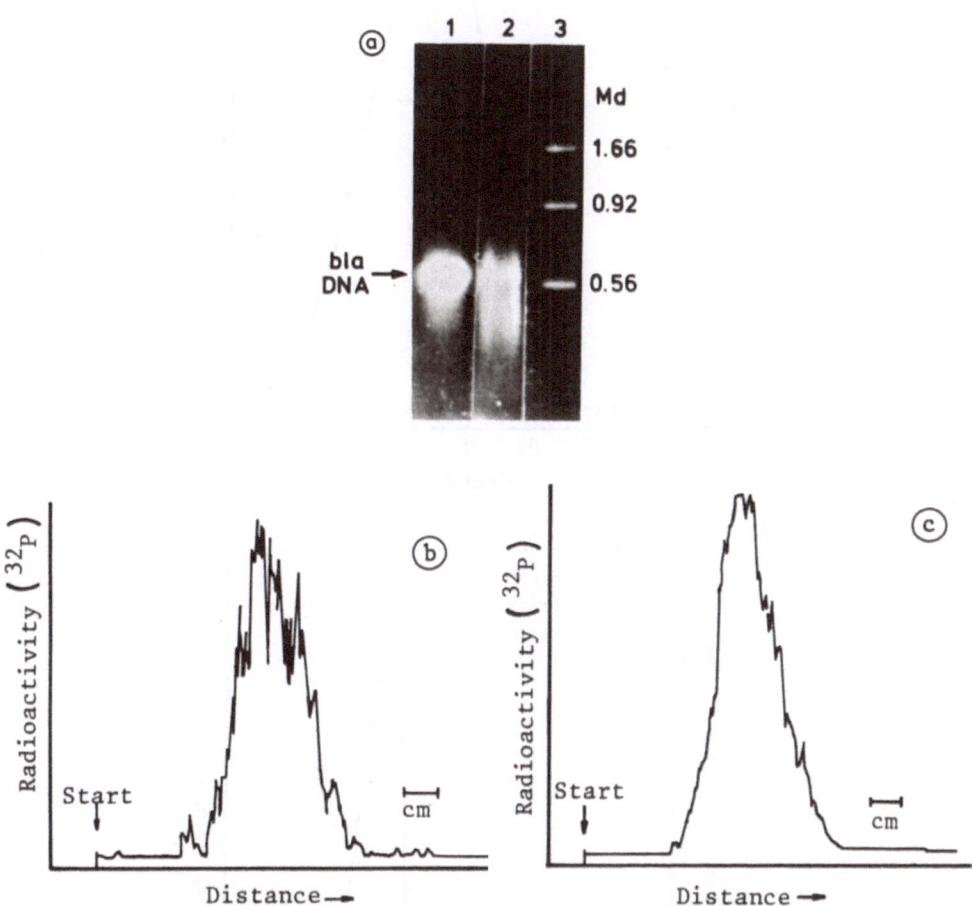

Fig. 1.   Electrophoretic analysis of the bla gene before and after
           sonication. (a) The autoradiogram of the agarose gel after
           electrophoresis (1% agarose, Loening buffer system, 20 V,
           overnight). Lane 1 and lane 2 show the ^{32}P-labelled DNA
           fragment containing the bla gene before and after sonica-
           tion, respectively. Lane 3 shows the HaeIII digest of
           M13 DNA serving as molecular weight standards. (b) and
           (c) show the radioactivity scan of lanes 1 and 2,
           respectively (Wong et al., 1980).

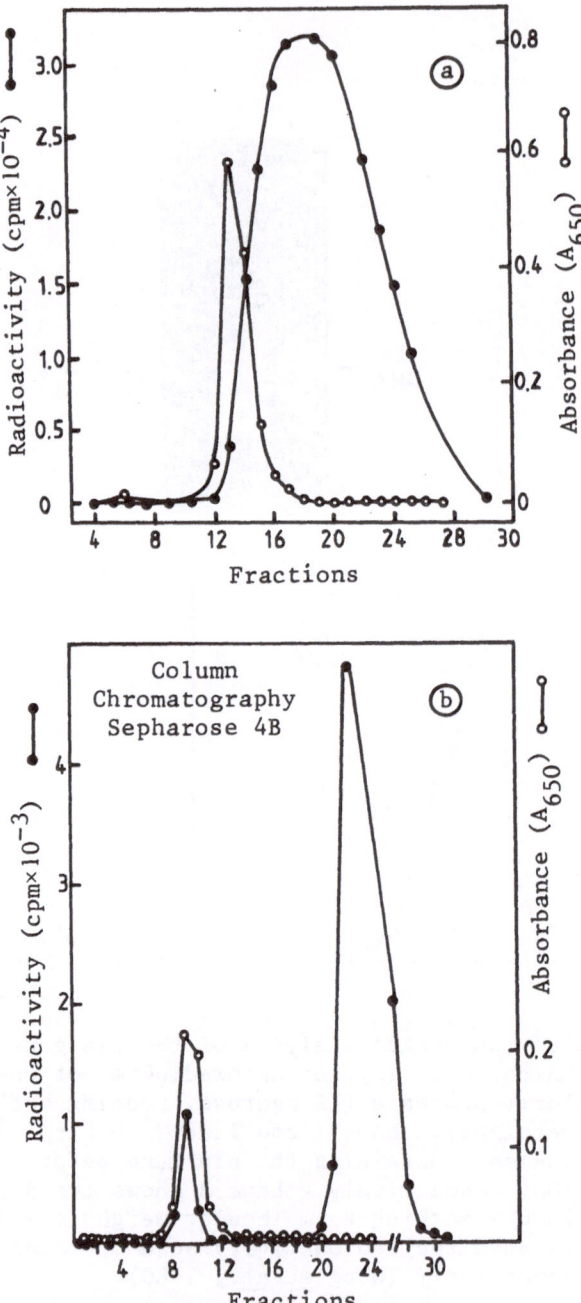

Fig. 2.   Chromatographic resolution of liposomes and ^{32}P-labelled
          DNA fragment on Sepharose 4B column. Liposome-DNA sus-
          pensions were applied onto the Sepharose 4B column and

eluted with 0.1 M NaCl/KCl containing Hepes (5 mM), pH 7.4
Fractions (3 ml) were collected and monitored for radioactivity and absorbance at 650 nm. The elution profiles
obtained for liposomes containing the ^{32}P-labelled DNA
before and after DNase I digestion are shown in (a) and
(b), respectively (Wong et al., 1980).

Similar observations were made with the injection liposomes
having entrapped the pBR322 plasmid (Sené and Nicolau, 1981).

Table 1 shows the uptake or the liposome-entrapped bla gene
into Hela cells (Wong et al., 1980).

Table 1. Liposome-mediated incorporation of bla gene DNA into cells

System	Input (^{32}P, cpm)	Incorporation into 10^7 cells[a]	
		^{32}P, cpm	% of input
^{32}P DNA in liposomes	128674	3182	2.5
^{32}P DNA in buffer	164400	174	0.1

[a]10^7 chick embryo cells were incubated for 2 h at 37°C with
DNA (2 μg with traces of nick-translated radioactive DNA)
which was either entrapped in liposomes or dissolved in buffer.
Cells were subsequently treated with DNase I for 30 min at
37°C, and then washed with PBS and finally monitored for radioactivity.

The figures of 2.5% was obtained by counting the radioactivity
of the cells incubated with the DNA-loaded liposomes. It may not
actually represent the number of intact DNA molecules having penetrated into the host cells as it is very difficult to make absolutely
sure that:
i) no DNA-loaded liposomes are still adsorbed on the cell
surface,
ii) all the radioactive DNA which has not penetrated into the
cell has been hydrolyzed by DNase and washed out. Line 2 of Table I
indicates that 0.1% of free DNA remains associated with the cells
under these conditions.

In an attempt to enhance the DNA-uptake by the cells we have
prepared liposomes entering the cells by an energy-dependent mechanism

Table 2. Liposome-mediated uptake of ^{32}P-DNA by Hela cells in exponential growth.

Liposomes	^{32}P-DNA total uptake (cpm)	^{32}P-DNA uptake in nuclear extract	Nuclear uptake as % of total uptake
A. Endocytosis (phagocytosis and pinocytosis)			
PC	1064	418	39
PC-cytochalasin B (50 g/ml)	192	58	
B. Endocytosis + Fusion (?)			
PC-PS (9:1)	860	240	28
PC-PS + Cytochalasin B (50 g/ml)	550	140	25

Mechanism of entry of the PC-PS liposomes : ~ 36% endocytosis (energy dependent)
~ 64% fusion (?) or/and pinocytosis (energy independent)

Efficiency of nuclear uptake : A) Endocytosis ~39%
B) Fusion (?) and/or pinocytosis ~25%.

(PC-liposomes (endocytosis) and liposomes entering the cells by both energy-dependent and an energy independent mechanism (fusion ?) (PC-PS liposomes). The recent results of Szoka et al. (1980) suggesting that fusion is a rare event (if it takes place at all) in the liposome-culture cell interaction, raise once more the question as to the nature of this energy independent mechanism.

Using these two preparations of injection liposomes and incubating them with Hela cells as described we obtained the following uptake (Table 2, Sene and Nicolau, 1981). Table 2 shows the liposome mediated uptake of ^{32}P-DNA by Hela cells in exponential growth. In the cells treated with fluid, neutral liposomes, the inhibition of endocytosis with 50 μg ml^{-1} cytochalasin B leads to a dramatic drop in the amount of ^{32}P-DNA associated with the cell and, correspondingly, with the nucleus. When the cells are incubated with fluid, charged liposomes entering the cells by an energy-dependent and an energy independent mechanism (Poste and Papahadjopoulos, 1976a), the cytochalasin B treatment is significantly less efficient than in the former case.

It appears that with the PC liposomes the nuclear uptake of 30% of the whole cellular uptake of ^{32}P-DNA, whereas it is only 25% with the PC-PS liposomes. The inhibition of endocytosis with cytochalasin B indicates that over 85% of this entry pathway is inhibited for PC liposomes, by only 36% of the entry for PC-PS liposomes.

Table 3 (Sene and Nicolau, 1981) shows the results obtained with the two types of liposomes studied incubated with Hela cells synchronized in mitosis.

Table 3. Liposome-mediated uptake of ^{32}P-DNA molecules by synchronized Hela cells

Type of liposome	Cell cycle phase	Incorporation in cells cpm/10^7 cells	Associated with the nuclear fraction	
			cpm	% of cellular uptake
PC	Mitosis	3514	2547	72
	G_1	4868	1829	37
PC-PS	Mitosis	6454	2977	46
	G_1	4100	1660	40

Not only is the nuclear uptake of the 32P-labelled DNA more efficient with endocytotic liposomes, but also the expression of the gene, i.e., the production of the enzyme β-lactamase is more efficient when these liposomes are used (Sené and Nicolau, 1981).

We further tried to enhance the number of exogeneous DNA molecules reaching the cell nucleus. During the transition of the cells from the G_2 phase to mitosis, the nuclear membrane breaks down and chromatine condenses in chromosomes. It seemed therefore likely that in mitosis we should observe the highest association of the exogeneous DNA molecules with the nuclear DNA.

The cells were synchronized in Mitosis (M) and in the G_1 phase. It results that, although the global cellular uptake by endocytosis is reduced in mitotic cells, we find associated with the nuclear DNA 72-75% of the molecules transported into the cells by the PC liposomes. When other entry mechanisms of the liposomes are predominant, only ∼40% of the 32P-DNA is found associated with the nuclear DNA. There is little difference between the uptake by fusion or endocytosis in the exponentially growing cells or in the G_1 phase. An interesting feature of the uptake of liposomes in synchronized cells is that in mitotic cells the global cellular uptake by the energy independent mechanism is quite high, but the number of molecules associated with the nuclear DNA is less than 50% of the total. With endocytosis liposomes the fraction of exogeneous DNA molecules associated with the nuclear DNA is significantly higher (∼75%). This suggests that the lipid bilayer protects the DNA molecules in the latter case, at least part of the time of their migration to the nucleus, whereas in the former case the DNA molecules are completely exposed to the action of the cytoplasmic DNases for all the time.

Further data concerning the cell-cycle dependent uptake of DNA encapsulated in liposomes are presented elsewhere (Nicolau and Sené, 1981).

EXPRESSION OF A β-LACTAMASE ACTIVITY

Bacterial β-lactamase activity can be easily assayed by color change from yellow to red (O'Callaghan et al., 1972) due to the disruption of the β-lactam ring of cephalosporin. We measured a spectroscopic shift in extracts prepared from cells 14 h after liposome treatment and upon the addition of cephalosporin. Figure 3a, b, shows the results obtained with extracts from Hela cells. Extracts from normal Hela cells treated with the antibiotic show a maximum at about 400 nm, whereas the extracts from Hela cells having incorporated the bla gene show a shift to around 510 nm. Figure 3b shows the differential spectra of the Hela cells having incorporated the bla gene minus the controls. A maximum at 510 nm becomes clearly visible. Similar results were obtained with chick-embryo fibroblasts (leucose and mycoplasma-free SFP-VALD chickens, Lohmann Tierzucht, Cuxhaven,

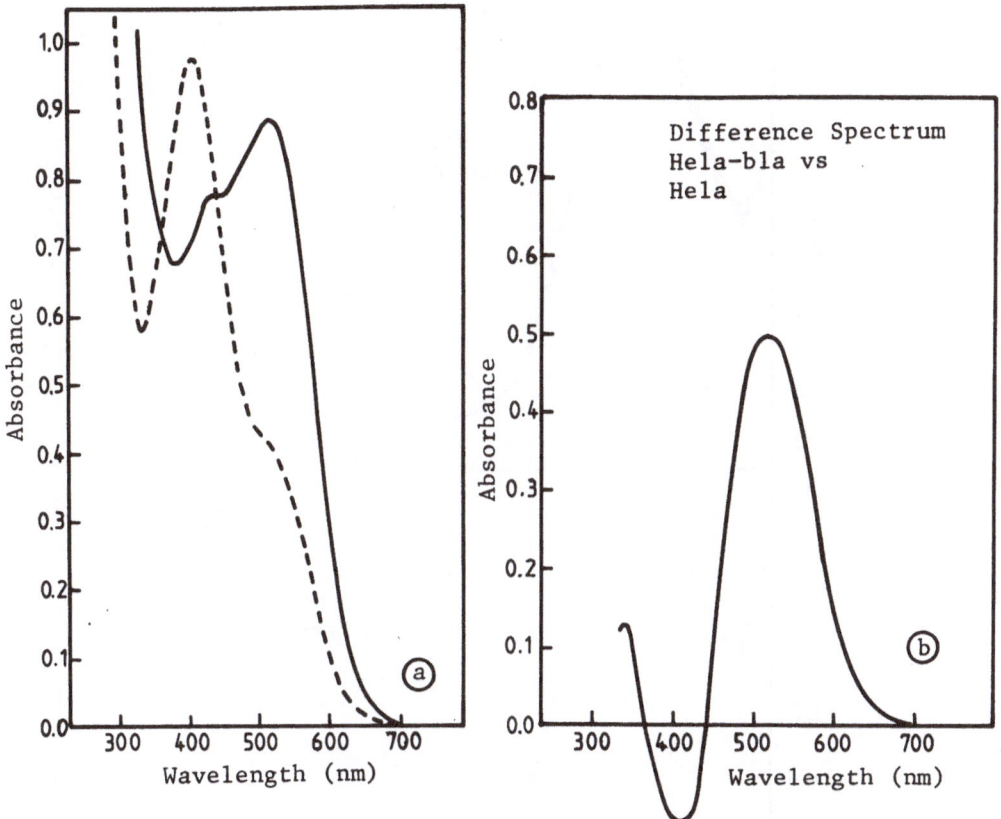

Fig. 3.   (a) Absorption spectra of cephalosporin (10^{-4} M in PBS,
pH 7.0) after reacting at 25°C with extracts from 10^{7}
Hela cells without (dashed line) and with (solid line) the
incorporated DNA fragment containing the bla gene.
(b) Difference spectrum of cephalosporin exposed to cell
extracts from the Hela cells with or without incorporated
bla gene.   (Wong et al., 1980).

FRG) and Detroit-6 (human bone marrow cells).   In order to rule out
that the incorporation of any DNA would produce the effect we had
detected in the spectra, a control experiment was performed in which,
instead of the bla gene or the pBR322 plasmid we used the conalbumin
gene inserted in a pBR322 plasmid lacking the sequence encoding for
the β-lactamase (Oudet, Sené and Nicolau, 1980, unpublished results).
The spectra are shown in Fig. 4a-c.

Results show that only the cells having incorporated the pBR322
plasmid or the bla gene react with cephalosporin in the way described,
thus indicating the appearance of a β-lactamase activity in these
cells. The conalbumin gene failed to generate such a reaction.

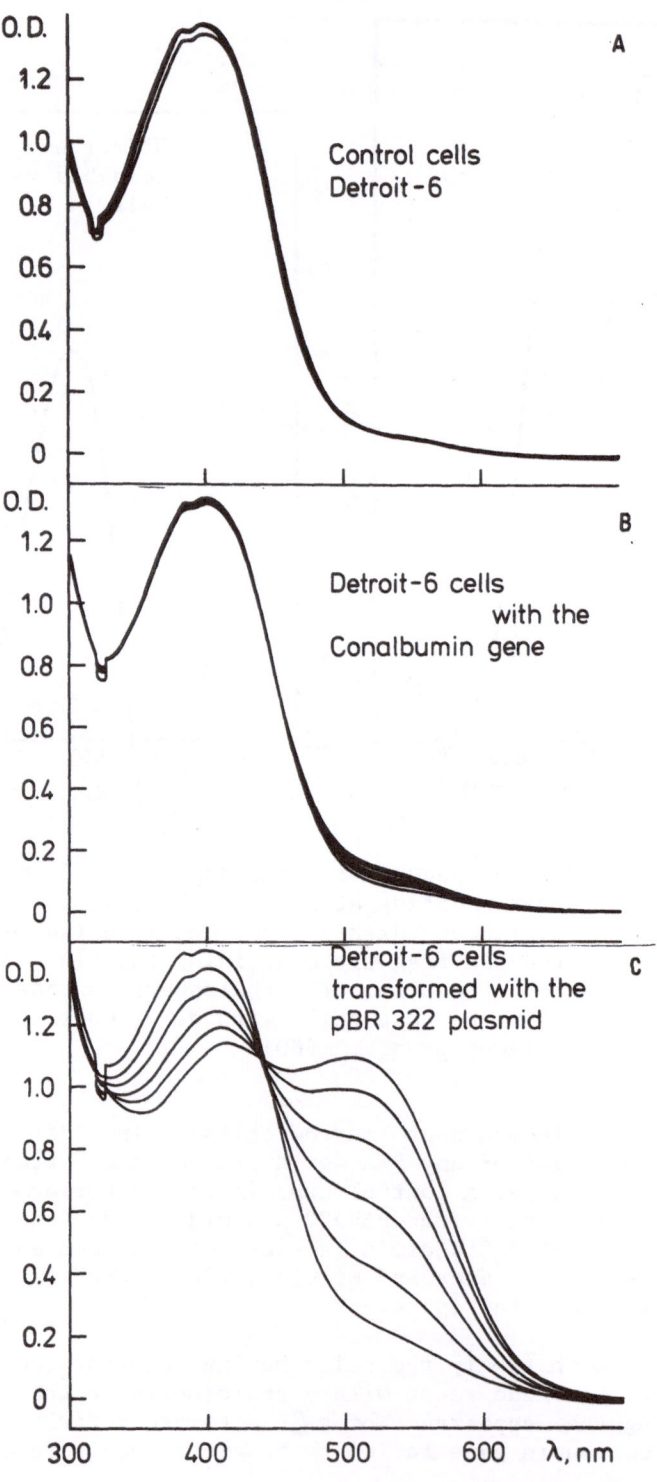

Fig. 4.   Absorption spectra of cephalosporin (10^{-4} M in PBS, pH
←———   7.0) after reaction at 37°C with extracts of Detroit-6
cells. a) Control Detroit-6 cells having incorporated
buffer-loaded ("empty") liposomes; b) Detroit-6 cells
having incorporated the liposome-entrapped conalbumin DNA;
c) Detroit-6 cells having incorporated the pBR322 plasmid
entrapped in liposomes. The spectra were recorded every
5 min during 30 min at 37°C.

To determine the degradation of ampicillin by a very different
method, we assayed its inhibitory effect of bacterial growth, in the
presence or absence of cell extracts. Ampicillin-sensitive E. coli
C600 bacteria grew normally at 37°C in LB medium supplemented with
both cell extracts and ampicillin (130 μg/ml). In control experiments,
however, neither extracts of DNA-liposome-untreated cells nor addition
of liposomes to the bacterial cultures allowed E. coli C600 to grow
in the presence of ampicillin. Moreover, when a bla-DNA fragment of
similar size was entrapped in liposomes and incorporated into cells,
the extracts of these cells neither showed a spectroscopic shift nor
permitted bacterial growth in the presence of ampicillin (Wong et al.,
1980).

Based on the presented results, the new phenotype can be
explained in different ways. In the case of the Hela cells it can
be explained by an ad hoc assumption that mycoplasmas or some other
microorganisms may be present in Hela cells and express the acquired
prokaryotic DNA. This explanation is unlikely at least for the CEC
derived from microbe-free eggs.

A far simpler explanation, which also accounts for several of
our control experiments and for the results with DNA fragments of
different genetic content, is the expression of the bla gene fragment
by the transcription and translation machinery of the eukaryotic
cells.

TRANSFORMATION RATE

1000 Detroit-6 cells having been transformed with the pBR322
plasmid and which had been found, both by the spectroscopic assay and
the electrofocusing test to express β-lactamase, were used for subcloning experiments. The subcloning was performed as batch-procedure,
i.e. 96 x 10 cells which were plated after having been transformed
with a DNA-fragment from the pBR322 plasmid which did not encode for
β-lactamase. The control cells were β-lactamase negative both by
spectrophotometry and electrofocusing.

Three weeks after seeding the cells were transferred to 25 cm^2
falcon flasks. The yields amounted to 55% for the pBR322 plasmid-
transformed cells and 29% for those transformed with the DNA fragments.

2-3 weeks after reaching confluence the cells extracts were prepared
from the plasmid transformed cells and from the controls and assayed
for β-lactamase by electrofocusing.

Out of 53 tested flasks containing the pBR322 plasmid transformed
cells, 3 showed a β-lactamase activity, though not a very strong one,
indicating that about 6% of the initially transformed cells were
expressing the enzyme, apparently in a stable manner. All the controls were negative.

An exhaustive checking of potential bacterial contamination of
the cells was performed at the Institut fur Mikrobiologie, Klinikum
Essen. No contamination whatsoever could be detected (Sené and
Nicolau, 1981).

CHARACTERIZATION OF THE EUKARYOTIC ENZYME

The isoelectric focusing pattern of the eukaryotic enzyme and
the bacterial enzyme are practically identical suggesting a great
similarity of structure of the two molecules (Sené and Nicolau,
1981). This is a fact which is difficult to explain at the present
time. In order to further characterize the eukaryotic enzyme, we
have measured the K_m values of the eukaryotic β-lactamases and compared them with the bacterial enzyme. The results are shown in
Table 4.

Table 4. Hydrolysis of cephalosporin by different β-lactamases

Source of β-lactamase	K_m, moles
E. coli	190 ± 20
LMTK-cells transformed with the bla gene	305 ± 20
LMTK-cells transformed with the pBR322 plasmid	310 ± 20

Here we observe a significant difference between the bacterial
and the eukaryotic enzyme. The measurement of K_m of the bacterial
enzyme, in a protein mixture, in order to mimic the cell extracts,
yielded similar results.

LEVEL OF EXPRESSION VS NUMBER OF DNA MOLECULES INCORPORATED

A correlation seems to exist between the enzymic activity of the eukaryote β-lactamase and the number of DNA molecules associated with the cells.

In an experiment aimed at checking this correlation, we introduced various amounts of radioactive pBR322 plasmid into the Hela cells and assayed the β-lactamase activity. The results are shown in Fig. 5. This dependence suggests that there might be a level of saturation for the incorporation of the exogeneous DNA which then is reflected in a somewhat constant remaining activity. This observation is of preliminary character but it is suggestive of the potentialities of the liposomes as DNA-carriers.

OTHER GENES

Several other transformation experiments with liposome-encapsulated DNA have been reported. The SV 40 DNA has been successfully employed by Fraley et al. (1981) and recently Schaefer-Ridder et al. (1981) succeeded the transformation of LMTK cells with the liposome-encapsulated recombinant plasmid pAGO carrying an active TK gene. The transformed phenotype (200 out of 10^6 cells) was stable under selective and non-selective conditions.

Table 5 (Schaefer-Ridder et al., 1981) gives the comparative efficiency of different transfection methods with the thymidine kinase gene.

Table 5.

Methods	% of TK$^+$ cells	Colonies per 10^6 cells
Liposomes	10	200
Ca-phosphate	3	500
DEAE-Dextran	0.1-1	0
Microinjection	50-100	(200-1000)[+]

[+]Data calculated for 10^6 cells.

Together with other colleagues in our laboratory, a number of collaborative studies have been initiated concerning the liposome-mediated transfer of genetic material in vitro (SV 40, conalbumin, thymidine kinase, β-globin, insulin) and in vivo. Despite certain obvious advantages over other methods of DNA transfer into cells,

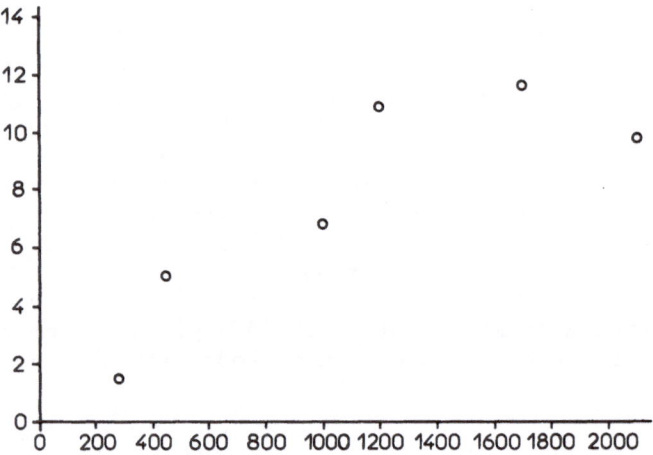

Fig. 5.   Enzymic activity (ΔOD510/1.59) of the eukaryotic
          β-lactamase in Hela cells vs the number of DNA
          molecules associated with the cell (assayed by
          measuring the radioactivity of a nicktranslated
          pBR322 plasmid).

the liposome method, used only in vitro would probably remain one
method among others.

It is our conviction that the major potentialities of the liposomes as DNA carriers reside in their capacity to be used in vivo.
Such experiments are being carried out presently in our laboratory.

CONCLUSIONS

We have described some of the work concerning the liposome
mediated gene transfer and the study of the expression of the transferred genes. From these results one can see that this process has
two components :

1) Transfer of the DNA into cells,
2) Expression of the transferred genes by the transcription and
translation machinery of the host cell.

Considerable progress has been achieved with the design and
preparation of efficient liposome carriers for DNA in several types
of cells ; by making use of the cell-cycle dependent properties of
the cells, high percentages of the incorporated DNA became associated
with the nuclear DNA.

The expression of the gene by the host cell transcription and
translation machinery is quite another problem. It has been possible
to express genes transferred by liposomes in bacteria (Fraley et al.,
1980), mycoplasma (Nicolau and Rottem, 1981) animal and human cells
in vitro (Fraley et al., 1980, Wong et al., 1980, Schaefer-Ridder et
al., 1981, Nicolau and Sene, 1981). The understanding of the
mechanism by which the exogeneous DNA reaches the nucleus, is or is
not integrated into the chromosomal DNA, the mechanisms of transcription and translation in case that a prokaryotic gene is expressed in
eukaryotic cells are far from being understood. They are all fascina-
ting directions of investigation.

One of the major interests in these studies is the use of liposomes in vivo in animal experiments. This seems to be one of their
strongest advantages which might give a new dimension to liposome
research.

REFERENCES

Deamer, D. and Bangham, A.C., 1976, Large volume liposomes by an
      ether vaporization method, Biochim, Biophys, Acta, 443:629.
Dimitriadis, G.T., 1978, Translation of rabbit globin mRNA intro-
      duced by liposomes into mouse lymphocytes, Nature, 274: 923.
Fraley, R.T., Fornari, C.S. and Kaplan, S., 1979, Entrapment of a
      bacterial plasmid in phospholipid vesicles : Potential for gene
      transfer, Proc. Natl. Acad. Sci. USA, 76: 3348.
Fraley, R.T., Subramani, S., Berg, P. and Papahadjopoulos, D., 1981,

      Introduction of liposome-encapsulated SV 40 into cells, J. Biol.
        Chem. 255: 10431.
Gersonde, K. and Nicolau, C., 1979, Improvement of the human red
        blood cell O_2 release capacity by lipid vesicle-mediated incor-
        poration of inositol hexaphosphate, Blut, 39: 1.
Gregoriadis, G. and Buckland, R.A., 1973, Enzyme-containing liposomes
        alleviate a model for storage disease. Nature, 244: 170.
Loening, V.E., 1967, The fractionation of high-molecular weight
        ribonucleic acid by polyacrylamide-gel electrophoresis. Biochem.
        J., 102: 251.
Lonberg-Holm, J., Gosser, L.B. and Shimshick, E.J., 1976, Interaction
        of liposomes with subviral particles of poliovirus type 2 and
        rhinovirus type 2, J. Virol., 19: 746.
Lurquin, P.F., 1979, Entrapment of plasmid DNA by liposomes and
        their interactions with plant protoplasts, Nucl. Acids Res.,
        6: 3773.
Mukherjee, A.B., Orloff, S., Butler, J.D., Triche, T., Lalley, P.
        and Schulman, J.D., 1978,   Entrapment of metaphase chromo-
        somes into phospholipid vesicles (lipochromosomes) :
        carrier potential in gene transfer, Proc. Natl. Acad. Sci. USA,
        75: 1361.
Nicolau, C. and Gersonde, K., 1979, Incorporation of inositol hexa-
        phosphate into intact red blood cells, I. Fusion of effector-
        containing lipid vesicles with erythrocytes. Naturwissenschaften
        66: 561.
Nicolau, C. and Sene, C., 1981, Cell-cycle dependence of the lipo-
        some mediated gene uptake by eukaryotic cells. Submitted for
        publication.
Nicolau, C. and Rottem, S., 1981, Expression of Tet[R] in M. capriolum
        after liposome-mediated transfer of the pBR322 plasmid.   In
        preparation.
O'Callaghan, C.H., Morris, A., Kirby, S.M. and Shingler, A.H., 1972,
        Novel method for detection of β-lactamase by using a chromogenic
        cephalosporin substrate. Antimicrob. Agents Chemother., 1: 283.
Poste, G. and Papahadjopoulos, D., 1976a, Lipid vesicles as carriers
        for introducing materials into cultured cells: Influence of
        vesicle lipid composition on mechanism of vesicle incorporation
        into cells, Proc. Natl. Acad. Sci. USA, 73: 1603.
Poste, G. and Papahadjopoulos, D., 1976b, Drug-containing lipid
        vesicles render drug-resistant tumour cells sensitive to actino-
        mycin D, Nature, 261: 699.
Poste, G., Papahadjopoulos, D. and Vail, W., 1976, Lipid vesicles as
        carriers for introducing biologically active materials into
        cells, in: "Methods in Cell Biology", vol. 14, D.M. Prescott,
        ed., Academic Press, New York.
Schaefer-Ridder, M., Wang, Y. and Hofschneider, P.H., 1981, Liposomes
        as gene carriers: High efficiency transformation of mouse L
        cells by the thymidine kinase gene, Science (in press).
Sene, C. and Nicolau, C., 1981, Liposome-mediated gene transfer in
        eukaryotic cells in: "Liposome, drugs and Immunocompetent

Cell Functions", C. Nicolau and A. Paraf, ed., Academic Press, London.

Singleton, W.S., Gray, M.S., Brown, M.L. and White, J.L., 1965, Chromatographically homogeneous lecithin from egg phospholipids, J. Am. Oil Chem. Soc., 42: 53.

Szoka, F., Jacobson, K., Derzko, Z. and Papahadjopoulos, D., 1980, Fluorescence studies on the mechanism of liposome-cell interactions in vitro, Biochim. Biophys. Acta, 600: 1.

Wilson, T., Papahadjopoulos, D. and Taber, R., 1977, Biological properties of poliovirus encapsulated in lipid vesicles: antibody resistance and infectivity in virus-resistant cells. Proc. Natl. Acad. Sci. USA, 74: 3471.

Wong, T.K., Nicolau, C. and Hofschneider, P.H., 1980, Appearance of β-lactamase activity in animal cells upon liposome-mediated gene transfer, Gene, 10: 87.

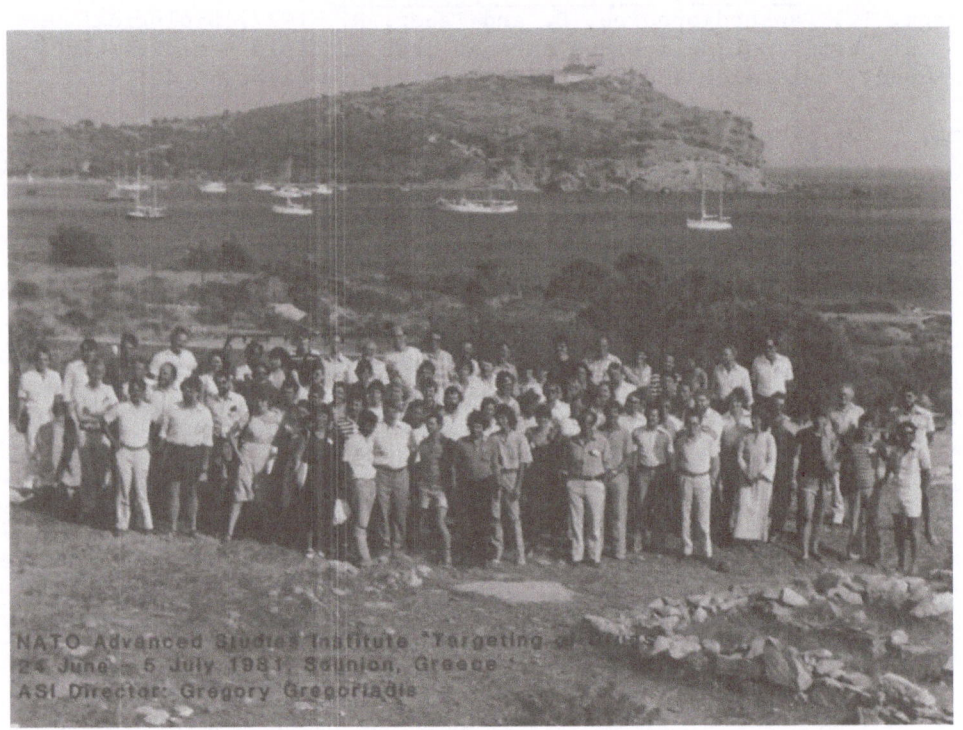

NATO Advanced Studies Institute 'Targeting of Drugs'
24 June – 5 July 1981, Sounion, Greece
ASI Director: Gregory Gregoriadis

CONTRIBUTORS

Alving, C.R., Department of Membrane Biochemistry, Walter Reed Army
    Institute of Research, Washington, DC 20012, USA.

Arnon, R., Department of Chemical Immunology, The Weismann Institute
    of Science, Rehovot 76100, Israel.

Balboni, P.G., Istituto di Microbiologia, Via L. Borsari 46, I-44100
    Ferrara, Italy.

Barbanti-Brodano, G., Istituto di Microbiologia, Via L. Borsari 46,
    I-44100 Ferrara, Italy.

Baurain, R., Laboratory of Physiological Chemistry, Universite
    Catholique de Louvain and International Institute of Cellular
    and Molecular Pathology, Brussels, Belgium.

Beigel, M., The Hebrew University of Jerusalem, Institute of Life
    Sciences, Jerusalem, Israel.

Belitsky, P., Department of Virology, Dalhousie University, Halifax,
    N.S., Canada.

Blair, H., Department of Biochemistry, Dalhousie University,
    Halifax, N.S., Canada.

Blumenthal, R., Section of Membrane Structure and Function,
    Laboratory of Mathematical Biology, National Cancer Institute,
    NIH, Bethesda, Maryland, 20205, USA.

Bucana, C., Cancer Metastasis and Treatment Laboratory, NCI-Frederick
    Cancer Research Center, Frederick, MD 21701, USA.

Busi, C., Istituto di Patologia Generale, via San Giacomo 14,
    I-40126 Bologna, Italy.

Connors, T.A., MRC Toxicology Unit, Medical Research Council
    Laboratory, Woodmansterne Road, Carshalton, U.K.

Cree, T.C., University of Wisconsin, Department of Human Oncology,
    WCCC Madison, WI 53792, USA.

Davies, A.J.S., Institute of Cancer Research, Royal Cancer Hospital,
    Chester Beatty Research Institute, Fulham Road, London SW3 6JB,
    England.

Deprez-De Campeneere, D., Laboratory of Physiological Chemistry,
    Université Catholique de Louvain and International Institute of
    Cellular and Molecular Pathology, Brussels, Belgium.

Doré, J.F., Inserm U218, Centre Léon Berard, 28 Rue Laënnec, 69373,
    Lyon Cedex 2, France.

Edwards, D., Institute of Cancer Research, Royal Cancer Hospital,
    Chester Beatty Research Institute, Fulham Road, London SW3 6JB,
    England.

Eytan, G., Department of Biology, Technion, Israel Institute of
    Technology, Haifa, Israel.

Fiume, L., Istituto di Patologia Generale, Via San Giacomo 14,
    I-40126 Bologna, Italy.

Fraley, R., Monsanto Company, St. Louis, Missouri 63166, USA.

Gerlier, D., INSERM U218, Centre Léon Berard, 28 Rue Laënnec, 69373,
    Lyon Cedex 2, France.

Ghose, T., Department of Pathology, Dalhousie University, Halifax,
    N.S., Canada.

Gipp, J.J., University of Wisconsin, Department of Human Onocology,
    WCCC Madison, WI, 53792, USA.

Gregoriadis, G., Division of Clinical Sciences, Clinical Research
    Centre, Watford Road, Harrow, Middx. HA1 3UJ, UK.

Heath, T., Department of Pharmacology, University of San Francisco,
    CA 94143, USA.

Henkart, P.A., Immunology Branch, National Cancer Institute, NIH,
    Bethesda, Maryland, 20205, USA.

Ihler, G.M., Texas A and M College of Medicine, College Station,
    Texas, 77843, USA.

Juliano, R.L., The University of Texas Medical School at Houston,
    Department of Pharmacology, Houston, Texas 77025, USA.

Kirby, C., Division of Clinical Sciences, Clinical Research Centre,
    Watford Road, Harrow, Middx. HA1 3UJ, U.K.

Kulkarni, P., Department of Pathology, Dalhousie University, Halifax, N.S., Canada.

Large, P., Division of Clinical Sciences, Clinical Research Centre, Watford Road, Harrow. Middx. HAI 3UJ, U.K.

Leserman, L.D., Centre d'Immunologie, INSERM-CNRS de Marseille-Luminy, Case 906, 13288 Marseille Cedex g, France.

Loyter, A., The Hebrew University of Jerusalem, Institute of Life Sciences, Jerusalem, Israel.

Magin, R.L., Department of Electrical Engineering, University of Illinois at Urbana-Champaign, Urbana, Illinois 61801, USA.

Margel, S., Departments of Chemical Immunology and Plastic Research, The Weizmann Institute of Science, Rehovot 76100, Israel.

Martin, F., Department of Pharmacology, University of San Francisco, CA 94143, USA.

Masquelier, M., Laboratory of Physiological Chemistry, Université Catholique de Louvain and International Institute of Cellular and Molecular Pathology, Brussels, Belgium.

Mattioli, A., Istituto di Patologia Generale, Via San Giacomo 14, I-40126 Cologna, Italy.

Mayhew, E., Department of Experimental Pathology, Roswell Park, Memorial Institute, Buffalo, New York 14203, USA.

Mazurek, N., Departments of Chemical Immunology and Plastic Research, The Weizmann Institute of Science, Rehovot 76100, Israel.

Meehan, A., Division of Clinical Sciences, Clinical Research Centre, Watford Road, Harrow, Middx. HA1 3UJ, U.K.

Nicolau, C., Centre de Biophysique Moleculaire, CNRS, 45045 Orleans Cedex, France.

Norvell, S., Department of Surgery, Dalhousie University, Halifax, N.S., Canada.

Papahadjopoulos, D., Cancer Research Institute and Department of Pharmacology, University of San Francisco, CA 94143, USA.

Pecht, I., Departments of Chemical Immunology and Plastic Research, The Weizmann Institute of Science, Rehovot 76100, Israel.

Petrank, A., Departments of Chemical Immunology and Plastic Research, The Weizmann Institute of Science, Rehovot 76100, Israel.

Pirson, P., Laboratory of Physiological Chemistry, Université Catholique de Louvain and International Institute of Cellular and Molecular Pathology, Brussels, Belgium.

Poste, C., Smith,Kline and French Laboratories, Philadelphia, PA 19101 and Department of Pathology and Laboratory Medicine, University of Pennsylvania, Philadelphia, PA 19104, USA.

Rustum, Y.M., Department of Experimental Therapeutics and Grace Cancer Drug Genter, Roswell Park Memorial Institute, Buffalo, New York 17203, USA.

Ryman, B.E., Department of Biochemistry, Charing Cross Hospital, Medical School (University of London), Hammersmith, London W6 8RF, UK.

Sekeris-Pataryas, K., Biology Division, Nuclear Research Center, Democritos, Aghia Paraskevi, Attiki, Greece.

Sené, C., Max Planck Institut für Strathlenchemie, 4330 Mulheim a.d. Ruhr, FRG.

Senior, J., Division of Clinical Sciences, Clinical Research Centre, Watford Road, Harrow, Middx HA1 3UJ, UK.

Straubinger R., Department of Pharmacology, University of San Francisco, CA 94143, USA.

Szoka, F., Department of Pharmacy, University of California, San Francisco, CA 94143, USA.

Thorpe, P.E., Institute of Cancer Research, Royal Cancer Hospital, Chester Beatty Research Institute, Fulham Road, London SW3 6JB, England.

Trouet, A., Laboratory of Physiological Chemistry, Université Catholique de Louvain and International Institute of Cellular and Molecular Pathology, Brussels, Belgium.

Vakirtzi-Lemonias, C., Biology Division, Nuclear Research Center Democritos, Aghia Paraskevi, Attiki, Greece.

van Nieuwmegen, R., Medical Faculty, Free University, Postbox 7161, 1007 MC Amsterdam, The Netherlands.

van Rooijen, N., Medical Faculty, Free University, Postbox 7161, 1007 MC Amersterdam, The Netherlands.

Vaughan, K., Department of Chemistry, Saint Mary's University, Halifax, N.S., Canada.

Weinstein, J.N., Section of Membrane Structure and Function, Laboratory of Mathematical Biology, National Cancer Institute, NIH, Bethesda, Maryland, 20205, USA.

Wieland, Th., Max Planck Institut fur Medizinische Forschung, Jahnstrasse 29, D-69 Heidelberg, FRG.

Yatvin, M.B., University of Wisconsin, Department of Human Oncology, WCCC Madison, WI 53792, USA.

Abrin
  antibody bound, 89
A chain
  antibody conjugates, 91
Actinomycin D, 236–240
  liposome-entrapped
    effect on actinomycin D-
      resistant Ridgway
      osteosarcoma, 239
    effect on Ridgway osteo-
      sarcoma, 236–238
  uptake by tumours, 240
Adenine-9-β-D-arabinofuranoside
  conjugates with desialylated
      fetuin, 5,8,12
  interaction with hepatocytes,
      8
Adriamycin
  complexes with DNA, 32, 33
  in-vivo activity of conjugate
      with antibody, 45
Albumin
  aggregated, 2
  conjugates, 10
  lactosaminated, 10
  linkage with daunorubicin, 22
  linkage with doxorubicin, 22
  in liposomes, 303–308,310,
      314,327.
β-Amanitin
  antiserum against, 1
  inhibitory effect, 2
  effect on hepatocytes, 2
  receptor for, 10
β-Amanitin – albumin conjugate
  effect on sinusoidal cells, 2
  mechanism of action 2,

  toxicity, 2
  toxicity to macrophages, 2
  uptake by cells, 2
Anthracyclines
  linkage to protein, 26
Antibodies
  anti-TAA, see Anti-TAA antibodies,
  as anti-tumour drug carriers, 31
  as carriers of cytotoxic
      agents, 32,56–60
  conjugated to toxin, 83–93
  induction of antibodies against,73
  monoclonal
    against colorectal carcinoma,91
    against experimental murine
      tumours, 33
    against human melanoma, 71
    anti-38C leukaemia, 34
    anti-YAC, 34
    anti-3LL, 34,42
    distribution in vivo, 43
    drug conjugates with, 46,47
    in drug targeting, 70–73,
      104, 318
    enhancement of immunogenicity
      with liposomes, 318, 319
    liposomes bearing, 186, 318
  pharmacokinetics of labelled, 73
Antibody-bound radionuclides
  diagnostic use, 74
  therapeutic activity, 75,76
  in tumour therapy, 74
Antibody-drug conjugates
  activity, 38
  function of antibody, 84
  chemotherapeutic index, 55
  with chlorambucil, 56–62

Antibody-drug conjugates (cont.)
  with daunomycin
    activity, 36,37,58,61,62
    binding procedures, 34
    mode of action, 42,44
  with daunomycin-dextran, 61,62
        (see also Daunomycin-
          dextran conjugate)
  dextran bridge in, 43
  with cis-diamino platinum
        dihydrochloride, 38
  with diphtheria toxin, 58,59,60
  with adriamycin, 34,58
  methodology, 34,35,38
  with methotrexate, 35,57-62,65
  with neocarzinostatin, 58
  with PDM, 61
  with ricin, 59,60
  with trenimon, 58,65
  tumour inhibition, 57-62
  uptake by YAC cells, 43-42
Antibody-toxin conjugates,83-93
        (see Toxin-antibody
          conjugates)
Anti-TAA antibodies
  fragments
    antigenicity, 70
    clearance through kidney, 70
    transcapillary passage, 70
    imaging with, 70
    disadvantages for target-
          ing, 70
  targeting with, 69
  tumour localisation, 66,67
Ara-A, see Adenine-9-β-D-arabino-
          furanoside
Ara-AMP, 10
Ara-C (see Cytosine arabinoside)
Asialofetuin-primaquine con-
          jugates
  antimalarial activity, 28
Azide
  effect on uptake of liposomes
          by cells, 193

Bacteriophage lambda
  as a cloning vehicle, 148
  dimensions, 148

entrapment in erythrocytes,
          148, 149
Bleomycin
  in liposomes, 178
Boron
  targeting, 68

Carboxyfluorescein
  hydrophobic impurities, 187
  leakage from liposomes,
    effect of lipid
          composition, 156-160
    on heating, 203
  in liposomes, 156,185,206
  as a marker of liposomes, 186
  purification, 187
Cell receptors, 105
Chlorambucil
  alkylating activity, 56
  bound to anti-tumour globulins
    clinical trial, 56
    endocytosis, 56
    therapeutic activity, 56,57
Cholera toxin, (see also Liposome-
          entrapped drugs)
  in liposomes
    immunoadjuvant effect, 308,
          338,347,348
Cis-dichlorodiamineplatinum (II)
  partitioned into the lipid phase
          of liposomes
    clearance from the circula-
          tion, 231
    uptake by tumours, 231,232
  release from heat-sensitive
          liposomes, 231
Colchicine
  uptake by Crithidia fasciculata
          as liposome-entrapped, 366
Concanavalin A
  as drug carrier, 33
Crithidia fasciculata
  interaction with liposomes
    effect of cell cycle, 362
    effect of liposomal compo-
          sition, size and
          charge, 365,366
    effect of metabolic inhibit-
          ors, 362

Crithidia fasciculata (cont.)
    kinetics, 362
  plasma membranes
    composition, 363
    properties, 361,362
Cromoglycate disodium
  action, 112, 114
  bound to microspheres, 114-121
Cytochrome-C
  entrapment in reconstituted
        viruses, 127
Cytosine arabinoside (see also
        ara-C)
  complexed with albumin
    injection of mice, 3
  effect on L1210 leukaemia, 100
  in liposomes
    effect on lung DNA syn-
        thesis, 296-298
  phase transition release, 210
  treatment of L1210 leukaemia,
        249-257
  toxicity studies, 251,252
Cytostatic drugs
  affinity for tumours, 102,104
  combination therapy, 99
  phase-specific, 99
  sites of action, 98
  synergism, 99

Daunomycin
  antibody-bound, 32,33,36,37,
        41,45
  complex with concanavalin A, 33
  complex with DNA, 32,33
  complex with melanotropin, 33
  conjugated to dextran, 47,61,62
  conjugated to Fab dimers, 39
Daunomycin-dextran conjugate
  cytotoxic activity, 48-50,
        61,62
  preparation, 48
  toxicity, 48
Daunorubicin
  clearance, 23
  linkage to DNA, 22

  linkage to protein, 22
Daunorubicin-albumin complex
  chemotherapeutic activity, 24-26
  clearance, 23
  lysosomal hydrolysis, 24
  stability in serum, 24
Desialylated fetuin, 27
Dextran
  advantages as a carrier, 50
  as a blood volume expander, 50
  as a bridge for drug-antibody
        linkage, 46,47
  as drug carrier, 31,102
Dictyostelium discoideum
  interaction with liposomes
    kinetics, 357-360
    mechanism, 360,361
  properties, 356,357
Digoxin
  as a target for liposomes, 242
Diphtheria toxin
  antibody-bound, 88
Diphtheria toxoid
  in liposomes, 311,308
DNA
  carried by erythrocytes, 145-151
  degradation by nucleases within
        erythrocytes, 150
  encoding for β-lactamase
    assay, 396-398
    expression in cells via
        liposomes, 402-405
    transformation rate via
        liposomes, 405,406
  entrapment in reconstituted
        viruses, 127
  erythrocyte-carried, 151
  in liposomes
    criteria for entrapment, 396-399
    delivery to cells, 378,379-381
    infectivity 375,379-381
    interaction with cells,
        393-395,399-402
    mechanism for cellular up-
        take, 399-401
    preparation, 394,396
  synthesis

DNA (continued)
  synthesis (continued)
    inhibition, 3,6,10
DNP-Cap-PE
  synthesis, 186
Doxorubicin
  linkage to DNA,22
Drug carriers
  antibodies, 20
  DNA, 20
  glycoproteins, 20
  hormones, 20
  liposomes, 20
  lysosomotropic criteria, 21,22
  nanocapsules, 20

Ectromelia virus
  infection of hepatic cells, 3
  infected mice, 3,4,8,10
  ingestion by Kupffer cells, 3
  replication, 3
Endotoxin
  in association with liposomes,
        314
Erythrocytes
  as drug carriers, 145
  encapsulation of virus T2, 147
  entrapment of virus
        particles, 147,148
  entrapped viruses
    clearance from
        circulation, 151
    survival, 151
  fusion with recipient
        cells, 149
  incorporation of free DNA, 147
  life-span in mice, 151
  loaded with magnetic iron, 146
  resealed, 145
  as slow-release capsules for
        drugs, 146
Erythrocyte ghosts
  as drug carriers, 126

Fab dimers
  daunomycin conjugate, 39
Fc-receptors, 185
Ferritin
  entrapment in reconstituted
        viruses, 127

Fetuin
  desialylated
    in liposomes, 4
    trifluorothymidine-bound, 4
    uptake by parenchymal cells, 4
Fibronectin
  effect on liposome uptake by
        macrophages, 295
Fluorescence microscopy, 193
5-Fluorodeoxyuridine
  conjugated to albumin, 3
  injection of mice, 3

Gelonin
  antibody bound, 91
Gene transfer
  methods, 146,147
Glucantime, see Meglumine anti-
        moniate
γ-Glutamyl transferase
  in tumours, 104
Glycolipids
  antimalarial properties, 341-344
Glycoproteins
  as drug carriers, 1-12
  hepatocyte-selective, 26
Gross cell surface antigen (see
        also Liposome-entrapped
        drugs)
  in liposomes, 327,329,330
  preparation, 328-330

Hepatitis B, 3,12
  treatment, 3,5
Hepatitis B surface antigens
  in liposomes, 311,316,327
High density lipoproteins
  effect on liposomes, 209,228
Hydantoins, 106
Hyperthermia-mediated drug
        release, 224

IgG
  entrapment in reconstituted
        viruses, 127
Imaging
  with radionuclides, 74
Immunoadjuvant effect
  of liposomal adenovirus
        proteins, 308,309

Immunoadjuvant effect (continued)
  of liposomal cholera
        toxin, 308,338
  of liposomal diphtheria
        toxoid, 308,310,311,327
  of liposomal γ-globulin,
        303-308,314,327
  of liposomal β-glucuronidase,
        308
  of liposomal Gross cell surface
        antigen
    mechanism, 332-335
    role of antigen incorpora-
        tion in liposomes, 332
    role of liposomal phospho-
        lipid, 332,334,335
    role of macrophage-stimulat-
        ing agents, 331
  of liposomal hepatitis B
        surface antigen, 308,
        311,316,327
  of liposomal influenza virus
        haemagglutinin, 308
  of liposomal influenza virus
        neuraminidase, 308
  of liposomal lipid A, 308,338,
        344,348-350
  of liposomal serum albumin,
        308,327
Immunomodulators
  in liposomes, 261-279
Intermediate density lipoproteins
  effect on phase transition
        release, 209
Inulin
  in liposomes, 159
Ipoemanol, 106

Kappa chain
  coating of lymphocytes, 178
  target for liposomes, 178

Leishmaniasis
  causative organism, 338
  clinical picture, 338
  occurrence, 338
Leukemia
  7,12-dimethylbenzanthracene-
        induced, 33

Leukemia (continued)
  L1210
    treatment with liposomal
        cytosine arabinoside,
        249-257
    effect of 'empty'
        liposomes, 255
Lipid A
  as immunoadjuvant, 338
  in liposomes, 338 (see also
        Liposome-entrapped drugs)
Lipoproteins
  effect on phase transition
        release, 209
Liposomes
  access to lysosomes, 200
  advantages as a carrier, 155-163
  antibody-bearing
    antibody availability, 176,179
    binding to cells, 194
    effect of papain, 176,179
    Fab availability, 179
    methodology, 176
    stability in serum, 176
    targeting to lymphocytes,
        178,180,185
  antimalarial properties
    enhancement of primaquine
        action, 342-344
    glycolipid components, 341-344
    mechanism, 341-344
  "antigen-suicide" technique, 319
  as carriers, see Liposome-
        entrapped drugs
  cells
    interaction with, 126,355-357,
        361-363,378-381
    localisation in macrophages, 264
    uptake by, 193,197,198
    lymphocytes, 313,315
  cholesterol content
    cholesterol free, 156-165
    cholesterol rich, 156-165
    control of liposomal
        permeability, 375
    effect on leakage of drugs,
        156,163
    effect on pore formation, 159,
        160

Liposomes (continued)
  cholesterol content (cont.)
    in immunoadjuvant effect
        312,313
  clearance
    from circulation, 230
    control, 165
    after intravenous
        injection, 167,168
    after intraperitoneal
        injection, 169-171
  covalent coupling
    to antibodies, 382-384
    to F(ab')₂, 382
    to haptens, 315
    to immunoglobulins, 186
    to macromolecules, 187
    to proteins, 311,312
  effect of,
    antigen concentration on
        immunoadjuvant
        properties, 306,307
    antigen exposure on immuno-
        adjuvant properties,
        309,210
    apolipoproteins on phase
        transition release,
        208,210
    azide on uptake by cells,
        193,198
    blockade of reticuloendo-
        thelial system on
        uptake, 290-292
    cholesterol content on pore
        formation, 159-160
    cholesterol content on re-
        tention of drugs,
        163,375
    2-deoxyglucose on uptake by
        cells, 193-198
    endotoxin on immunoadjuvant
        properties, 315
    glycerol on uptake by
        cells, 197
    high density lipoproteins,
        208,209,228
    lipid A on immunoadjuvant
        properties, 315
    lipoprotein on phase trans-
        ition release, 207-209

    liposomal cholesterol on leak-
        age of drugs, 156
    lysolecithin on immunoadjuvant
        properties, 315
    papain on antibody coated, 176,
        179
    phospholipid component on up-
        take by liver and spleen
        165
    phospholipid packing on leakage
        of drugs, 156
    polyethylene glycol on uptake by
        by cells, 197
    serum, 156-157,205
    serum components on phase
        transition release, 200,207
    serum on temperature
        sensitive, 205
    sphingomyelin on stability, 229
    storage on leakage of drugs,
        171-175
    whole blood, 158
  fluorochrome staining, 311
  half-life
    dependence on phospholipid
        component, 165,167
  hapten-bearing
    interaction with Ig-bearing
        myeloma cells, 186
    binding to tumour cells, 190
  immune reactions against, 302,303
  immunoadjuvant effect, 327-335
  immunoadjuvant properties
    advantages, 317
    cells involved, 312,313
    cellular response, 316
    effect of antigen concentrat-
        ion, 306, 307
    effect of antigen exposure,
        309,310
    effect of endotoxin, 315
    effect of lipid A, 315
    effect of lysolecithin, 315
    enhancement, 313-316
    humoural response, 316
    impairment, 315
    mechanism, 303,305
    role of liposomal cholesterol,
        312,313
    role of lymphocytes, 312,313

Liposomes (continued)
  immunoadjuvant properties
        (continued)
    role of macrophages, 312
    T-cell dependent
        response, 316
  immunogenicity
    in conjunction with lipid
        A, 344
    in rabbits, 346
    in rodents, 346
  in immunology,
    immunopotentiation, 344
    immunosuppression, 344,348,
        349
    role of macrophages, 344
  impact in biomedical research,
        301
  interaction
    with cells, 126,355-357,361-
        363,378-381
    with Fc receptors, 190
    with plasma, 229
    with endotoxin, 315
    with lymphocytes, 312,313,
        315
    with Crithidia fasciculata,
        356,361-363
    with Dictyostelium discoid-
        eum, 356,357
    with Pseudomonas aeruginosa,
        356
  leakage of drugs
    effect of liposomal
        cholesterol, 156,163,375
    effect of phospholipid
        packing, 156
    effect of sphingomyelin, 229
    effect of storage, 171-175
    in vitro, 155-163
    in vivo, 163
    at phase transition, 207,
        209-211
  localisation in the lungs
    mechanism, 268-271
    optimal conditions, 268
    role of monocytes, 268
  lymphocytes
    effect on their mitogenic
        reaction, 313

lymphocytes (continued)
    affinity for, 313
    changes in lymphocyte
        structure, 313
    capping, 313
    role in immunoadjuvant
        properties, 312, 313
    inhibition of proliferation,
        315
  medical applications, 235-246
  as models for membrane
        research, 223
  multilamellar
    phase transition solute
        release, 209,211
  opsonization, 190,193,196
  phagocytosis
    assessment, 187
    antibody-mediated, 345
    complement-mediated, 345
  preparation, 310
    heat-sensitive, 225
    entrapping efficiency,
        376,377
    temperature-sensitive, 205
  receptor endocytosis, 200
  retention of drugs
    effect of liposomal cholest-
        erol, 163,375
    effect of sphingomyelin, 229
    in vivo, 163
    in vitro, 155-163
  reverse phase evaporation -
        made
    advantages, 375
    control of vesicle size, 375
    cytosine arabinoside, 252-254,
        256
    efficiency of entrapment,
        375,376-378
    homogeneity, 378
    phase transition release,
        209-211
  sensitized, 315
  small unilamellar
    diameter, 156
    phase transition solute
        release, 209-211
  targeting
    with antibodies, 176,381-384

Liposomes (continued)
  targeting (continued)
    with Fab', 375
    with F(ab')₂, 375,382
    with glycolipids, 381
    influencing factors, 155-163,
      175-181
    to lymphocytes, 178,180,185
    with monoclonal antibodies,
      318,384
    problems, 319,320
    with secondary antibodies,
      242-246
  temperature sensitive, 203-219
    advantages, 218
    disadvantages, 218
    drug release, 206
    effect of serum, 205
    multilamellar, 204
    preparation, 205
    unilamellar, 204
  transcapillary passage, 230
    tumour detection, 236,242-246
  uptake
    by cells, 193,197,198
    by liver and spleen, 165
    by reticuloendothelial
      system, 290-294
  in vaccines, 337-350,317-319
    advantages, 317,318
    disadvantages, 318,319
  vesicle size
    control, 375
Liposome-entrapped drugs
  actinomycin D, 236-238,249
  adriamycin, 249
  adenovirus proteins
    immunoadjuvant effect, 208,
      309
  albumin
    immunogenicity, 303-307,
      308,327
  antigens
    exposure on liposomal
      surface, 309
    Forssman, 345
    Gross virus-associated cell
      surface, 308,327,329,330
    hepatitis B surface antigens,
      308,311,316,327

antigens (continued)
    immunogenicity, 303
    interaction with antibody,312
    methods of incorporation, 303
    tumour-associated, 327
    uptake by spleen, 313
  bleomycin, 178
  carboxyfluorescein, 156-160,
      185-187,203,206
  cholera toxin, immunoadjuvant
      effect, 308,338
  colchinine, uptake by Crithidia
      fasciculata, 366
  cytosine arabinoside,
    as aerosol spray, 293
    clearance from lungs, 296,297
    effect on DNA synthesis on
      lungs, 296,298
    localization in lungs, 296
    phase transition release, 210
    therapeutic efficacy, 249-258
    uptake by tumour in vivo, 212-
      216
  DNA, 375,378-382,393-395,399-405
  daunomycin, pharmacokinetics of,
      236
  cis-dichlorodiamine platinum
      (II), 231
  diphtheria toxoid
    immuno adjuvant effect, 308,
      310,311,327
  genes, 393-395,399-402
  β-glucuronidase
    immunoadjuvant effect, 308
  horse radish peroxidase, 308,310
  immunomodulators
    macrophage activation
      factors, 265-279
    muramyl dipeptide, 265-267,
      271-278
  influenza virus haemagglutinin
    immunoadjuvant effect, 308
  influenza virus neuraminidase
    immunoadjuvant effect, 308
  intraperitoneal injection, 171
  intravenous injection, 169,170
  inulin, 159
  lipid A
    composition, 344

Liposome-entrapped drugs (cont.)
  lipid A (continued)
    immunoadjuvant effect, 308,
        338,344,348-350
    toxicity, 350
  lymphokines
    activation of tumouricidal
        lung macrophages,
        265-267
    stimulation of host resist-
        ance to metastases,
        276-278
    therapy of lung metastases,
        271-275
  meglumine antimoniate
    treatment of visceral leish-
        maniasis, 338,339,340
  melphalan
    clearance from blood, 163,165,
        173,177
    intraperitoneal injection,
        171
    intravenous injection, 170
    release from liposomes,
        161,162
  methotrexate
    clearance from blood, 214,225
    leakage from liposomes, 187
    effect on myeloma cells, 190
    phase transition release, 210
    targeting with monoclonal
        antibodies, 384-386
    therapeutic effect, 249
    toxicity, 386
    effect on tumour cells, 195,
        204,216,218
    uptake by tumour in vivo,
        212-216
  polyvinylpyrrolidone,159
  primaquine
    anti-malarial effect, 340,341
  m-RNA, 393
  stibogluconate, 338
  sucrose, 159
  therapeutic index, 236,249
  vincristine,
    clearance from blood, 164,
        165,173,177
    release from liposomes, 161,
        162

Liquid-crystalline phase trans-
    ition temperature, 205
Liver
  sinusoidal cells as targets, 2
Low density lipoproteins
  effect on phase transition
    release, 209
Lymphatic leukemia, 33
Lymphoma
  Moloney virus induced, 33

Macrophages, 262-279
  activated
    intravenous transfusion, 262
    tumouricidal properties,
        262,267
  activation
    with lymphokines, 262,266
    with microorganisms, 262
    with muramyl dipeptide, 264,
        267
    with parasites, 262
    mouse peritoneal, liposome
        uptake by, 286-290
    problems, 264
    with surface components of
        microorganisms, 262
Macrophage-activation factors
  cell receptors, 265
  entrapment in liposomes, 265
Malaria
  chemotherapy,
    with chloroquine, 341
    with primaquine, 341
  life cycle
    role of erythrocytes, 340
    role of hepatic parenchymal
        cells, 341
    role of liver, 340
  treatment with primaquine-
    desialylated fetuin
    complex, 27
Meglumine antimoniate, 338
Melanotropin
  as drug carrier, 33
Melphalan
  leakage from liposomes upon
    storage, 172-174
  liposomal clearance from blood
    after storage, 175

Melphalan (continued)
  release from liposomes
    effect of cholesterol, 160-
      162
    effect of serum, 160-162
  uptake by cells, 100
Methotrexate
  albumin-bound, 32
  fibrinogen-bound, 32
  immunoglobulin-bound, 32,45,57,
    65
  in liposomes, (see Methotrexate
    in liposomes)
Methotrexate in liposomes
  effect on Ridgway osteo-
    sarcoma, 238
  release from heat-sensitive
    liposomes
    clearance from circulation,
      224-227
    uptake by tumours, 224-229
  targeting with monoclonal
    antibodies, 384-386
Methoxsalen, 106
Methyl hydrazine
  albumin-bound, 32
  fibrinogen-bound, 32
Micelles
  as drug carriers, 232
Microspheres
  in cell labeling, 109-111
  chemistry, 109-111
  composition, 109-111
  Fc receptor labeling, 114
  fluorescent, 111
  immunomicrospheres, 111
  magnetic, 146
  polyacrolein, 117
  polyaldehyde, 111
  size, 111
Monoclonal antibodies (see
        Antibodies)
Muramyl dipeptide
  in liposomes
    activation of tumouricidal
      lung macrophages,
      265-267
    stimulation of host
      resistance to meta-
      stases, 276-278

therapy of lung metastases,
    271-275
Myeloma cells
  murine MOPC, 315
  as targets, 185

Nitrogen mustards, 100,101,102

Opsonins
  effect on liposome uptake by
      tissues, 294

Pentostam, (see Sodium stibo-
      gluconate)
Phase transition release
  in vitro, 207
  in vivo, 211
Phosphatidyl ethanolamine
  coupled to immunoglobulin, 186
Plasmacytoma
  mineral oil-induced, 33
Plasmids
  entrapment in reconstituted
      viruses, 127
Plasmodium berghei
  chemotherapy, 26
  treatment with primaquine, 26
  treatment with primaquine-
      desialylated fetuin complex,
      27
Plasmodium ovale
  chemotherapy, 26
  treatment with primaquine, 26
Plasmodium vivax
  chemotherapy, 26
  treatment with primaquine, 26
Polyethylene glycol
  stimulation of liposome uptake
      by cells, 197
Poly(L-lysine)
  as a drug carrier, 102
  methotrexate-bound, 102
Polyvinylpyrolidone
  in liposomes, 159
Porphyrins
  as agents for phototherapy of
      tumours, 102
  as carrier molecules, 102
Primaquine
  antimalarial activity, 28

Primaquine (continued)
  linkage to desialylated
          fetuin, 27
  liposomal
    activity, 27
    toxicity, 27
    treatment with, 27,341
Pro-drugs
  0-glucuronide of aniline
          mustard, 102
  mechanism of action, 101
  p-phenylenediamine mustard, 101
  selectivity, 101
D-Propanolol, 106
Proteins
  as drug carriers, 104
  erythrocyte-carried, 151
Pseudomonas aeruginosa
  drug-resistant strain, 369,370
  interaction with liposomes, 368
  resistance to antibiotics, 368

Radionuclides
  therapeutic activity of anti-
          body bound, 75,76
Ricin
  antibody bound, 90
Ridgway osteosarcoma
  effect of liposomal actino-
          mycin D, 239
RNA-polymerase B
  inhibition, 1,2

Sarcoma 180 tumour, 231
Sendai virus
  reconstituted
    as drug carrier, 125
    as hybrid vesicles, 128-132
    F protein-promoted cell
          fusion, 135
Sodium stibogluconate
  in liposomes, 338
Sucrose
  in liposomes, 159
Sulphadiazene
  as a drug carrier, 101

Targeting
  of antiprotozal drugs, 19
  of antitumour drugs, 19

of liposomes (see Targeting of
          liposomes)
of radionuclides, 55,74
Targeting of liposomes
  with glycoproteins, 204
  hyperthermia-mediated, 223-232
  with immunoglobulins, 204
  with lectins, 204
  problems, 204
Tetrapeptide spacer arm, 23,26
Toxin-antibody conjugates
  with abrin, 89-92
  chemistry, 87
  cytotoxicity, 88-91
  with diphtheria toxin, 88,89
  in drug targeting, 83-93
  function of the toxin, 86
  with gelonin, 91
  with ricin, 90,91
Trifluorothymidine,
  conjugates with desialylated
          fetuin, 4
Trypanosomes
  antigenic variation, 361
  tumour markers
    as targets, 68,69
Tumour-specific antigens
  existence, 32

Vaccines (see also Immuno-
          adjuvant effect)
  liposomes in, 337-350
Very low density lipoproteins
  effect on liposomal phase
          transition release, 209
Vesicles, (see Liposomes)
Vincristine
  in liposomes
    clearance from blood after
          storage, 175
    leakage upon storage, 172-174
  release from liposomes
    effect of cholesterol, 160-162
    effect of serum, 160-162
Viruses
  reconstituted
    as drug carriers, 126
    entrapped in erythrocytes, 151
    fusion with cells, 126-140
    fusogenic, 126

Viruses (continued)
  reconstituted (continued)
    implantation of membrane
        proteins, 132-134
    phagocytosis, 139
    proteolytic activity, 130
Vitamin E, 106